DIAGNOSTIC ASSESSMENT IN CHILD AND ADOLESCENT PSYCHOPATHOLOGY

DIAGNOSTIC ASSESSMENT IN CHILD AND ADOLESCENT PSYCHOPATHOLOGY

Edited by

David Shaffer
Christopher P. Lucas
John E. Richters

Foreword by Professor Sir Michael Rutter

THE GUILFORD PRESS
New York   London

© 1999 The Guilford Press
A Division of Guilford Publications, Inc.
72 Spring Street, New York, NY 10012
http://www.guilford.com

Printed in the United States of America

This book is printed on acid-free paper.

Last digit is print number: 9 8 7 6 5 4 3 2 1

Library of Congress Cataloging-in-Publication Data
available from the Publisher

ISBN 1-57230-502-9

To Joy and Bill Ruane.
Their support of assessment
and other research with children and adolescents
has and will affect countless children and their parents
and has been central to the success of many
important research projects.

About the Editors

✦

David Shaffer, MB, FRCP, FRCPsych, is Irving Philips Professor of Psychiatry at Columbia University College of Physicians and Surgeons, New York, and at the New York State Psychiatric Institute. He has been influential in the development of both the ICD and DSM diagnostic systems for children and adolescents. He created the widely used Children's Global Assessment Scale (C-GAS) and developed and led the NIMH-DISC through a series of revisions, culminating in the now widely used NIMH DISC-IV. He is a Founder Member of the Academy of Medical Sciences in London and has received the American Psychiatric Association's Agnes Purcell McGavin Award, the American Mental Health Fund Prize for Research in Psychiatry, and the Award for Research in Suicide from the American Suicide Foundation.

Christopher P. Lucas, MB, ChB, MMedSc, MRCPsych, is Assistant Professor of Psychiatry at Columbia University College of Physicians and Surgeons, New York, and at the New York State Psychiatric Institute. He received a Scientist Development Award for Clinicians (K20) from the National Institute of Mental Health in 1995 to study the measurement of child psychopathology and has been involved in the computerization and testing of a number of psychiatric instruments, most recently the NIMH-DISC. His research interests lie in the field of psychiatric nosology and the experimental study of reliability and validity of measurement of psychopathology in children and adolescents. He is the author of the DISC Predictive Scales and the Multimedia Adolescent Suicide Interview (MASI).

John E. Richters, PhD, is a developmental psychologist at the National Institute of Mental Health, where he has served as Chief of the Disruptive Disorders Program and Assistant Chief of the Child and Adolescent Disorders Research Branch. Dr. Richters has conducted research and published numerous scientific articles and book chapters on a wide range of topics concerning the assessment, classification, diagnosis, etiology, and treatment of psychopathology in childhood. He is also a coeditor, with David Reiss, Marion Radke-Yarrow, and David Scharff, of *Children and Violence*, published in 1993 by The Guilford Press. Dr. Richters is a recipient of the American Psychological Association's Boyd McCandless Young Scientist Award for Distinguished Early Scientific Career Contributions to Developmental Psychology, and currently serves on the editorial boards of *Applied Developmental Science and Development* and *Psychopathology*.

Contributors

✧

Adrian Angold, MRCPsych, Department of Psychiatry and Behavioral Sciences, Center for Developmental Epidemiology, Duke University Medical Center, Durham, North Carolina

Robert F. Belli, PhD, Institute of Social Research and Department of Psychology, University of Michigan, Ann Arbor, Michigan

Hector R. Bird, MD, Department of Clinical Psychiatry, Division of Child and Adolescent Psychiatry, College of Physicians and Surgeons, Columbia University, New York, New York; Department of Child and Adolescent Psychiatry, New York State Psychiatric Institute, New York, New York

Milagros Bravo, PhD, Behavioral Sciences Research Institute and Department of Graduate Studies in Education, University of Puerto Rico, San Juan, Puerto Rico

Glorisa Canino, PhD, Behavioral Sciences Research Institute and Department of Pediatrics, School of Medicine, University of Puerto Rico, San Juan, Puerto Rico

Patricia Cohen, PhD, Department of Epidemiology, Joseph L. Mailman School of Public Health, and Department of Psychiatry, College of Physicians and Surgeons, Columbia University, New York, New York; Department of Epidemiology of Mental Disorders, New York State Psychiatric Institute, New York, New York

Edwin H. Cook, Jr., MD, Laboratory of Developmental Neuroscience and Departments of Psychiatry and Pediatrics, University of Chicago, Chicago, Illinois

Ronald E. Dahl, MD, Child and Adolescent Sleep and Neuroendocrine Laboratory, Western Psychiatric Institute and Clinic, Pittsburgh, Pennsylvania; Departments of Psychiatry and Pediatrics, University of Pittsburgh Medical Center, Pittsburgh, Pennsylvania

Lorah Dorn, PhD, Department of Nursing and Psychiatry, University of Pittsburgh School of Nursing, Pittsburgh, Pennsylvania

Prudence W. Fisher, MS, Department of Psychiatry, Division of Child and Adolescent Psychiatry, College of Physicians and Surgeons, Columbia University, New York, New York; Department of Child and Adolescent Psychiatry, New York State Psychiatric Institute, New York, New York

Elizabeth L. Hart, PhD, Department of Psychiatry, Yale University School of Medicine, New Haven, Connecticut

Stephen P. Hinshaw, PhD, Clinical Psychology Training Program, and Department of Psychology, University of California at Berkeley, Berkeley, California

Stephanie Kasen, PhD, Department of Psychiatry, College of Physicians and Surgeons, Columbia University, New York, New York; Department of Epidemiology of Mental Disorders, New York State Psychiatric Institute, New York, New York

Ronald C. Kessler, PhD, Department of Health Care Policy, Harvard University Medical School, Boston, Massachusetts

Markus J. P. Kruesi, MD, Institute for Juvenile Research and Department of Psychiatry, Division of Child and Adolescent Psychiatry, University of Illinois–Chicago, Chicago, Illinois

Benjamin B. Lahey, PhD, Department of Psychiatry and Psychology, University of Chicago School of Medicine, Chicago, Illinois

Christopher P. Lucas, MB, ChB, MMedSc, MRCPsych, Departments of Psychiatry, Division of Child and Adolescent Psychiatry, College of Physicians and Surgeons, Columbia University, New York, New York; Department of Child and Adolescent Psychiatry, New York State Psychiatric Institute, New York, New York

Wendy D. Marans, MS, Child Study Center, Yale University, New Haven, Connecticut

Daniel K. Mroczek, PhD, Department of Psychology, Fordham University, Bronx, New York

Joel T. Nigg, PhD, Department of Psychology, Michigan State University, East Lansing, Michigan

Brian Rabian, PhD, Department of Psychology, University of Southern Mississippi, Hattiesburg, Mississippi

Richard Rende, PhD, Department of Psychology, Rutgers University, The State University of New Jersey, Piscataway, New Jersey

Neal D. Ryan, MD, Department of Psychiatry, University of Pittsburgh School of Medicine, Pittsburgh, Pennsylvania; Department of Psychiatry, Western Psychiatric Institute and Clinic, Pittsburgh, Pennsylvania

David Shaffer, FRCP, FRCPsych, Department of Pediatric Psychiatry, Babies Hospital, Columbia–Presbyterian Medical Center, New York, New York; Departments of Psychiatry and Pediatrics, College of Physicians and Surgeons, Columbia University, New York, New York; Department of Child and Adolescent Psychiatry, New York State Psychiatric Institute, New York, New York

Wendy K. Silverman, PhD, Child and Family Psychosocial Research Center and Department of Psychology, Florida International University, Miami, Florida

Fred R. Volkmar, MD, Child Study Center, Yale University, New Haven, Connecticut

Myrna M. Weissman, PhD, Department of Psychiatry, College of Physicians and Surgeons, and Department of Epidemiology, School of Public Health, Columbia University, New York, New York; Division of Clinical and Genetic Epidemiology, New York State Psychiatric Institute, New York, New York

Foreword

✦

This volume is greatly to be welcomed because it provides a clear account of the numerous ways in which methods of psychopathological assessment have advanced over the last dozen years or so, and because it outlines some of the challenges that remain to be met. In order to provide adequate coverage of methods of assessment, it does not deal with the broader diagnostic issues that constituted a major portion of its predecessor, the 1988 volume *Assessment and Diagnosis in Child Psychopathology*, which was published at the time that the major systems of psychiatric classification were being revised. However, these broader issues provide the essential background to the measurement advances, as well as setting the agenda for the research needed over the next dozen years.

This volume takes forward our understanding of the strengths and limitations of the two main types of structured interviews: respondent-based methods that rely on careful design of hierarchical questioning to obtain yes–no answers on predetermined behaviors, and interviewer-based methods designed to obtain detailed descriptions of actual behavior that may be rated according to carefully operationalized criteria. Four chapters describe the questionnaires that are available for measuring both general psychopathology and specific symptom patterns. It is assumed, on solid grounds, that both dimensional and categorical approaches have an important place, although the interconnections between them are not discussed in detail. Four critically important issues that received only very limited attention in the earlier volume are: the subject matter of chapters on the assessment of the functional impairment deriving from psychopathology, on obtaining a systematic family history, on retrospective recall (essential in the study of connections between child and adult disorder), and on the meaning of cultural variations and how they should be dealt with. Biological resources still have limited diagnostic utility in ordinary clinical practice, but that situation is about to change in the years ahead, and the two chapters on this topic provide valuable signposts on what may prove to be of value.

As I look ahead to a future version of this text, there are several areas in which research advances should provide the basis for new chapters. Most obviously, ways need to be found to appreciate why the agreement between informants is usually modest and why the correlates of different accounts are often so different. It is clear that there are important psychosocial risk factors for psychopathology, but improvements are needed in both their conceptualization and their measurement. Observational and psychometric approaches are likely to prove of growing importance in the assessment of cognitive (including social-cognitive) risk factors, as well as in the assessment of scholastic impairment, which shows such strong association with some forms of psychopathology. Since the earlier volume, the topic of comorbidity (meaning the co-occurrence of supposedly separate disorders) has received increasing recognition because of its high frequency, but further research is much needed in order to elucidate its meaning. The interconnections between dimensions and categories continue to be important, but their investigation is only just beginning. Most of all, there has come an awareness that the boundaries of many of the traditional "severe" diagnoses extend more broadly than has hitherto been appreciated. Genetic research, as well as other types of study, has opened up new avenues for the study of diagnostic validity.

It is obvious that all of these issues can be studied only if adequate measures are available. That is where this volume really comes into its own. There is no better account of the "tools of the trade" that may be used in both clinical research and clinical practice. But, more than that, the book provides a clear and insightful account of many of the key conceptual and methodological considerations that need to be borne in mind in using the measures, and in developing new and better measures. In this way, the chapters combine readily understandable "state-of-the-art" overviews and thoughtful guidelines on how the field may move ahead. The volume is thus a "must" for practitioners and investigators.

PROFESSOR SIR MICHAEL RUTTER, FRS
Professor of Developmental Psychopathology,
Institute of Psychiatry, London, England

Preface

✧

It has been a privilege to edit this book, and we have been fortunate to enlist the participation of many leaders in the field to give their evaluations of various aspects of the standardized assessment of psychopathology in children and adolescents. Their work provides a representative snapshot of the science of assessment at the turn of the century.

This book' predecessor, the 1988 volume *Assessment and Diagnosis in Child Psychopathology,* edited by Michael Rutter, A. Hussain Tuma, and Irma S. Lann, was a widely used reference. A comparison with that volume provides interesting insights into how this field has changed over the past years. It is clear that assessment in the late 1990s is alive and moderately well.

Perhaps the most notable changes have been technological. The field has benefited from a great deal of technical research on how questions should be structured, on the limits of reliable recall, and on contextual influences. Instruments of all kinds can now be computerized to a greater or lesser extent, depending on the type of instrument, resulting in reduced handling of data, fewer errors, and less expense. There are excellent contributions addressing each of these topics in this book.

It is also clear that measurement is living in the shade of the blockbuster classification systems DSM-IV and ICD-10. These systems are shaping the range and nature of the phenomena that most investigators are seeking to measure. Their emphasis on operationalizable, key criteria is narrowing the difference between instruments; it has almost certainly led to better reproducibility as measured by test–retest reliability and has led to a new focus on, and interest in, scoring algorithms, how these algorithms should be modified by impaired function, and the need for them to be transparent and not in a "black box."

Although these developments are all of great value, they should not blind us to certain costs or to the many areas where measurement is still poorly developed. We know next to nothing about what to look for in preschoolers or how best to measure it. The criteria for younger children that have found their way into DSM and ICD are by no means comprehensive. Their manifestation may vary according to how they are operationalized using different assessment techniques; they are rarely pathognomonic, either of any specific psychiatric disorder or of disorder in general; and, of greatest concern, there are very few studies that can tell us whether the phenomena that have been chosen as criteria are indeed the best predictors of cause and course.

Our ability to check the value of criteria, either of a diagnostic construct or of the way that construct is rendered by a particular instrument, is caught in the circular problem of assessment. Standardized diagnostic techniques were developed precisely because clinical experts are fallible and inconsistent, both with each other and with themselves over time. The standards against which we must measure validity must come from large-scale, longitudinal studies that use a broad array of measures that extend beyond the existing repertoire used by DSM-IV and ICD-10, and that examine the predictive validity of different formulations of disorder.

It is vitally important that the fields of measurement and its first cousin, classification, remain creative and not confined to technological fine tuning. There is a need for heuristic research. The relationship between measurement and classification is a two-way street. Classification systems might tell us what to measure, but they, too, need nourishment from new data on the different values of phenomena that go beyond those now passed down to us—in what threatens to be a pattern of conservatism that may promote consistency at the expense of validity.

We look forward to a future edition of this book that will not only tell us how to measure better, but will also inform us about what is most important to measure.

Contents

✧

I

MEASURES FOR ASSESSING GENERAL PSYCHOPATHOLOGY

✧

1

Respondent-Based Interviews

✧

DAVID SHAFFER
PRUDENCE W. FISHER
CHRISTOPHER P. LUCAS

The process of establishing a psychiatric diagnosis has traditionally required (1) a knowledge of the clinical features of the condition; (2) a systematic inquiry with the patient, and/or with those who know the patient well, about past and current behavior, emotions, and thoughts; (3) observations of the patient's behavior and language; and, for some diagnoses, (4) the results of specific tests (e.g., tests of language, learning, or intelligence). Each of these elements has required professional expertise until recently. However, the development of operationalized, criterion-based diagnoses for both the *Diagnostic and Statistical Manual of Mental Disorders* (DSM) and the *International Classification of Diseases* (ICD) systems has made the clinical features of many diagnoses broadly known and, at some level, understandable to the intelligent layperson. The process of describing disorders in lucid operational terms has also promoted the development of the respondent-based interview (RBI) technique, which allows interviewers with no clinical training to elicit defining information for many important symptoms. Skilled observations of behavior, interpretation of language cues, and the administration of specialized tests remain the province of the clinician, but not all diagnoses require such expertise. Clinical observation and interpretation are very important in, say, the differential diagnosis of psychotic or complex mood disorders, but they may be less important for common mood and anxiety disorders, and almost unnecessary for the attention-deficit and disruptive behavior disorders. Indeed, the latter are often characterized by overt behaviors that are rarely witnessed by a clinician.

3

The implications of these developments should not be underestimated. We argue in this chapter that the accuracy of many diagnoses made with RBIs is comparable to those made by a clinician. This factor, taken together with the significant cost advantages, the breadth of diagnostic coverage afforded by the RBI approach, and the opportunities for standardization, open exciting new possibilities for clinical research and preventive activities.

TYPES OF DIAGNOSTIC ASSESSMENT

The four ways in which information about symptoms and clinical phenomena can be recorded are the RBI, the symptom questionnaire, the interviewer-based interview (IBI), and the clinician rating scale.

An RBI is a precise script that obtains clinically relevant information through carefully worded and ordered questions that are read to the informant as written. The answers given to these questions are restricted to a few predefined alternatives. Because the respondent is required to interpret the questions and decide on a reply without the assistance of the interviewer, the instruments are referred to as "respondent-based interviews" (Angold et al., 1995). They could as well be considered "author-based," since the questions represent the instrument author's interpretation of how to define and ask about a particular clinical phenomenon.

The predefined questions and limited response options of RBIs resemble those of closed-ended symptom questionnaires, such as the Child Behavior Checklist (Achenbach, 1994) or the ACQ Behavior Checklist (Achenbach, Conners, & Quay, 1983). However, questionnaires usually obtain less detailed information about symptoms and have a simpler, more "linear" format (i.e., one question is followed by the next, with few if any branches or skips). Because of the simplicity of their structure, symptom questionnaires do not require the direction of an interviewer and are usually self-administered. In contrast, the typical RBI includes many contingencies; that is, the response to a given question is used to determine whether further elaboration is needed or whether questions can be directed to a new topic. For example, if the answer to a question about experiencing depression is "yes," it will lead to further questions about duration and frequency, whereas if it is "no," the interview will proceed to questions about a different symptom. The additional data obtained from these elaborations are used to determine whether a reported symptom is *clinically* significant (i.e., whether it matches the criteria laid down in the large standard classification systems, such as ICD and DSM). Another example of how the data are used to decide the course of the interview is that if a certain number of symptoms are endorsed, the interview script will lead to questions that relate to the whole diagnosis, such as impairment or treatment, rather than to elaborations of single symptoms.

Although the contingencies of the RBI resemble the normal iterative process of the clinical interview, they are too complex for the interviewee to navigate without assistance. As a result, the order and content of the questions need to be directed by a trained interviewer or by a computer. With advances in computer technology, the operational differences between symptom questionnaires and RBIs have narrowed. Highly structured interviews can now be directed by a computer instead of an interviewer and, like questionnaires, can be self-completed. Similarly, standardized responses can be readily extracted to provide scales for use in dimensional analyses, which are traditionally the province of questionnaires.

IBIs differ from RBIs in several respects (see Angold & Fisher, Chapter 2, this volume). They are entitled "interviewer-based" instruments because of the interviewer's all-important role in their administration. The interviewer has the option of varying the order or wording of questions, and respondents need not limit their responses to "yes," "no," or "sometimes." Fuller descriptions of the symptomatic phenomena can be given, and, using his/her clinical knowledge, the interviewer can interpret the response and rate it in a standard format. However, this flexibility comes at a cost: interviewers using IBIs require extensive training and periodic observation to guard against rating drift. Each interview may also need to be recorded and edited by an expert after administration to check interrater reliability, all of which is time-consuming and costly.

Clinician-completed rating scales or diagnostic checklists, such as the Hamilton Depression Rating Scale (Hamilton, 1960) and the many DSM checklists created by hospitals and individual clinics, are often used to standardize a clinician's opinions or conclusions after completion of a clinical evaluation. However, such a procedure is in some sense a "black box," because it does not reveal how the information was collected, interpreted, or put together to enable the clinician to reach a conclusion.

HISTORY

IBIs for child and psychiatric disorders were first developed over 30 years ago (Rutter & Graham, 1968). However, it was not until the development of the criterion-based DSM-III nosological system (American Psychiatric Association, 1980) that RBIs became possible. The first highly structured diagnostic interview, the Diagnostic Interview Schedule (DIS) for adults (Robins, Helzer, Croughan, & Ratcliff, 1981), was developed for a large epidemiological field study—the Epidemiologic Catchment Area study (Robins & Regier, 1991)—carried out in the United States in 1980. A sister version of that instrument, the Diagnostic Interview Schedule for Children (DISC; Costello, Edelbrock, Dulcan, Kalas, & Klaric, 1984), was subsequently developed, and versions of that interview are now the most widely administered RBIs for children (Shaffer et al., 1993, 1996; Shaffer, Fisher, Lucas, Dulcan, & Schwab-Stone, in press).

COMPARISONS BETWEEN RESPONDENT- AND INTERVIEWER-BASED INTERVIEWS

Advantages of an RBI

The main advantages of RBIs over IBIs are as follows:

1. The potential for standardization and reliability is greater for an RBI. The form of the interview is set and unvarying. Its structure, wording of questions, and arrangement of diagnostic algorithms can, in principle, be changed and improved by repeated testing and modification. By contrast, the reliability and validity of an IBI are subject to human variations in skill, thoroughness, quality of training, and editing, as well as to the vagaries of the assessor's mood, temperament, and patience. Both RBIs and IBIs are bound by the arbitrary operationalization of complex and at times subtle criteria within the major nosological systems. In turn, the process of operationalization is limited by the clarity, precision, and scope of these criteria.

2. An RBI's rigid script and limited range of response options are features that lend themselves well to extensive computerization—and, with that, ease of administration and a multitude of data management efficiencies. The essential features of IBIs (their flexibility in phrasing questions, and the use of the respondent's own descriptions as a basis for rating) limit the extent to which they can be computerized.

3. RBIs are less expensive to use; they cost less to administer. They can be administered by a lay interviewer instead of a clinician—or, least expensively of all, they can be self-administered by a respondent using a computer in visual, auditory, or combined modes. A computerized interview "cleans" data as it goes with built-in checks for out-of-range or incompatible answers, reducing the cost and the need for postadministration editing. Finally, the task of training is confined to the operation of the computerized program and to training on the limitations of the procedure, all of which can be effectively provided in a manual.

With the advent of computerized self-administration, one can foresee routine comprehensive screening and triage of children or teens who are being admitted to high-risk settings in which there are few clinicians available, such as correctional facilities, youth shelters, or busy community clinics. Other cost-saving examples abound. Large-scale screening projects could be carried out in high schools, with many students being assessed at the same time in a classroom, supervised only by a small staff whose task would be to set up multiple computers, download and review the data, and (most importantly) refer those who might need intervention to a case manager. A clinic could incorporate an RBI into a telephony program to carry out previsit screening and triage. In research projects, telephony programs could allow subjects to be interviewed conveniently and spare the cost of home or lab visits.

Limitations of an RBI

1. With its rigid format, an RBI can do little to address invalid responses given by a respondent who misunderstands a question. By contrast, clinical interviewers using an IBI are free to rephrase a question until they judge that it has been understood, to ask for examples, and to use clinical experience to check that the example given matches the target symptom.

2. IBIs offer a better opportunity to classify atypical phenomena. This is important because RBIs tend, for reasons of economy, to choose only one way of operationalizing a given symptom. Although the designers of these instruments intend that the most common and stereotypical symptom be described, all clinicians are familiar with unusual presentations of symptoms that may not be included in the authoring process. The accurate placement of a symptom may only emerge when a subject is asked to describe the symptom at greater length, and this cannot be done with an RBI.

3. IBIs are potentially shorter to administer and more acceptable to the respondent, because the interviewer can use his/her clinical judgment to abbreviate an inquiry and insert pauses in the interview.

WHAT KIND OF DIAGNOSIS?
THE PROBLEM OF CASENESS

It is clear that there are many children and adolescents in the community who, though symptomatic, function well; they and their caregivers do not seek treatment and have no plans to do so. In the Methods for Epidemiology in Children and Adolescents (MECA) study, a substantial number of subjects met diagnostic criteria but were functioning well (Shaffer et al., 1996). This phenomenon was especially common in children and adolescents with anxiety diagnoses, but it was also found with other disorders (see Table 1.1).

Should such children be regarded as having a mental disorder? DSM-IV (American Psychiatric Association, 1994) requires that a diagnosis of a mental disorder be accompanied by impairment or distress. This approach to diagnosis is quite different from that used in other fields of medicine, where such conditions as hypertension or the early stages of cancer are clearly seen as "abnormal," even though they do not cause symptoms or impairment. Given this peculiarity of psychiatric nosology, it is important that an RBI in-

TABLE 1.1. Percentage of Children Aged 9–17 Meeting DSM-III-R Diagnostic Criteria (on DISC-2.3) at Various Levels of Impairment

Diagnosis	Criteria Regardless of CGAS	Criteria and CGAS ≤ 70: Mild	Criteria and CGAS ≤ 60: Moderate	Criteria and CGAS ≤ 50: Severe
Any anxiety				
P	21.0	7.7	4.6	2.0
Y	23.7	10.0	4.4	1.9
C	39.5	18.5	9.6	4.3
Simple phobia				
P	11.7	3.7	2.1	1.0
Y	11.2	4.7	1.9	0.9
C	21.6	9.5	4.7	2.1
Social phobia				
P	7.9	3.7	2.3	1.2
Y	8.5	4.2	1.9	1.0
C	15.1	3.8	1.9	0.8
Agoraphobia				
P	1.6	0.7	0.4	0.3
Y	5.1	2.6	1.1	0.4
C	6.5	3.8	1.9	0.8
Separation anxiety				
P	2.5	1.6	0.8	0.3
Y	3.1	1.7	1.1	0.5
C	6.5	4.1	2.4	1.1
Overanxious				
P	4.3	2.5	1.2	0.6
Y	5.4	3.3	1.5	0.6
C	11.4	8.0	4.4	2.1
Any depression				
P	3.9	3.1	2.3	1.2
Y	6.0	4.7	2.3	1.3
C	8.8	7.5	4.5	2.6
Major depression				
P	3.1	2.6	1.9	1.1
Y	4.8	3.8	1.8	0.9
C	7.1	6.1	3.8	2.1
Any disruptive				
P	8.1	5.8	3.7	1.7
Y	7.1	5.7	3.0	1.6
C	14.3	11.8	7.2	3.9
Attn. def. hyp. dis.				
P	4.5	2.9	1.9	1.2
Y	2.2	1.6	0.8	0.5
C	6.5	4.9	3.3	2.0

(*continued*)

TABLE 1.1. *(continued)*

Diagnosis	Criteria Regardless of CGAS	Criteria and CGAS ≤ 70: Mild	Criteria and CGAS ≤ 60: Moderate	Criteria and CGAS ≤ 50: Severe
Opp. Def. Dis.				
P	4.4	3.9	2.7	1.2
Y	2.2	2.1	1.4	0.9
C	7.1	6.6	4.7	2.6
Conduct dis.				
P	1.4	1.1	0.9	0.5
Y	4.4	3.6	2.1	1.1
C	5.8	5.1	3.2	2.1

Note. The subjects ($n = 1,285$) were from the community sample of the MECA study. CGAS, Children's Global Assessment Scale; P, parent interview only; Y, youth interview only; C, information combined across parent and youth interviews. From Shaffer et al. (1996). Copyright 1996 by Lippincott Williams & Wilkins. Reprinted by permission.

clude an assessment of impairment. There are several ways of doing this (see Bird, Chapter 7, this volume):

1. A single global measure, such as the Children's Global Assessment Scale (Shaffer et al., 1983), can be used. Such measures are simple and reliable, but if more than one diagnosis is present, one cannot attribute the source of the impairment; therefore, it is not useful for meeting DSM diagnostic criteria.

2. Measures of impairment can be used that clearly represent the consequences of the most common symptoms of a diagnosis. For example, in separation anxiety disorder, questions to assess impairment might include queries about loss of schooling, interference with peer relations, distress felt by the child, and a deterioration in the relationship between child and parents. However, all of these impairments could be attributable to, say, the child's refusal to attend school, and it is not clear how this should be resolved. Conversely, some disorders affect fewer functional domains than others—for example, bulimia nervosa or encopresis (in part because they have fewer symptoms and narrower modes of presentation). Does this mean that severe bulimia nervosa should be counted as less impairing than, say, mild attention-deficit/hyperactivity disorder (ADHD)? Such difficulties in selecting which areas of impairment to include in the RBI and how to weigh their differential impact make this approach problematic.

3. A standardized set of impaired domains can be used for each diagnosis. This is the approach used in DSM-IV, which requires impairment in either social, occupational, or academic functioning. It is also the approach used in the DISC-IV (discussed later in this chapter). It is not entirely satis-

factory, because, as indicated above, some disorders are inherently less likely than others to impair certain domains of functioning. However, it has the advantage of circumventing the difficult and arbitrary task of weighting different forms of impairment. Although such a set of domains used to assess impairment is far from complete, it represents a reasonable working compromise; its principal limitation is that describing impairments without specifying from which symptoms they arise probably increases the likelihood of confounding one domain with another.

PREPARING AND TESTING
A RESPONDENT-BASED INTERVIEW

The ideal RBI would (1) provide coverage of all relevant diagnoses and aspects of the diagnoses, (2) be reliable, and (3) optimize validity. However, these goals are not necessarily compatible. For example, an investigator may quite reasonably want to obtain information about the date of onset and offset of an episodic condition, or about whether symptoms experienced many years previously met diagnostic criteria. Unfortunately, such complicated information may be beyond the respondent's ability to recall or beyond the author's ability to describe in a way that the respondent understands. The conventional approach to this problem is to take the position that good reliability and validity must take precedence over the user's wish list. However, how much reliability and how much validity are really necessary? It is important to avoid pessimism and not to prejudge what can and cannot be done. When proposals for an RBI were first voiced, there were many who felt that this would be a travesty of the clinical process and that it could not and should not be done. In practice, something *was* done—and, using results of careful empirical testing as a basis for change, researchers have discovered methods to refine what was previously thought impossible into an instrument with high reliability and validity.

Psychometric Testing

Until an RBI has been field-tested, it is no more than a "work in progress." What kind of field testing is required? In what context should it be carried out? And if unreliability is found, what might be its cause, and what can be done about it?

Types of Reliability

Interrater Reliability

Agreement between interviewers, or "interrater reliability," is a useful procedure for determining whether different users follow the same procedures, interpret the same responses in a similar way, and/or use techniques that elicit similar, relevant information. It is therefore an index of successful training in all of these areas. However, it has little value in the assessment of an RBI, because the RBI gives little opportunity for the variations in procedure or interviewer interpretation that interrater reliability is best designed to identify. Early investigations of highly structured instruments such as the DIS (Robins et al., 1981) and the DISC (Costello, Edelbrock, Kalas, & Dulcan, 1984) went to some lengths to examine whether ratings obtained by clinicians and nonclinicians were systematically different. These studies were essentially asking whether clinicians and nonclinicians differed in their ability to read accurately and stick to the script. Not surprisingly, they did not.

Test–Retest Reliability

Despite the rigid prescription of the order and content of questions and answers, respondents may answer a given question inconsistently when it is put to them on two different occasions. This is troublesome, because it suggests that at least one of the replies is incorrect. This phenomenon is captured by the assessment of "test–retest reliability" (Anastasi, 1988); such an assessment usually consists of administering and then readministering the instrument under similar conditions. Poor test–retest reliability of an RBI can result from a number of sources, all of which need to be considered when one is analyzing the causes of an unreliable part of an interview. Sources of unreliability include the following:

1. *Nature of the sample.* Reliability of categorical diagnoses has been thought to be greatest in either patients with no symptoms or those with a severe disorder. In these instances, a small number of changes in response to individual questions or symptoms are unlikely to result in a reclassification of the patient's status. Patients with a mild disorder who meet a number of criteria just above or just below the diagnostic threshold pose a greater challenge. A changed response to a single question could change whether a diagnosis is present or absent. For this reason, reliability is nearly always higher in a clinical than in a community sample. However, a recent study on the Diagnostic Interview for Children and Adolescents suggests that high levels of psychopathology contribute to low test–retest reliability (Granero Pérez, Ezpeleta Ascaso, Doménich Massons, & de la Osa Ch200, 1998).

Testing the correlation between two continuous measures is less sensitive to the threshold effect described above. However, one should avoid concluding too much from a higher intraclass correlation (a measure used to determine the strength of two continuous variables), because the statistical relationship between kappa and the intraclass correlation coefficient (ICC) will always result in a higher ICC (on the order of 0.1 to 0.2) than kappa (the measure of agreement between categorical measures).

Even if the instrument is to be used in community studies, it should be tested in both a community and a clinical sample, because it is unlikely that a sufficient number of cases of the less common disorders will be found in a community sample. Conversely, community testing is valuable even if the instrument is designed to be used primarily in clinical settings and for uncommon conditions such as psychosis or mania, because it will tell the investigators whether it is detecting false positives.

2. *Sample size.* Power considerations are important. Kappa, the usual measure of reliability, is sensitive to prevalence and may mean little if derived from a very small sample (Fleiss, 1981), because if prevalence is low, a change in the diagnostic status of a single subject from one time to another will have a disproportionate effect on this statistic. For this reason, many investigators require at least five examples of the disorder at Time 1 or Time 2 before using kappa to measure reliability. Caution must be used in evaluating test–retest reliability estimates obtained from small studies, because the 95% confidence intervals for estimates of kappa will not be less than 0.3 unless sample sizes are on the order of several hundreds.

3. *General cognitive effects.* Many cognitive factors are involved in answering an interview question—for example, comprehension, information retrieval, estimation and judgment, and response formulation (Tanur, 1992; Sudman, Bradburn, & Schwarz, 1996). Comprehension can be influenced by receptive language ability, age, and question complexity/clarity (Breton et al., 1995; Fallon & Schwab-Stone, 1994). Children find it difficult to estimate time duration and frequency within a time frame (e.g., "How many times a month did you do this?"). Questions that require self-reflection and/or comparison with others (Fallon & Schwab-Stone, 1994; Granero Pérez et al., 1998) are also difficult to answer. Moreover, replies may be influenced by the time available to respond and by the respondent's reactions to the interviewer's behavior; nonverbal cues and social desirability considerations may influence the time and thought given to a question (Jorm, Duncan-Jones, & Scott, 1989).

4. *Confusion effect.* If a question is ambiguous, long, or complicated; if it has multiple components; or if it is written in language that is beyond a respondent's comprehension due to age, literacy, education, or intelligence, it may be confusing to the respondent. The respondent may focus on and respond to different elements of the questions on initial and subsequent retesting, resulting in different answers across testing situations. Reliability is likely to be greatest if questions are short (Breton et al., 1995) and are stated in simple, age-appropriate language that vividly conveys the essence of the phenomenon. However, not all long questions reduce reliability. Long questions that include multiple concepts are problematic, but long questions that clarify the interviewer's intention (e.g., by addressing an example) may actually improve reliability (Lucas et al., 1998; Sudman et al., 1996).

5. *Timing effect.* Unreliability in a clinical subject may be due to the first

interview's being conducted at the time of maximum distress or help seeking. Under such conditions, the respondent may bring forward information to support the request for help.

6. *Educational effect.* As the interviewee answers more and more questions, his/her understanding of the purpose of the interview may change. He/she may decide that the interviewer is only interested in serious problems, or, conversely, that the interviewer is interested in quite minor problems. In this way the interviewee may, between the start and the end of an interview or between the initial and retest interviews, alter his/her threshold for giving a positive (or negative) response. A lengthy RBI educates the respondent about the nature of psychopathology and about what represents a symptom. A variant of the educational effect is found in the avoidant effect (see below).

7. *Avoidant effect.* The interviewee may learn that whenever he/she gives a positive response, additional questions are asked, and that this lengthens the interview. If this matters to respondents—for example, if they perceive the interview experience as too stressful, lengthy, boring, or tiring—they may consciously or subconsciously alter their response pattern, and limit the number of positive replies toward the end of the interview or on reinterview (Lucas, 1992). It is possible that measures with a branching structure, such as the Composite International Diagnostic Interview (CIDI; World Health Organization, 1995) or the DISC (Shaffer et al., in press), may be particularly affected where initial probes (stems) are followed by more detailed questions (contingents).

8. *Mood effect.* An interviewee's current mood can influence his/her recall and disposition to label a recalled feeling as normal or abnormal. If this mood varies between interviews, one would also expect a response change (Jensen, Traylor, Xenakis, & Davis, 1988).

9. *Therapeutic effect.* The process of the RBI may lessen anxiety or improve mood, with the result that fewer symptoms are reported at reinterview.

10. *Memory effect.* It is common for people to remember events as occurring more recently than they did. The determinants of this phenomenon, also called "telescoping," are not known; however, it is reasonable to believe that they might operate most strongly during an initial interview, when (as a form of social expectancy effect) there is a perceived expectation that the respondent has something to report.

11. *Embarrassment effect.* Reliability may be low for questions that address socially undesirable behaviors or emotions. These questions are likely to be influenced by subtle interviewer effects, with some interviewers facilitating and others discouraging embarrassing revelations. Authors should be cautious about dealing with this problem by using coy language or ambiguous euphemisms, because these, by adding to the "confusion effect," may make a difficult situation worse. There is some evidence that a self-completion format will increase the endorsement rate for embarrassing questions

(Turner et al., 1998), which could be an added consideration favoring the use of RBIs.

12. *Threshold effect.* Small changes in symptom levels in cases at or near the diagnostic threshold will have a disproportionate effect on reliability (Jensen et al., 1995).

13. *Motivational effect.* Certain subjects (e.g., clinical subjects) or informants (e.g., adults) may be inclined to answer more or less assiduously on each occasion (Jensen et al., 1995).

Few of these effects have been tested experimentally. Recent work (Lucas et al., in press) has attempted to parse out specific features of RBIs associated with unreliability.

Attenuation

Unreliability in measurement hinders all psychiatric research. Discrepant reporting in a test–retest paradigm is usually from positive to negative, rather than in the opposite direction; that is, subjects report fewer symptoms on retesting. This phenomenon is called "attenuation" and has been viewed as a particular problem for self-report questionnaires and respondent-based interviews (Costello, Burns, Angold, & Leaf, 1993), although it is seen in all forms of repeated psychiatric inquiry (Andreasen et al., 1981; Helzer et al., 1985; Anthony et al., 1985; Lucas, 1992). Its pervasiveness has led to the suggestion that this is not simple measurement error, but represents a systematic bias in reporting (Jensen et al., 1995; Ribera et al., 1996). In general, attenuation is greater in community subjects, child informants, and less severe cases (Jensen et al., 1995). Using the Spanish DISC in an Hispanic population, Ribera et al. (1996) noted that "[for every] instance in which kappas were < 0.4, there was evidence of significant attenuation" (p. 198).

Attenuation is probably due to some combination of the factors listed above (Robins, 1985; Fallon & Schwab-Stone, 1994; Lucas, in press). It is not known when attenuation "bottoms out" (i.e., how many readministrations are necessary for response rates to reach a point of asymptote or stability), nor whether, in a situation in which test–retest reliability is low, responses given the first time are more or less correct than responses given on retest. The answers to these questions may well be content-, informant-, or method-specific, but they undoubtedly deserve greater study.

The type of question that is most likely to attenuate is a "stem question" that is placed early in the interview (i.e., a question asked of everyone that, depending on a subject's response, generates contingent questions). As noted earlier, other types of questions that frequently attenuate are questions with long, multiple constructs and questions that require an assessment of timing, duration, or symptom frequency. In addition, symptoms that are not readily visible to others (e.g., questions about mood states or other subjective feelings) are likely to attenuate more if asked of a parent informant about a youth than of the youth himself/herself. Jensen et al. (in press) demonstrated a "location" effect by examining endorsement rates of a standard section whose position in the interview was altered by means of a counterbalanced design. Regardless of content (mood or behavior symptoms), sections given first were endorsed more often at first administration and declined most between first and second interviews. This finding is compatible with an "education" or "avoidant" effect, whereby interviewees make a conscious effort to avoid further questions and/or become better educated about the nature and purpose of the interview as they proceed into the interview.

If mindset, lack of appreciation of the task, or fatigue with the process are mediating processes in unreliability, then experimental approaches incorporating graphic aids and questioning strategies need to be developed to minimize these problems and to better educate the respondent before the first interview or to devise less fatiguing tests.

Clinical Validity

Valid Representation of Criteria

Many of the key "symptoms" of common child psychiatric disorders are normal when they occur at certain ages, or are only considered to be symptoms when they occur excessively or go on for too long a time. This has resulted in the DSM and ICD classification systems' requiring symptoms to occur above a minimum frequency, for longer than a certain period, or before or after a certain age. Because for many behaviors there are few age-based norms, and normal frequency counts are not readily available, the designers of classification systems are faced with a problem that they address by using such vague adverbs as "often," "severe," or "age-appropriate."

When faced with vaguely written criteria, the author of an RBI must either leave the decision as to what these adverbs mean to the untutored opinion of the respondent, or develop his/her own numerical rules. This may not be a bad thing, because in setting frequency thresholds, the author, like the modern nosologist, is contributing actively to a heuristic process; the arbitrarily operationalized criteria can be supported or refuted in future research. It is possible to avoid the need for radical rewrites of the interview by offering various frequencies, durations, and so forth as response options, so that items can be recalibrated with revisions of the diagnostic algorithm rather than with extensive revisions of the instrument.

The process of writing questions to address sensible but arbitrary criteria is difficult, and clinically experienced investigators often hold divergent views. In the preparation of the DISC (see below), it was helpful to convene a committee of such investigators to prepare the first draft.

Measuring Validity

Some of the ways in which the validity of an RBI can be tested include the following:

1. Investigators can determine whether known patients have more symptoms/diagnoses than nonpatients do.
2. The extent of agreement between the conclusions of an experienced and well-qualified clinician and the determination made by the RBI can be determined. If a symptom has been endorsed on the RBI, it is important to determine whether the patient is referring to something that most clinicians would regard as the target symptom, criterion, or diagnosis. This approach provides information about whether the questions in the RBI are over- or undersensitive with reference to the clinical criteria, and it may also provide anecdotal information about whether the questions elicit unintended information. However, this approach will work if only one crucial variable is changed at a time—for example, if the clinician bases his/her conclusions on information from the same specified informant, and not on the opinion generated by a committee that has access to information from multiple sources. The limitations of this approach lie in the quality of the criterion (i.e., a single clinician's opinion). The problems of establishing a diagnostic standard are legion and have been discussed elsewhere (Shaffer et al., 1993).
3. The most demanding, and in some ways the least helpful, approach to testing validity is to compare the data obtained from a single informant with some aggregate of information obtained from multiple informants— such as that presented at the usual clinical case conference, in which data from the child, the parent, the school teacher, previous clinical notes, and the results of any tests are combined. Although comparisons of this kind may indicate the relationship between information from one source and from multiple sources, they have limited value as a guide to developing or improving the RBI.

THE DIAGNOSTIC INTERVIEW SCHEDULE FOR CHILDREN: A FAMILY OF INSTRUMENTS

The National Institute of Mental Health (NIMH) Diagnostic Interview Schedule for Children (NIMH DISC or DISC) is an RBI designed to assess over 30 of the most common psychiatric diagnoses in children and adolescents, according to the DSM and ICD diagnostic systems. The instrument was originally designed to be administered by "lay" (clinically untrained) interviewers, following a brief training period, in large-scale epidemiological surveys of children and adolescents; it is now being used in many clinical studies, screening projects, and service settings as well. The DISC comprises two interviews: the DISC-P, to be administered to parents or knowledgeable caretakers about their children, and the DISC-Y, to be administered directly to youth.

History

The impetus for developing the DISC came in 1979 as an initiative by NIMH that called for an instrument that could be used in large-scale surveys of children and adolescents to determine the rate of mental disorders in U.S. youth. The first version of the interview, the DISC-1, was based on DSM-III, and its content and structure were originally outlined by an NIMH committee convened in 1980 that included Keith Conners, Barbara Herjanic, and Joaquim Puig-Antich. Extensive further development and field testing in a clinical sample was undertaken by Costello and Dulcan (Costello, Edelbrock, Dulcan, Kalas, & Klaric, 1984). The design of the DISC-1 reflected a cautious transition from the semistructured to the fully structured approach. It included many "write-ins," used by the interviewer to describe a symptom in the respondent's words; these necessitated a good deal of postinterview coding. Symptoms were grouped by the environment in which they occurred (e.g., home, school, etc.) on the assumption that this was how they would be best conceptualized by the respondent, and also in order to eliminate redundancy from criteria shared between different diagnoses. Finally, the instrument was designed to be highly sensitive, with generally low thresholds for defining a behavior or feeling as abnormal.

This last feature led to problems with apparently implausibly high prevalence rates. A validity study (Costello, Edelbrock, Kalas, & Dulcan, 1984) showed poor correspondence between diagnoses obtained from a single-informant DISC and case conference diagnoses (the latter were based on information derived from multiple sources). These findings were misinterpreted as showing that the DISC-1 was invalid, whereas they probably reflected poor agreement between informants (see above).

The next version of the instrument, the DISC-R, was prepared in 1985 and was nearly compatible with DSM-III-R (a draft of the final criteria was used in its preparation). It was developed by modifying questions found unreliable in Costello and colleagues' sample or questions that had a very high prevalence rate in an unreferred community population (Shaffer et al., 1993). A high prevalence in the community sample was considered an indication for revision, based on the reasoning that if the prevalence of a symptom exceeded 20% in a community population, the instrument was probably picking up a mixture of normal and pathological states. The revision process used to develop the DISC-R established a precedent of iterative change based on previous empirical study, upon which all subsequent versions of the DISC have been built.

The DISC-R was designed without "skips." Information was obtained about every symptom, so that it could be used for diagnostic symptom scales. Many of the DISC-1's open-ended questions were deleted to minimize the need for postinterview coding. Some disorders, including pervasive developmental disorders, were considered to require clinical observation and/or formal testing, and therefore were omitted as inappropriate for a respondent-based interview. Most symptoms were grouped by diagnosis rather than by setting, and this allowed for subsequent diagnostic modular organization. The DISC-R also included a graphic "time line" as a memory aid for important time frames. Field trials conducted on a clinical population (Shaffer et al., 1993; Schwab-Stone et al., 1993; Piacentini et al., 1993) showed the DISC-R to have better test–retest reliability than the DISC-1. These trials also showed that the test–retest reliability of the DISC-R was greater than that obtained by clinicians using an instrument prepared to provide definitions of symptoms, suggested questions, and standardized rating scales to denote the definite or questionable presence or absence of individual symptoms. This finding of greater reliability for the DISC-R over the clinician ratings illustrated how, even with substantial structure, clinicians who are often used as the criteria against which measures are judged themselves rarely meet the standards of diagnostic reliability expected in research instruments.

DISC-R field trial data were used in 1989 to create the DISC-2.1, in which unreliable questions were again revised; modular organization of diagnoses was extended, so that groups of related diagnoses were contained and could be used independently of the others; and the psychosis section, which had proved difficult to use, was modified to include two screening questions that, if not endorsed, led to a "skip-out" of the section. Finally, a process of elaboration was initiated that has continued through all subsequent versions of the DISC. Questions were added to assess factors of age at first episode, precipitating stressors suggestive of an adjustment disorder, impairment associated with the current episode, and treatment history. The DISC-2.1 was field-tested at three sites on 97 clinical cases and 278 community children and adolescents aged 9 to 17 (Jensen et al., 1995). Low-incidence diagnoses, such as anorexia nervosa and obsessive–compulsive disorder, were examined through collaborative agreements with specialized clinical settings (Fisher et al., 1993). Findings from these trials were used in 1991 to develop the DISC-2.3 (Shaffer et al., 1996). Scoring algorithms were constructed that permitted a diagnosis to be established either on symptom criteria alone or together with a specified level of diagnosis-specific impairment. A Spanish-language version of the DISC-2.3 was prepared for the Puerto Rico site of the MECA study (Bravo, Woodbury-Farina, Canino, & Rubio-Stipec, 1993), and used for Spanish-speaking subjects/informants.

In 1992, NIMH established the DISC Editorial Board (DEB) to oversee further development of the instrument and maintain its standardization. The first task of the DEB was to oversee the development of the NIMH DISC-IV (discussed below). The DEB continues to be charged with interpreting the findings from methodological and research studies as a basis for amending the interview and its algorithms.

The NIMH DISC-IV

The current version of the instrument, the DISC-IV, was developed to be compatible with DSM-IV and ICD-10 and to be retrocompatible with DSM-III-R. Another important difference from previous versions is that the DISC-IV includes assessment for three time frames: the present (past 4 weeks), the last year, and "ever." The present-state assessment is thought to be the most accurate, because it minimizes the risk of bias due to telescoping. It is useful for providing information on point prevalence, and is also valuable for clinicians who need to know about a youth's current state. The 1-year time frame, although less accurate than a brief current time frame, is widely used. One-year prevalence is (or should be) higher than point prevalence; it is therefore especially useful in risk factor research, since it provides a larger number of cases. Clinicians routinely ask for lifetime history of disorders, even though the evidence for accurate recall is not good and tends to be influenced by present mental state (Pulver & Carpenter, 1983; Bromet, Dunn, Connell, Dew, & Schulberg, 1986; Dohrenwend, 1990). Although salient symptoms may be recalled, it is unlikely that all of the symptoms that are required to make up a diagnosis will be remembered. Moreover, unless a disorder was severe, it is even less likely that the frequency and duration of the symptoms will be remembered. All in all, this makes the accurate retrospective assignment of diagnosis highly speculative. The whole-life component of the DISC-IV is therefore heuristic and should be used with caution until empirical research defines the domains in which it is valid.

The Parent and Youth Interviews

All versions of the DISC have been prepared with parallel forms for youth aged 9 to 17 (DISC-Y) and for parents or knowledgeable caretakers of youth aged between 6 and 17 (DISC-P). The types and ranges of behaviors and symptoms covered in the parent and youth versions are generally similar, although the pronouns differ. If a question in the DISC-Y refers to a thought or feeling, the question in the parent interview will ask for observable manifestations of the thought (e.g., "Did he seem ___?" or "Did he say that he felt ___?"). Modified versions of the DISC-P for parents of children under age 6, and of the DISC-Y for older teens and young adults, are currently in development.

Scope and Organization of the DISC-IV

The DISC-IV covers DSM-IV and DSM-III-R criteria for over 30 diagnoses, as well as ICD-10 diagnostic criteria for most of these. Like the DISC-

2.1 and DISC-2.3, the DISC-IV is organized into six diagnostic modules, but each diagnosis is fully "self-contained" to allow users to drop diagnostic sections without affecting the scoring of other sections (see Table 1.2 for a list of diagnoses). To enable users to arrive at this modular organization, certain symptoms (e.g., irritability, restlessness, concentration problems) are asked about more than once over the whole interview. Having single rather than grouped, multidiagnosis modules is advantageous, in that a research project requiring information on only a small number of diagnoses from separate modules can efficiently customize the interview.

Some diagnostic sections have been written to be compatible with "adult" interviews. For example, the questions in the schizophrenia section were adapted from the CIDI (World Health Organization, 1995), and the use questions for the substance use disorders were made compatible to those contained in the DIS (for adults) (Robins, Cottler, Bucholz, & Compton, 1996).

The diagnostic sections are followed by an elective whole-life module, which assesses whether a child or adolescent has had any diagnosis not currently present in the past year, since his/her fifth birthday.

Question Structure

Questions contained in the DISC-IV have been carefully designed to be read *exactly* as written. There are very few open-ended responses allowed; most re-

TABLE 1.2. List of Diagnoses Covered in the DISC-IV

Anxiety disorders	Mood Disorders
Social phobia	Major depressive episode
Separation anxiety disorder	Dysthymic disorder
Specific phobia	Manic episode
Panic disorder	Hypomanic episode
Agoraphobia	
Generalized anxiety disorder	Schizophrenia
Selective mutism	
Obsessive–compulsive disorder	Attention-deficit and disruptive behavior
Posttraumatic stress disorder	disorders
	Attention-deficit/hyperactivity disorder
Miscellaneous disorders	Oppositional defiant disorder
Anorexia nervosa/bulimia nervosa	Conduct disorder[a]
Elimination disorders[a]	
Tic disorders[a]	Substance use disorders
Pica[a]	Alcohol abuse/dependence
Trichotillomania[a]	Nicotine dependence
	Cannabis abuse/dependence
	Other substance abuse/dependence

[a]Whole-life assessment included in core interview.

sponses are limited to "yes" and "no," although a few offer an additional "sometimes" or "somewhat" choice or a closed-ended frequency option.

The DISC-IV contains approximately 3,000 questions that fall into four categories:

1. About 10% are "stem" questions. These are sensitive, broad questions that address essential aspects of a symptom. All stem questions are asked of everyone.

2. About 45% of the questions are "contingent" questions, which are asked only if a previous question is answered positively. Contingent questions are used to determine whether the symptoms meet some very specific characteristics of a diagnostic criterion (e.g., frequency, duration, intensity). An example of a stem–contingent arrangement is shown in Figure 1.1. This stem–contingent structure allows the DISC-IV to build symptom and criterion scales for most diagnoses.

3. Approximately 25% are diagnosis-dependent questions about age of onset, impairment, and treatment, which are only asked if a number of diagnostic criteria have been endorsed (usually just over half of those required for a diagnosis).

4. About 15% are questions that are part of the elective whole-life module.

Measurement of Impairment

As discussed earlier, DSM-IV (American Psychiatric Association, 1994) requires that a psychiatric diagnosis only be assigned if the symptoms give rise

---

3. In the last year—that is, since you started ninth grade—was there a time when you often felt grouchy or irritable and often in a bad mood, when even little things would make you mad?

IF YES,   A. Was there a time in the last year when you felt grouchy or irritable for a long time each day?

IF NO, GO TO Q 4
B. Would you say that you felt that way for **most of the day**?
C. Was there a time when you felt grouchy or irritable **almost every day**?

IF NO, GO TO Q 4
D. In the last year, were there two weeks in a row when you felt grouchy or irritable almost every day?

IF NO, GO TO Q 2
E. Now, what about the **last four weeks**?
Since you came home from Camp Treetop, have you often felt grouchy or irritable and in a bad mood?

FIGURE 1.1. Sample DISC-IV question (major depressive episode—irritable mood).

to impairment or distress. To meet this requirement, the DISC-IV includes a standard series of questions addressing six domains of impairment (impact on relations with parents/caretakers, participation in family activities, participation in peer activities, academic/occupational functioning, relationships with teachers/boss, and self-distress about symptoms). The impairment questions are asked of subjects endorsing a minimal number of symptoms. Each domain of impairment has two parts. The first part assesses whether impairment is present, and the second measures severity or frequency. For example, for major depressive disorder, the questions assessing impairment in academic function read:

> When the problems were worst, did feeling sad or depressed make it difficult for you to do your schoolwork or cause problems with your grades?
>
> IF YES, How bad were the problems you had with your schoolwork because you felt this way? Would you say: very bad, bad, or not too bad?

Algorithms have been developed to allow investigators to specify the number (or nature) of the impairment items required for a diagnosis.

Scoring, Diagnostic Algorithms, and Symptom Scales

The DISC-IV is typically scored by algorithms that apply Boolean logic (i.e., "ands" and "ors") to combine the answers to component questions. These algorithms are programmed in SAS (SAS Institute, 1990). Algorithms have been prepared to score the parent and youth interviews separately (the "single-informant" algorithms), as well as to combine information across the parent and youth interviews (the "combined" algorithms). These latter algorithms use an "or" rule, which scores a criterion present if it is endorsed by either a parent or a youth. In addition, algorithms to assess "caseness" (as defined by meeting symptomatic criteria plus demonstrating a significant degree of impairment) have been prepared and are being tested, as are algorithms to score the interview according to the ICD-10 and the earlier DSM-III-R diagnostic criteria.

In addition to the diagnostic algorithms, symptom and criterion scales for most diagnoses can be obtained with the SAS scoring program. A symptom scale for a diagnosis contains all of the key stem questions for that diagnosis. Criterion scales are essentially counts of the criteria for a diagnosis, built from combinations of stem and contingent items that make up each criterion. Analyses have been done on test data to indicate which cutoff scores best predict diagnosis.

The DISC-IV interview can be hand-scored, although this is inadvisable, as it is an error-prone and complicated procedure.

Computerization

The DISC-IV is an ideal candidate for computerization, given the highly structured nature of the interview, the limited response options, the complicated branching and skipping instructions, and the need for the interviewer to keep close track of an informant's answers to numerous symptoms in order to ask onset and impairment questions correctly. Given the complexity of the NIMH DISC-IV, it is recommended that investigators using more than a single diagnostic module use a computer-assisted program to aid administration. Although use of a computer program does not reduce administration time, it reduces training time, cuts down on interviewer and editor error, and eliminates data entry costs (Shaffer et al., in press).

The computer-assisted version of the NIMH DISC-IV is the C-DISC-4.0, which is owned and distributed by the Division of Child and Adolescent Psychiatry at Columbia University. The C-DISC-4.0 is available in both English and Spanish versions (see below) and can be run from DOS or Windows. The application program incorporates the SAS single-informant scoring algorithms, and generates a diagnostic and symptom report based on the algorithm within minutes of the completion of an interview. Some data management functions are also incorporated into the software. However, if a user wants to combine information across informants, require impairment, or generate the symptom and criterion scale scores, it is necessary to download ASCII data from the C-DISC-4.0 application and read this into the SAS algorithm programs.

In 1997, Columbia University was awarded a contract by NIMH with the primary purpose of providing unlimited copies of the C-DISC-4.0 for projects supported by the U.S. Department of Health and Human Service (DHHS) for a license fee negotiated with the DHHS. The license fee provides for access to technical support in the use of the application and program updates. The application is also available to non-DHHS public health investigators and clinical and commercial users. Through the university, graduate students and educators will be provided the program at a modest fee.

Spanish Version of the DISC-IV

Under the direction of an International Spanish Advisory Group sponsored by the NIMH, Glorisa Canino and her colleagues at the University of Puerto Rico have undertaken the official Spanish translation of the NIMH DISC-IV in accordance with the guidelines set down by the DEB.

Administration Time

The administration time for the complete NIMH DISC-IV averages about 70 minutes per informant in a community population, and about 105 minutes in a clinical population. Administration can be shortened by dropping diagnostic sections that are not of interest for a particular setting or study. New DISC derivations (see below) are being planned that will have an appreciably shorter administration time.

Training

Training sessions instruct trainees about the conventions and rules for administering the DISC-IV, the use of time lines, and identification of the "active" parts of symptom questions. Trainees are also taught techniques for nondirective presentation of questions, and are shown how to use the computer software. Trainers provide demonstrations, round-robin exercises, and videotape models, and trainees are observed giving practice interviews. Training users in administration of computer-assisted versions of the NIMH DISC-IV can be completed in 2 or 3 days, depending upon trainees' experience in administering RBIs. Training users to administer the paper DISC-IV takes an additional 2 to 3 days.

Performance of the DISC-IV in a Clinical Sample

Although psychometric testing of the NIMH DISC-IV is not yet complete, partial results concerning the performance of the interview from a sample of 82 children and adolescents (aged 9 to 17) and 84 parents recruited from child psychiatric outpatient clinics have been presented (Fisher et al., 1997; Shaffer et al., in press). Sixty percent of the sample was nonwhite and/or Hispanic, and all subjects were fluent in English. Lay interviewers were trained for 2 to 4 days on DISC-IV administration. The DISC-IV (including the optional whole-life module) was administered twice, with an interval between administrations of 3 to 10 days (mean = 6.6 days); the C-DISC-4.0 computerized application was used. The interviewers were blind to responses given by the other informants and at the other testing session (four interviews per subject).

Test–Retest Reliability

Test–retest reliability for selected diagnoses can be found in Table 1.3. Data from a comparable sample (Jensen et al., 1995) using the DISC-2.1 are also shown for comparison purposes. The NIMH DISC-IV compares favorably with earlier versions of the instrument, even though it takes longer to administer and is significantly more complex, given that diagnoses are assessed for multiple time frames.

TABLE 1.3. Test–Retest Reliability (Kappa) of the DISC-IV (Past Year) in a Clinical Sample Aged 9–17

| | DISC-IV[a] | | | DISC-2.1[b] | |
	Parent (n = 84)	Youth (n = 82)	Combined	Parent (n = 97)	Youth (n = 97)
Attn.-def./hyp. dis.	.79	.42	.62	.69	.59
Opposit. def. dis.	.54	.51	.59	.67	.46
Conduct dis.	.43	.65	.55	.70	.86
Any anxiety disorder[c]	—	—	—	.58	.39
Specific phobia	.96	.68	.86	—	—
Social phobia	.54	.25	.48	—	—
Separation anx. dis.	.58	.46	.51	—	—
Generalized anx. dis.	.65	—	.58	—	—
Major depressive episode	.66	.92	.65	.69[d]	.38[d]

[a]The data are from Fisher et al. (1997).
[b]The data are from Jensen et al. (1995).
[c]Includes DSM-III-R simple phobia, social phobia, separation anxiety disorder, overanxious disorder, panic disorder, etc.
[d]These numbers (from DISC 2.1) are for depression and/or dysthymia. DISC-IV numbers are for Major depressive episode only.

Administration Time and Acceptability to Informants

In this clinical sample, the administration time for the DISC-IV varied greatly, because administration time is dependent upon how many symptoms are endorsed. Administration of the DISC-P ranged from just over 1 hour (62 minutes) to 4 hours (283 minutes), with a mean time of about 2 hours (115 minutes). The DISC-Y was slightly faster, ranging from under 1 hour (48 minutes) to nearly 3 hours (169 minutes), with a mean time of 113 minutes. Administration time in community subjects is likely to be significantly shorter, in view of the higher properties of subjects who are diagnosis-negative.

After completion of the first DISC-IV interview, parents and youth were given questionnaires to assess their reaction to the interview. These forms were completed privately, and responses were put in a sealed envelope. As shown in Table 1.4, at the end of this lengthy interview, only a small minority seemed to find the experience unpleasant.

Sensitivity of the DISC-2.1 in a Clinical Sample

To date, there are no published validity data on the DISC-IV. In an investigation using an earlier version of the DISC (DISC-2.1) in a clinical sample,

TABLE 1.4. Three-Site DISC-IV Reliability Study

	Parent %	Child %
Acceptability ratings of DISC-IV reliability protocol[a]		
Was interview interesting, boring, or neither?		
Interesting	73.6	47.6
Boring	6.9	17.1
Neither	17.2	19.5
Don't know	2.3	15.9
Was interview too long, too short, or right length?		
Too long	41.9	55.4
Too short	1.2	2.4
About right	51.2	36.1
Don't know	5.8	6.0
Do you feel more comfortable, more upset, or same (as before the interview)?		
More comfortable	20.9	32.5
More upset	4.7	3.6
About the same	70.9	53.0
Don't know	3.5	10.8
Would you tell a friend to participate?		
No	26.6	27.3
Yes	65.8	59.7
Don't know	7.6	13.0
Acceptability of computerized version[b]		
If had choice, would prefer interviewer to use:		
Computer	32.5	44.7
Paper and pencil	1.3	3.9
Don't care	64.9	44.7
Don't know	1.3	6.6

Note. Data from Shaffer et al. (in press).
[a] $n \approx 84$ parents and 82 children.
[b] $n \approx 77$ parents and 76 children.

Fisher et al. (1993) examined the sensitivity of the DISC-2.1 for certain uncommon psychiatric disorders (i.e., major depressive, obsessive–compulsive, psychotic, tic, and substance use disorders). Subjects were recruited from centers specializing in the treatment of each of the uncommon disorders, and their diagnosis had been confirmed by senior clinicians at each center, so that the centers' diagnoses served as the criterion measures. Overall findings showed that the DISC-2.1 had good to excellent sensitivity (range = .73 to 1.0) for these disorders. Used alone, the DISC-P was generally more sensitive than the DISC-Y.

Performance of the DISC-2.3 in a Community Sample

Data on the reliability and validity of the DISC-IV in community subjects have been collected by investigators from the NIMH sponsored Unmet Needs, Outcomes, and Costs for Children and Adolescents study and are currently being analyzed (W. Narrow, personal communication, 1999). The most recently published psychometric information on the DISC in a community sample comes from the MECA study (Schwab-Stone et al., 1996), which used the DISC-2.3 with a sample of 247 parent–child pairs (the children were aged 9 to 17). Slightly over half of the youth were judged on the Time 1 DISC-2.3 interview to be "symptom-rich" (the remainder had no disorder at Time 1). Although lay interviewers administered the initial interviews, clinicians administered the retest interviews.

Reliability

Overall, the DISC-2.3 showed parent diagnoses (i.e., diagnoses based on the parent interview only) to have moderate to good diagnostic reliability, as did the diagnoses assigned on the basis of combined parent and child information. Reliability for the diagnoses obtained with the child interview was less good (see Table 1.5), with the exception of conduct disorder. Most of the unreliability in the DISC-2.3 seemed to be a result of the "attenuation effect" described earlier (Lucas et al., in press).

Reliability may appear misleadingly low when applied to categorical diagnoses. A change in a single response can bring a case to above or below the diagnostic threshold. To determine whether this was so, the data from the MECA exercise were used to calculate the reliability (in terms of ICCs) of the symptom and criterion scales for the DISC-2.3. As expected, the symptom and criterion scales had better reliability than did the categorical diagnoses for most disorders (see Table 1.5).

Validity

The MECA study examined validity for the DISC-2.3 (Schwab-Stone et al., 1996), in an exercise designed to determine whether information elicited on the DISC corresponded to "clinically meaningful" symptomatology. As noted above, clinicians administered the DISC-2.3 at Time 2. During the administration, they were instructed to tag any question where a subject's behavior (verbal and nonverbal cues) might indicate an ambiguous response, such as a marked hesitation or a puzzled look. Tagged questions and every criterion that had been endorsed became the focus of a further, third inquiry, where these questions were asked more clinically. A format such as the following was used: "You told me that you had _____. Could you tell me some more about that?" or "When I asked you _____, you seemed unsure about

TABLE 1.5. Test–Retest Reliability of DISC–2.3 in a Community Sample

| | Diagnostic reliability[a] (Kappa statistics) | | | Scale reliability (ICCs) | | | | | |
| | | | | Symptom counts | | | Criterion counts | | |
	Parent	Youth	Parent and youth combined	Parent	Youth	Parent and youth combined	Parent	Youth	Parent and youth combined
Attention-def./hyp. dis.	.60	.10	.48	.57	.30	.95	.61	.27	.82
Opposit. def. disorder	.68	.18	.59	.83	.40	.77	.81	.57	.42
Conduct disorder	.56	.64	.66	.83	.83	.83	.79	.70	.73
Any anxiety dis.[b]	.56	.39	.47	—	—	—	—	—	—
Overanxious disorder	.60	.28	.52	.73	.40	.46	.71	.44	.55
Separation anx. dis.	.45	.27	.49	.75	.42	.61	.67	.46	.61
Social phobia	.45	.33	.44	.63	.44	.24	.61	.44	.58
Simple phobia	—	—	—	.69	.53	.72	.69	.53	.71
Panic disorder	—	—	—	.43	.11	.22	.46	.04	.12
Agoraphobia	—	—	—	.64	.49	.53	.66	.35	.40
Major depressive episode	.55	.37	.45	.66	.56	.64	.51	.40	.49

[a]Data from Schwab-Stone et al. (1996).
[b]Includes social phobia, agoraphobia, panic, overanxious disorder, generalized anxiety disorder, and separation anxiety disorder.

your reply. Can you tell me more about that?" The clinician then made a rating based on the answers to this inquiry, which was then compared with his/her original DISC-2.3 ratings. For most diagnoses, agreement between the DISC-2.3 and the final clinical rating was moderate to very good for both the parent and youth interviews, separately and combined. Exceptions to this were the parent report of separation anxiety disorder and the youth report of ADHD, both of which were poor.

POTENTIAL APPLICATIONS
FOR RESPONDENT-BASED INTERVIEWS

The need for inexpensive, convenient instruments for establishing psychiatric diagnoses is not confined to large-scale field research. There are very few trained clinicians available in rural and inner-city areas of the United States, as well as in most of the Third World. In many other areas, available clinicians have had inadequate training in diagnostic methods or are under such time and/or financial pressures that their ability to perform comprehensive diagnostic evaluations is reduced. In all such situations, the availability of RBIs can be a boon. However, many of the complex requirements of a research instrument reduce clinical utility (e.g., ascertainment of symptom presence in several time frames, and inquiry about symptom details when it has already been ascertained that the diagnosis could not be present). It was with this need in mind that our research group began preparing an abbreviated instrument, the "Quick DISC." In this modified, time-saving instrument, symptoms that have a strong negative predictive value are ascertained first, so that if none are endorsed the interview skips to the next diagnostic module. In addition, the presence of symptoms is assessed for the current month only.

In China—a developing-world setting in which patients speak many different dialects and languages—an English-language version of the DISC is being used as a prompt for psychiatric nurses, who translate the questions into the appropriate dialect or language (P. Leung & T. P. Ho, personal communication, 1997). Although it is likely that the highly standardized elements of the RBI would be lost under such circumstances, its ability to serve as a script for partially trained clinicians remains of value.

Many of the advantages that RBIs hold for research investigators are also advantages in nonresearch settings, such as clinical and public health contexts: the lessening of reliance on skilled clinicians, the potential for increased reliability, and the capacity for computerization.

1. *Clinical applications.* Although the decision on whether or how to treat a patient depends on more than a simple DSM or ICD diagnosis, an RBI can prove useful for a clinician. When it is used as part of the initial diagnostic

workup, it can allow the clinician to save precious time by delegating part of the evaluation task to a nonclinician—or, better still, to the patient himself/herself when a self-completion mode is used. The clinician can then focus his/her inquiry on the context and contingencies of the reported symptoms. Use of the RBI results can also improve compliance with existing diagnostic systems by specifying the extent to which the symptoms adhere to the standardized diagnostic criteria. Finally, these results can become part of a computerized database against which the performance of the individual and/or the clinic at large can be gauged.

2. *Public health applications.* Youth at high risk for a psychiatric disorder are regularly assessed by social welfare agencies. They attend shelters for runaways and the homeless, are interviewed by probation officers, or are incarcerated in juvenile detention centers and prisons. The treatable psychiatric disorders that many of these children and adolescents suffer from may go unrecognized because of a shortage of clinicians to identify their condition. The routine implementation of low-cost RBIs, ideally in the self-completion format, could change this situation radically.

REFERENCES

Achenbach, T. M. (1994). Child Behavior Checklist and related instruments. In M. E. Maruish (Ed.), *The use of psychological testing for treatment planning and outcome assessment* (pp. 517–549). Mahwah, NJ: Erlbaum.

Achenbach, T. M., Conners, C. K., & Quay, H. C. (1983). *The ACQ Behavior Checklist.* Burlington: University of Vermont, Department of Psychiatry.

American Psychiatric Association. (1980). *Diagnostic and statistical manual of mental disorders* (3rd ed.). Washington, DC: Author.

American Psychiatric Association. (1994). *Diagnostic and statistical manual of mental disorders* (4th ed.). Washington, DC: Author.

Anastasi, A. (1988). *Psychological testing* (6th ed.). New York: Macmillan.

Andreasen, N. C., Grove, W. M., Shapiro, R. W., Keller, M. B., Hirschfield, R. M. A., & McDonald-Scott, P. (1981). Reliability of lifetime diagnosis. A multicenter collaborative perspective. *Archives of General Psychiatry, 38,* 400–405.

Angold, A., Prendergast, M., Cox, A., Harrinton, R., Simonoff, E., & Rutter, M. (1995). The Child and Adolescent Psychiatric Assessment (CAPA). *Psychological Medicine, 25,* 739–753.

Anthony, J. C., Folstein, M., Romanoski, A. J., Von Korff, M. R., Nestadt, G. N., Chahal, R., Merchant, A., Brown, C. H., Shapiro, S., Kramer, M., & Gruenberg, E. M. (1985). Comparison of the lay Diagnostic Interview Schedule and a standardized psychiatric diagnosis: Experience in eastern Baltimore. *Archives of General Psychiatry, 42,* 667–675.

Bravo, M., Woodbury-Farina, M., Canino, G. J., & Rubio-Stipec, M. (1993). The Spanish translation and cultural adaptation of the Diagnostic Interview Schedule for Children (DISC) in Puerto Rico. *Culture, Medicine and Psychiatry, 17,* 329–344.

Breton, J. J., Bergeron, L., Valla, J. P., Lepine, S., Houde, L., & Gaudet, N. (1995). Do children aged nine through eleven years understand the DISC Version 2.25 questions? *Journal of the American Academy of Child and Adolescent Psychiatry, 34*(7), 946–956.

Bromet, E. J., Dunn, L. O., Connell, M. M., Dew, M. A., & Schulberg, H. C. (1986). Long-term reliability of diagnosing lifetime major depression in a community sample. *Archives of General Psychiatry, 43*(5), 435–440.

Costello, A. J., Edelbrock, C. S., Dulcan, M. K., Kalas, R., & Klaric, S. H. (1984). *Report on the Diagnostic Interview Schedule for Children (DISC).* Washington, DC: National Institute of Mental Health.

Costello, A. J., Edelbrock, C. S., Kalas, R., & Dulcan, M. K. (1984). *The NIMH Diagnostic Interview Schedule for Children (DISC): Development, reliability, and comparisons between clinical and lay interviewers.* Unpublished manuscript.

Costello, E. J., Burns, B. J., Angold, A., & Leaf, P. J. (1993). How can epidemiology improve mental health services for children and adolescents? *Journal of the American Academy of Child and Adolescent Psychiatry, 32,* 1106–1113.

Dohrenwend, B. P. (1990). "The problem of validity in field studies of psychological disorders" revisited. *Psychological Medicine, 20*(1), 195–208.

Fallon, T., & Schwab-Stone, M. (1994). Determinants of reliability in psychiatric surveys of children aged six to twelve. *Journal of Child Psychology and Psychiatry, 35*(8), 1391–1408.

Fisher, P. W., Lucas, C., Shaffer, D., Schwab-Stone, M. M., Dulcan, M., Graae, F., Lichtman, J., Willoughby, S., & Gerarld, J. (1997). *Diagnostic Interview Schedule for Children, Version IV (DISC-IV): Test–retest reliability in a clinical sample.* Poster presented at the 44th Annual Meeting of the American Academy of Child and Adolescent Psychiatry, Toronto, Canada.

Fisher, P. W., Shaffer, D., Piacentini, J., Lapkin, J., Kafantaris, V., Leonard, H., & Herzog, D. (1993). Sensitivity of the Diagnostic Interview Schedule for Children, 2nd edition (DISC–2.1), for specific diagnoses of children and adolescents. *Journal of the American Academy of Child and Adolescent Psychiatry, 32*(3), 666–673.

Fleiss, J. L. (1981). *Statistical methods for rates and proportions* (2nd ed.). New York: Wiley.

Granero Pérez, R., Ezpeleta Ascaso, L., Doménech Massons, J. M., & de la Osa Chapparo, N. (1998). Characteristics of the subject and interview influencing the test–retest reliability of the Diagnostic Interview for Children and Adolescents, Revised. *Journal of Child Psychology and Psychiatry, 39*(7), 963–972.

Hamilton, M. (1960). A rating scale for depression. *Journal of Neurology, Neurosurgery and Psychiatry, 23,* 56–61.

Helzer, J. E., Robins, L. N., McEvoy, L. T., Spitznagel, E. L., Stoltzman, R. K., Farmer, A., & Brockington, I. F. (1985). A comparison of clinical and Diagnostic Interview Schedule diagnoses: Physician reexamination of lay interviewed cases in the general population. *Archives of General Psychiatry, 42,* 657–666.

Jensen, P., Roper, M., Fisher, P., Piacentini, J., Canino, G., Richters, J., Rubio-Stipec, M., Dulcan, M., Goodman, S., Davies, M., Rae, D., Shaffer, D., Bird, H., Lahey, B., & Schwab-Stone, M. (1995). Test–retest reliability of the Diagnostic Interview Schedule for Children (DISC 2.1). Parent, child, and combined algorithms. *Archives of General Psychiatry, 52,* 61–71.

Jensen, P. S., Traylor, J., Xenakis, S. N., & Davis, H. (1988). Child psychopathology rating scales and interrater agreement: 1. Parents' gender and psychiatric symptoms. *Journal of the American Academy of Child and Adolescent Psychiatry, 27,* 442–450.

Jensen, P. S., Wantanabe, H. K., & Richters, J. E. (in press). Who's up first? Testing for order effects in structured interviews using a counterbalanced experimental design. *Journal of Abnormal Child Psychology.*

Jorm, A. F., Duncan-Jones, P., & Scott, R. (1989). An analysis of the retest artifact in longitudinal studies of psychiatric symptoms and personality. *Psychological Medicine, 19,* 487–493.

Lucas, C. P. (1992). The order effect: Reflections on the validity of multiple test presentations. *Psychological Medicine, 22,* 197–202.

Lucas, C. P., Fisher, P., Piacentini, J., Zhang, H., Jensen, P., Shaffer, D., Dulcan, M., Schwab-Stone, M., Regier, D., & Rubio-Stipec, M. (in press). Features of interview questions associated with attenuation of symptom reports. *Journal of Abnormal Child Psychology.*

Lucas, C. P., Zhangh, H., Mroczek, D., Fisher, P., Shaffer, D., Lahey, B., Dulcan, M., Canino, G., Bourdon, K., Narrow, W., Xu, L., & Friman, P. (1998). *The DISC predictive scales: Efficiently screening for diagnoses.* Poster presented at the 1998 meeting of the Academy of Child and Adolescent Psychiatry, Anaheim, CA.

Piacentini, J., Shaffer, D., Fisher, P., Schwab-Stone, M., Davies, M., & Gioia, P. (1993). The Diagnostic Interview Schedule for Children—Revised Version (DISC-R): III. Concurrent criterion validity. *Journal of the American Academy of Child and Adolescent Psychiatry, 32*(3), 658–665.

Pulver, A. E., & Carpenter, W. T. (1983). Lifetime psychotic symptoms assessed with the DIS. *Schizophrenia Bulletin, 9*(3), 377–382.

Ribera, J., Canino, G., Rubio-Stipec, M., Bravo, M., Bauermeister, J. J., Alegria, M., Woodbury, M., Huertas, S., Guevara, L. M., Bird, H. R., Freeman, D. H., & Shrout, P. (1996). The Diagnostic Interview Schedule for Children (DISC-2.1) in Spanish: Reliability in a Hispanic population. *Journal of Child Psychology and Psychiatry, 37*(2), 195–204.

Robins, L. N. (1985). Epidemiology: Reflections on testing the validity of psychiatric interviews. *Archives of General Psychiatry, 42,* 918–924.

Robins, L. N., Cottler, L., Bucholz, K., & Compton, W. (1996). *The Diagnostic Interview Schedule, Version 4.* St. Louis, MO: Washington University.

Robins, L. N., Helzer, J. E., Croughan, J., & Ratcliff, K. S. (1981). The National Institute of Mental Health Diagnostic Interview Schedule: Its history, characteristics, and validity. *Archives of General Psychiatry, 38*(4), 381–389.

Robins, L. N., & Regier, D. A. (Eds.). (1991). *Psychiatric disorders in America: The Epidemiologic Catchment Area Study.* New York: Free Press.

Rutter, M., & Graham, P. (1968). The reliability and validity of the psychiatric assessment of the child: I. Interview with the child. *British Journal of Psychiatry, 114*(510), 563–579.

SAS Institute. (1990). *SAS/STAT user's guide, Version 6* (4th ed., Vol. 2). Cary, NC: Author.

Schwab-Stone, M., Fisher, P., Piacentini, J., Shaffer, D., Davies, M., & Briggs, M. (1993). The Diagnostic Interview Schedule for Children—Revised Version (DISC-R): II. Test–retest reliability. *Journal of the American Academy of Child and Adolescent Psychiatry, 32*(3), 651–657.

Schwab-Stone, M. E., Shaffer, D., Dulcan, M. K., Jensen, P. S., Fisher, P., Bird, H. R., Goodman, S. H., Lahey, B. B., Lichtman, J. H., Canino, G., Rubio-Stipec, M., & Rae, D. S. (1996). Criterion validity of the NIMH Diagnostic Interview Schedule for Children, Version 2.3 (DISC-2.3). *Journal of the American Academy of Child and Adolescent Psychiatry, 35*(7), 878–888.

Shaffer, D., Fisher, P., Dulcan, M. K., Davies, M., Piacentini, J., Schwab-Stone, M. E., Lahey, B. B., Bourdon, K., Jensen, P. S., Bird, H. R., Canino, G., & Regier, D. A. (1996). The NIMH Diagnostic Interview Schedule for Children, Version 2.3 (DISC–2.3): Description, acceptability, prevalence rates, and performance in the MECA study. Methods for the Epidemiology of Child and Adolescent Mental Disorders Study. *Journal of the American Academy of Child and Adolescent Psychiatry, 35*(7), 865–877.

Shaffer, D., Fisher, P., Lucas, C. P., Dulcan, M., & Schwab-Stone, M. E. (in press). NIMH Diagnostic Interview Schedule for Children, Version IV (NIMH DISC-IV): Description, differences from previous versions, and reliability of some common diagnoses. *Journal of the American Academy of Child and Adolescent Psychiatry.*

Shaffer, D., Gould, M. S., Brasic, J., Ambrosini, P., Fisher, P., Bird, H., & Aluwahlia, S. (1983). A Children's Global Assessment Scale (CGAS). *Archives of General Psychiatry, 40,* 1228–1231.

Shaffer, D., Schwab-Stone, M., Fisher, P., Cohen, P., Piacentini, J., Davies, M., Conners, C. K., & Regier, D. (1993). The Diagnostic Interview Schedule for Children—Revised Version (DISC-R): I. Preparation, field testing, interrater reliability, and acceptability. *Journal of the American Academy of Child and Adolescent Psychiatry, 32*(3), 643–650.

Sudman, D., Bradburn, N. M., & Schwarz, N. (1996). *Thinking about answers: The application of cognitive processes to survey methodology.* San Francisco: Jossey-Bass.

Tanur, J. M. (1993). *Questions about questions: Inquiries into the cognitive bases of surveys.* New York: Russell Sage Foundation.

Turner, C. F., Ku, L., Rogers, S. M., Lindberg, L. D., Pleck, J. H., & Sonenstein, F. L. (1998). Adolescent sexual behavior, drug use, and violence: Increased reporting with computer-survey technology. *Science, 280,* 867–873.

World Health Organization. (1995). *Composite International Diagnostic Interview, Version 2.0.* Geneva: Author.

2

Interviewer-Based Interviews

✧

ADRIAN ANGOLD
PRUDENCE W. FISHER

In this chapter, we consider a diverse group of diagnostic interviews for use with children and adolescents and their parents that have been in reasonably widespread use for a number of years, and for which some published psychometric data are available. This group includes the Anxiety Disorders Interview Schedule for Children (ADIS-C); the Child and Adolescent Psychiatric Assessment (CAPA); the Child Assessment Schedule (CAS); the Diagnostic Interview for Children and Adolescents (DICA) and its close relative, the Missouri Assessment of Genetics Interview for Children (MAGIC); and the various versions of the Schedule for Affective Disorders and Schizophrenia for School-Age Children (K-SADS). All of these interviews enable their users to make *Diagnostic and Statistical Manual of Mental Disorders*, fourth edition (DSM-IV) diagnoses, and all have components for assessing psychosocial impairment resulting from psychiatric symptoms and disorders.

SOME GENERAL COMMENTS ON THE NEED FOR STRUCTURED PSYCHIATRIC INTERVIEWS

Interviews are vital tools in all forms of clinical medical diagnosis, and they have a particularly prominent position in psychiatry. All structured interviews used in psychiatry have their roots in the clinical interview conducted by individuals with special training in psychiatry, clinical psychology, social work, and nursing. When it became clear that clinical training was sufficiently varied that colleagues of the same discipline, working in the same establishment, were often unable to agree about an individual's diagnosis even when they were presented with exactly the same information, researchers concluded that this situation needed to be remedied and began to develop structured interviews (Cantwell, 1988; Gould, Shaffer, Rutter, & Sturge, 1988; Remschmidt, 1988).

The literature on medical decision making had already demonstrated that clinicians suffer from a number of information collection biases that are detrimental from a diagnostic point of view: (1) They tend to come to diagnostic determinations before they have collected all the relevant information; (2) they tend then to collect information selectively to *confirm* those diagnoses ("confirmatory bias"); (3) they tend to ignore disconfirmatory information; (4) they combine information in idiosyncratic ways; and (5) they tend to base their judgments on the most readily available cognitive patterns (the "availability heuristic"). Further problems arise because of a tendency to see correlations where none exist ("illusory correlation") and, conversely, to miss real correlations (see Achenbach, 1985, for a helpful introduction to the basics of the medical decision-making literature).

The existence of these problems set some clear directions for the development of structured interviews:

1. Structure information coverage, so that all interviewers will have collected all relevant information from all subjects.

2. Define the ways in which relevant information is to be collected.

3. Make a diagnosis only after all relevant confirmatory and disconfirmatory information has been collected.

4. Structure the process by which relevant confirmatory and disconfirmatory information is combined to produce a final diagnosis.

For instance, one of the first structured diagnostic interviews, the Present State Examination (PSE; Wing, 1974) provided a list of symptoms to be inquired about, gave detailed definitions of those symptoms, required interviewers to question until they could determine whether the symptom as defined was present or not, and developed a computerized diagnostic algorithm to standardize the final stages of diagnostic decision making. Now, as then, all structured interviews attempt to achieve these four goals in one way or another.

INTERVIEWER- AND RESPONDENT-BASED INTERVIEWS

A basic distinction has arisen between two different strategies for structuring information coverage and defining ways to collect relevant information. These two methods have been dubbed "interviewer-based" (or sometimes "investigator-based") and "respondent-based" (Angold et al., 1995). This distinction comes down to a difference in *what* is structured, or the level at which information is structured. In an interviewer-based interview, the mind of the interviewer is structured. In essence, the interview schedule serves as a tool to guide the interviewer in determining whether symptoms are present, but the interviewer makes the decisions on the basis of information provided by the child or adult. In order to reduce idiosyncrasies in these interviewer judgments, definitions of symptoms are provided, and the interviewer is expected to question until he/she can decide whether the symptoms described meet these definitions. Interviews of this sort were the first to be developed, since they sprang naturally from clinical practice. Early examples of this type of interview were the PSE (Wing, 1974) and the Reynard (Guze, Goodwin, & Crane, 1969) for adults, and the Isle of Wight Interview for children (Graham & Rutter, 1968; Rutter & Graham, 1968). In each of these cases, *clinicians* were expected to conduct the interviews, since it was felt that only they had the necessary training and experience to be able to decide about the presence or absence of symptoms, even when quite detailed definitions were provided.

Although the PSE and the Isle of Wight Interviews were used extensively in moderate-sized epidemiological surveys, it was clear that the use of clinician interviewers created both logistical and budgetary problems. Very large-scale epidemiological studies, such as the Epidemiologic Catchment Area study (Regier et al., 1984), mandated the use of nonclinician ("lay") interviewers. However, it was felt that such interviewers would be incapable of making the judgments required by interviewer-based interviews; thus respondent-based psychiatric interviews were developed, following the methodologies used by political and marketing surveys. In a respondent-based interview, it is the *questions* put to the subject that are structured, and the interviewer makes no decisions about the presence of symptoms. Prescribed questions are asked verbatim in a preset order, and the interviewee's responses are recorded with a minimum of interpretation or clarification by the interviewer. Information variance due to variability in interviewing style or content is thus minimized. The Diagnostic Interview Schedule was the paradigmatic example in adult psychiatry (Robins, Helzer, Croughan, Williams, & Spitzer, 1979). The original DICA was the first child interview of this sort (Herjanic & Campbell, 1977; Herjanic, Herjanic, Brown, & Wheatt, 1975), although it has progressively been transformed into an interviewer-based interview. The National Institute of Mental Health (NIMH) sponsored the development of the respondent-based Diagnostic Interview Schedule for Children (DISC), beginning in the early 1980s (Costello, Edelbrock, Dulcan, Kalas, & Klaric, 1984; Edelbrock & Costello, 1990). The obvious difficulty with such an interview is that although one knows exactly what has been asked in each interview, and exactly what was answered, there is no control over differences in how subjects interpret questions or respond to them.

It is important to be aware, however, that the goals of these two interviewing strategies are the same—to reduce information variance as much as possible. Strategies for data combination to produce diagnoses and scale scores have also shown considerable convergence, with computer scoring emerging as a key diagnostic method for both respondent-based and interviewer-based interviews. It is also important to bear in mind that all of the interviews considered here are moving targets. Interview developers and users are constantly modifying and updating them in response to changes in nosological systems, the requirements of particular studies, and increasing experience with the strengths and weaknesses of their own and others' measures.

It is perhaps worth noting here that respondent-based interviews have often been referred to as "highly structured," while interviewer-based interviews have been called "semistructured." These are misnomers, since the issue is not *how much* structure is present, but *what* is structured—the questions or the definition of symptoms.

However, the distinction between interviewer- and respondent-based interviews is not hard and fast in actual practice, because there has been considerable cross-fertilization between these approaches. For instance, the CAPA, which grew primarily from the interviewer-based tradition, includes a subset of questions that are to be asked of all subjects (as in a respondent-based interview), but then allows further questioning for clarification. On the other hand, the DICA, which had previously been regarded as a respondent-based interview, now requires interviewers to question much more flexibly, and should thus be regarded as an interviewer-based instrument. So it is perhaps best to consider interviews as lying at various locations along three dimensions: (1) degree of specification of questions, (2) degree of definition of symptom concepts, and (3) degree of flexibility in questioning permitted to the interviewers. Interviews that provide extensive definitions and require interviewers to make judgments lie at the interviewer-based end of the spectrum, whereas those that specify every question and allow no interviewer deviation from those questions lie at the respondent-based end of the scale. Figure 2.1 is a schematic representation of where each of the interviews discussed in this chapter lies, with the DISC included as a reference point.

A BRIEF INTRODUCTION TO THE INTERVIEWS

In this section, we present a very brief introduction to each of the interviews covered in this chapter, with a focus on their characteristic response formats.

Schedule for Affective Disorders and Schizophrenia for School-Age Children

The K-SADS family of interviews consists of a group of very diverse assessments. Indeed, the only features that all of the current versions of the

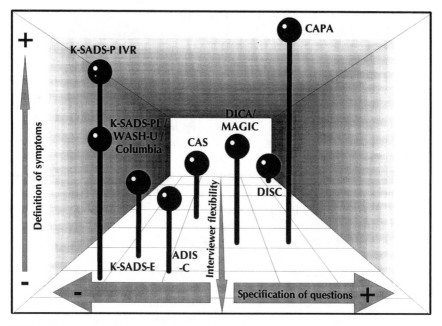

FIGURE 2.1. A graphic depiction of the relative degrees of definition of symptoms, specification of questions, and interviewer flexibility employed by the interviews described in this chapter.

K-SADS have in common are the name, the ability to make DSM-IV diagnoses, and the fact that all were designed to be administered *by clinicians.*

1. K-SADS-P IVR. The original version of the K-SADS was the K-SADS-P (Puig-Antich & Chambers, 1978), which was a downward extension of the adult Schedule for Affective Disorders and Schizophrenia, and which focused on the Research Diagnostic Criteria (Spitzer, Endicott, & Robins, 1978). Note that the "P" in its title stands for Present. It was designed for use with children aged 6–17, but did not include symptoms relevant to many childhood diagnoses. It was substantially revised to cover DSM-III-R (Ambrosini, Metz, Prabucki, & Lee, 1990) and DSM-IV. The version most recently developed by Ambrosini and colleagues is called the K-SADS-P IVR. The time frame for this interview is the "present episode" of any disorder. This version is closest conceptually to the original K-SADS-P in including quite detailed definitions of severity codings for each symptom. The modal form for these symptom codings is a 6-point scale, involving judgments about various combinations of intensity, duration, frequency, environmental responsiveness, psychosocial impairment, and observation.

2. K-SADS-E. The K-SADS-E (E for Epidemiologic; Orvaschel, Puig-

Antich, Chambers, Tabrizi, & Johnson, 1982) has, since its inception, collect-ed ratings of the present episode of any disorder *and* the *worst* past episode. It therefore combines the present-episode and lifetime time frames. This inter-view was never even remotely similar in format to the K-SADS-P, because it rated only the presence or absence of symptoms, rather than employing the carefully defined severity codings of the K-SADS-P. The latest edition is DSM-IV-compatible and allows the current *episode* (not individual symptoms) to be rated as "mild," "moderate," or "severe."

3. K-SADS-PL. A group in Pittsburgh has developed the K-SADS-PL (PL for Present and Lifetime) as a sort of cross between the K-SADS-P and the K-SADS-E (Kaufman et al., 1997; Shanee, Apter, & Weizman, 1997). Symptom ratings have been reduced to 3-point scales (typically "not at all," "subthreshold," and "threshold"), and fairly minimal anchoring definitions of each point are provided. An initial 82-item screen interview, which allows skipping of substantial symptom areas, is also available.

4. WASH-U-KSADS. Like the K-SADS-PL, the WASH-U-K-SADS (Geller, Zimerman, Williams, & Frazier, 1996) involves both present and life-time time frames. Rather brief definitions of symptoms are given, and level of severity is coded, but the severity codings are highly idiosyncratic and bear little relation to those in other versions of the K-SADS.

5. Columbia K-SADS. This version rates the current episode, the past 2 weeks, and the worst past episode. The symptom "definitions" provided are often simply restatements of the DSM-IV criteria, although sometimes (par-ticularly in relation to depression) a little more guidance is given. Symptom severity is typically rated on what appears to be a 6-point scale, like that of the K-SADS-P and K-SADS-P IVR; however, closer inspection reveals that two of the points are usually defined only as being "intermediate" between two other points. Thus, only four points (one being symptom absence) are really defined.

Although the various K-SADS interviews were developed for use by clinicians, some have also have been used with lay interviewers (see, e.g., Hodges, McKnew, Burbach, & Roebuck, 1987; Lewinsohn, Hops, Roberts, Seeley, & Andrews, 1993).

The K-SADS interviews differ from most interviews in directing that the parent should be interviewed first and then the child should be seen by the same interviewer, who is then expected to resolve any discrepancies be-tween the child's and the parent's reports. The interviewer then completes a single record representing his/her conflation of the two interviews. This pro-cedure obviously requires considerable clinical judgment, and is subject to the criticism that the process of combining the information is quite uncon-trolled, so that it is impossible to determine what specific information was ob-tained from each interviewee. This method also seems likely to bias the re-sults of the interview in favor of the parental reports (Angold et al., 1987), and some workers have preferred to score the interviews with the parent and the child separately (see, e.g., Weissman et al., 1987). When this is done, the usual high level of parent–child disagreement appears.

Child and Adolescent Psychiatric Assessment

The CAPA is one of an integrated group of instruments developed to assess a variety of risk factors for, manifestations of, and outcomes of child and adolescent psychiatric disorders in a coherent fashion. In addition to the usual symptom and impairment assessments, it also includes extensive ratings of the family environment and relationships, family psychosocial problems, and life events (including traumatic events and physical and sexual abuse). A separate module called the Child and Adolescent Impact Assessment (Angold et al., 1998; Messer, Angold, Costello, & Burns, 1996) measures the impact of the child's problems on the family, while the Child and Adolescent Services Assessment (Ascher, Farmer, Burns, & Angold, 1996; Farmer, Angold, Burns, & Costello, 1994) measures service use for mental health problems in multiple sectors and settings. Psychosocial impairment in 17 domains of functioning is measured both at the syndromic level and overall. In the interview with the child, 62 items reflecting the child's observed behavior are also coded.

In order to facilitate completion of the interview by nonclinicians, the CAPA provides a more molecular approach to symptom codings. Symptom definitions are provided in a glossary and on the schedule, and rules are specified to allow nonclinicians to code the intensity, frequency, duration, and date of onset of symptoms separately. For instance, with the symptom of depressed mood, rules for coding intensity specify the degree of intrusiveness of the symptom into other activities, the degree of uncontrollability, and the range of activities that must be affected for depressed mood to be regarded as being symptomatic. This approach has been shown to allow nonclinicians to make reliable judgments of symptom severity while using a highly flexible questioning format, with heavy emphasis on getting descriptions and examples of possible pathological emotions and behaviors to ensure that codings are not based on the informant's misunderstanding of what was being asked about (Angold & Costello, 1995; Angold et al., 1995; Costello, Angold, March, & Fairbank, 1998).

A special version of the CAPA has been developed for use with young adults (the Young Adult Psychiatric Assessment—YAPA), through the addition of the assessment of antisocial personality disorder, the removal of some items that are not relevant to this age group (e.g., the elimination disorders), and modifications to the assessment of impairment that take into account the different living and working situations of many young adults. Work on a version of the interview for use with the parents of preschool children is ongoing. In addition, a version with empirically derived screen items is available. This version allows sections to be skipped if screen symptoms are absent. A streamlined version for collecting data for twin studies is also available, and it includes a module for the lifetime assessment of certain disorders (Simonoff et al., 1997).

Diagnostic Interview for Children and Adolescents

The DICA began life as a respondent-based interview over 20 years ago (Herjanic & Campbell, 1977; Herjanic et al., 1975; Herjanic & Reich, 1982a, 1982b; Reich & Earls, 1987; Reich, Herjanic, Welner, & Gandhy, 1982; Welner, Reich, Herjanic, Jung, & Amado, 1987). Since then it has been progressively modified, so that its paper-and-pencil version is now a solidly interviewer-based interview (Ezpeleta et al., 1997; Ezpeleta, de la Osa, Doménech, Navarro, & Losilla, 1995; de la Osa, Ezpeleta, Doménech, Navarro, & Losilla, 1997; Reich, 1999). However, there is also a computer-based version of the DICA that remains fully respondent-based (Reich, Cottler, McCallum, Corwin, & VanEerdewegh, 1995). Both of these DICAs are radically different from the original DICA. In addition, the group responsible for the development of the DICA (of which Multi-Health Systems now owns the copyright) has produced a modification called the MAGIC. The biggest difference between the DICA and the MAGIC is that the MAGIC has a "specifications manual," which includes more specific guidance on how to elicit key features of symptoms, as well as various clarifications of coding instructions. In many ways, this manual constitutes a very attractively written glossary for the MAGIC. In other words, different congeners of the DICA run the gamut of interviewing styles, from fully respondent-based to interviewer- and glossary-based (Reich, 1999).

The DICA and the MAGIC have explicitly different versions for self-reports from children aged 6 (or 7) to 12 and adolescents aged 13 to 17. The differences between these versions concern differences in the wording of questions. The DICA has also been used with even younger children, although special training is required for its administration to children aged under 6 or 7, and the instructions to interviewers essentially tell them to ignore the usual questioning format laid out in the schedule and to use their own questions. The DICA and MAGIC also adopt a lifetime time frame.

Symptoms are typically coded on a 3-point scale ("no," "sometimes/somewhat," "yes") for items about emotional symptoms, and a 2-point scale ("no," "yes") for disruptive behaviors, with information about frequency sometimes being added. Impairment is measured at the syndrome level by three items asking about symptoms making it hard to "get along" with family, with friends, and at school, rated on 4-point scales ("not at all," "not too much," "somewhat," "quite a bit").

Child Assessment Schedule

The CAS is modeled after the traditional clinical interview with children, in that it is organized around thematic topics and provides ratings of many items that are not required if all one wants to do is to make ratings of the DSM criteria for disorders (Hodges, Cools, & McKnew, 1989; Hodges, Kline, Stern, Cytryn, & McKnew, 1982; Hodges et al., 1987; Hodges, Mc-Knew, Cytryn, Stern, & Kline, 1982; Hodges & Saunders, 1989; Hodges, Saunders, Kashani, Hamlett, & Thompson, 1990). The CAS now exists in child (7–12), adolescent, and parent report forms. Although originally developed for use by experienced clinicians (Hodges, Kline, et al., 1982), the CAS has now been used by lay interviewers in several studies. Symptoms are scored on a 4-point scale ("yes," "no," "ambiguous," "not scored"). This is followed by questioning about the onset and duration of positive symptoms. The items to be coded are defined in brief sentences, and the questions are not simply rephrasings of the codings; rather, each coding defines a concept, and the interviewer must make a judgment about the coding based on the answer to the question (plus any additional questions that may be thought necessary). However, the standard 4-point response coding is quite straightforward and much less complex than the codings required for the K-SADS-IVR interviews and the CAPA.

The CAS also has a 56-item section for recording observations of the child's behavior during the interview. Interviewers can use algorithms provided by the developer of the interview to generate diagnoses, but computerized scoring is recommended. These algorithms can also be used to generate symptom scales reflecting a number of areas of psychopathology. Short definitions of the material to be considered are provided on the schedule, as well as a key question pertaining to each item.

Psychosocial impairment is measured with a separate interview, the Child and Adolescent Functional Assessment Scale, which can also be used alone or with another diagnostic interview (Hodges & Wong, 1996, 1997; Hodges, Wong, & Latessa, 1998).

Anxiety Disorders Interview Schedule for Children

Despite its title, the ADIS-C also provides brief ratings of symptoms pertinent to other disorders. However, its coverage of the anxiety disorders is much more thorough (Silverman, 1991; Silverman & Eisen, 1992; Silverman & Nelles, 1988; Silverman & Rabian, 1995). The interview is designed for *clinician* use, and was derived from the adult ADIS (di Nardo, Moras, Barlow, Rapee, & Brown, 1993). Questions that should be asked are provided, and guidance is given about when to use additional questions. Most symptoms are scored on a simple 3-point scale ("yes," "no," "other"). However, in the anxiety section, a good deal of use is also made of 9-point scales (represented by a thermometer) ranging from "not at all" to "very, very much." Similar scales are used to rate "interference," which is the ADIS-C term for psychosocial impairment resulting from disorders. Skip structures are frequently employed, so many individuals will not be asked about all symptoms.

INTERVIEW TIME FRAMES

The K-SADS interviews, the ADIS-C, and the CAS all focus on a child's "current" status, though the definition of "current" is largely unspecified. The K-SADS-PL and K-SADS-E also explore lifetime histories of "worst" episodes. The DICA and MAGIC adopt a lifetime time frame as their standard format, but for some disorders an additional, shorter time frame is also included. For instance, the depression section of the MAGIC asks about the "past month," as well as whether the child has "ever" had symptoms. The CAPA covers a "primary period" of 3 months, but also asks whether certain uncommon symptoms (such as suicide attempts) have ever occurred.

SPECIFICATION OF QUESTIONS,
INTERVIEWER FLEXIBILITY,
AND THE DEFINITION OF SYMPTOMS

As Figure 2.1 shows, the interviews differ widely in the specification of questions. Of course, in a fully respondent-based interview like the DISC, all questions are completely specified and no others may be used. One also needs to bear in mind that interviews are constantly evolving in response to experience with them in practice, the demands of different studies and clinical settings for particular types of assessment, and changes in the nosologies they are designed to implement.

The ADIS-C, CAPA, DICA, and MAGIC all contain questions that, under most circumstances, should be asked as written in the schedule. These serve as introductions to topic areas. In each instance, additional questions are then asked as necessary, to allow the interviewer to determine exactly whether the symptom should be coded as being present. Many such questions are provided in the CAPA, and somewhat fewer are provided on the CAS (but it is not clear to what extent the "set" questions of the CAS are mandated for use); most guidance on this process for the DICA and MAGIC is provided in the MAGIC's specifications manual. All these interviews also provide at least some additional instructions about when to probe further. The K-SADS group of interviews provides a range of suggested questions, but no formal rules about when they are to be used or skipped. Interviewers are also expected to ask any additional questions necessary to clarify responses.

By "interviewer flexibility," we mean the degree to which an interviewer is expected or encouraged to use judgment in asking additional clarifying questions. In this respect, the K-SADS interviews (and perhaps the ADIS-C) may be seen as providing most flexibility, because they demand that judgments based on clinical experience be made; moreover the K-SADS interviews do not mandate the use of any particular questions. The problem question is "Flexibility to do what?" The answer is relatively clear in the case of the K-SADS-P IVR and the CAPA, where very detailed coding rules are provided at the symptom level. The task of the interviewer is to determine whether the criteria specified in the coding rules are met. However, with the other instruments, it often appears that the interviewer's job is to get the answer *to the original question*. Variable amounts of guidance on how to do so are provided—in considerable detail in the MAGIC's specifications manual, with little or no detail in the K-SADS-E or ADIS-C, or with brief symptom definitions in the CAS.

The K-SADS-P IVR and the CAPA provide detailed *definitional* glossaries at the symptom level, which means that the task of the interviewer is most clearly specified at the level of the *definition* of symptoms. The CAPA glossary also contains many procedural instructions on good ways to conduct questioning in general, and in relation to specific symptoms, but these are presented as being secondary to the definitional issues. The MAGIC's specifications manual can also be seen as being a glossary, but it is first and foremost a *procedural* manual; it is primarily about *how* to collect the information. In the course of this discussion of procedure, it also includes a good deal of definitional material, but it does not provide formal definitions of items in the way that the K-SADS-P IVR and the CAPA do.

On the other hand, all the interviews considered here differ from the DISC in that the interviewer's task is not to record answers to specific questions, but to question until he/she can make a clear *judgment* of the child's symptomatic status.

WHO CAN DO INTERVIEWER-BASED INTERVIEWS?

Although interviewer-based structured interviews were originally developed for use by clinicians (the ADIS-C, K-SADS, and CAS), it has become clear that nonclinician interviewers can be trained to make what are usually regarded as "clinical" judgments (Angold et al., 1995; Hodges et al., 1987). However, it is also apparent that this requires a continuing commitment to training and to quality control. When symptoms are clearly defined and distinguished from one another, it also becomes apparent that clinicians are not always clear or in agreement about psychopathological distinctions, so they also require training to fit them for structured interviewing. The point is that the interviewer-based approach requires simply that all interviewers be capable of eliciting the required information in an appropriate and efficient manner, and of making the appropriate judgments about symptom coding. Some nonclinicians are very good at this task, and (sad to say) some clinicians do it very poorly.

IN WHAT SITUATIONS CAN INTERVIEWER-BASED INTERVIEWS BE USED?

It is probably fair to say that clinicians do not enjoy doing respondent-based interviews very much, because the questions they can ask are so highly constrained (though we know of no direct studies of this question). If they add their own questions, then the advantages of using a respondent-based interview at all are lost, because an unstructured component has been added. On the other hand, training on an interviewer-based interview is usually of interest to clinicians, because it raises a host of issues about interviewing style and strategy that few have had time or encouragement to think through during their training. Thus, interviewer-based interviews may be particularly suitable for use in clinical assessments. Several leading centers now have a structured interview as a standard part of the clinical assessment; given the very unsatisfactory reliability of unaided clinical interviews, this may be the wave of the future. There also seems to be no question that interviewer-based interviews are suitable for clinical research studies, and both interviewer-based and respondent-based interviews have been widely used in such studies.

When it comes to general population studies, some have doubts about the place of interviewer-based instruments. Such studies provided the initial impetus for the development of respondent-based psychiatric interviews, but this impetus arose from the supposition that "lay" interviewers could not be trained to do interviewer-based interviews. However, recent advances in the quality of definitions of psychiatric symptoms associated with interviewer-based interviews have resulted in its being perfectly possible to train "lay" interviewers adequately, and to achieve levels of reliability as good as those found with respondent-based interviews. Indeed, at present, some of the largest ongoing community studies are using interviewer-based instruments (Costello et al., 1996; Lewinsohn et al., 1993; Simonoff et al., 1997). The only situation in which it seems likely that interviewer-based interviews would not be appropriate is a study of a national household probability sample. Such studies require the use of large numbers of interviewers scattered over an enormous geographical area, and it is unlikely that the necessary level of training and quality control required for interviewer-based interviews can be implemented in such a study.

Concerns have been expressed about the relative costs of training and quality control for interviewer-based versus respondent-based interviews, but when we compared the cost per subject interviewed, using figures from recently funded NIMH grants, we found the cost differential to be small or nonexistent. At present, it seems that decisions about whether to use an interviewer-based interview in any type of study should be made on the basis of which interview collects the information best suited to answering the questions under study, rather than on the basis of type of interview alone.

ADVANTAGES AND DISADVANTAGES OF INTERVIEWER-BASED INTERVIEWS

Interviewer-based interviews have four substantial theoretical and practical advantages: (1) If the interviews have been conducted and coded properly, the meanings of their ratings are precisely known; (2) they provide opportunities to cross-check discrepant or confusing information; (3) they enable the use of efficient open-ended questioning strategies; and (4) they allow the use of redundant questioning, which has been shown in adults to improve the quality of responses. However, these advantages carry with them three costs: (1) More intensive training must be provided to interviewers; (2) a higher level of quality control is required; and (3) the requirement for detailed symptom definitions means that numerous coding rules must be developed for each interview, and this has resulted in substantial differences among interviews in how symptoms are specified.

What Do the Codings Mean?

In an interviewer-based interview, a positive coding for a symptom means that it has been determined that the symptom as defined in the schedule is present. In a respondent-based interview, one knows only that a child or parent responded positively to a particular question. Consider a question such as the following (from the DISC-2.1): "Do you spend more time in the bath or shower than you should or wash your hands more than you need to?" It is up to the child to decide the meanings of "more than you should" and "more than you need to," and the child's decisions about these meanings may differ from those that would be made by psychopathologists. This problem has been documented with unusual symptoms that most children never experience, such as obsessive-compulsive or psychotic symptoms. Such symptoms have been greatly overreported when the DISC has been used (Breslau, 1987). When clinicians reviewed what the children said, it was obvious that what was being reported was not obsessive–compulsive disorder or psychosis. However, if an unstructured clinician review is added to the diagnostic process, one no longer knows exactly what factors went into the final rating, and one great advantage of the respondent-based interview is lost. Reliance on clinical experience is of relatively little help with this problem in most cases, because clinicians' internal meanings for these terms also vary widely. Over the last few years, one of us (Angold) has asked residents to tell him how often a child would have to be disobedient to meet the DSM-III-R criterion for oppositional defiant disorder "often actively defies or refuses adult requests or rules." Answers have ranged from once or twice a week to many times a day! Thus, this advantage of interviewer-based interviews is absolutely dependent on the clear specification of the decision rules for when a symptom is present and on the interviewers' adherence to those rules. On the other hand, there are also situations in which it can be expected that what the child and interviewer mean by a question will be the same. For instance, there is general agreement about what constitutes stealing, so there may be little advantage to the interviewer-based approach with a question like "Have you ever stolen anything?"

Cross-Checking Discrepant or Confusing Information

It is common in clinical practice to find that certain answers appear to contradict previously given information, or lead to uncertainty about whether a symptom is present. In an interviewer-based interview, one simply attempts to clarify the contradiction or confusion. The respondent-based approach provides no such mechanism for resolving such difficulties, since interviewers are not allowed to exercise their judgment about such matters. If a respondent-based interview is modified to allow interviewers to exercise their judgment in this, then one must be concerned about the rules for doing so and for coding the responses, and the interview can be said to have an interviewer-based component. In fact, this is the path that has been taken by the DICA over the last few years.

The Use of Open-Ended Questions

The distinction between open-ended and closed questions is not absolute, but open-ended questions are those that offer the chance to provide a wide range of answers or free-recall descriptions of phenomena, whereas closed questions call for one of a limited set of responses. For example, an open-ended question in response to being told by a child that he/she has received a bad school report might be "How did you feel about your bad grades?," whereas "Did your bad grades make you feel unhappy?" would be a closed question. If a child has just admitted to stealing, responding with "Tell me more about that" involves an open-ended question, whereas "What did you steal?" is a closed question. Basically, closed questions call for a yes–no answer or a date, frequency, duration, or other quite specific piece of information, whereas open-ended questions give a child the opportunity to provide a description of his/her feelings or behavior.

The work of Rutter, Cox, and their colleagues offers some direct guidance on the best ways to use these different sorts of questions with adults, and in the light of the literature on children's memory, there is little reason not to use a similar approach with children. Rutter, Cox, and colleagues concluded that, in general, most factual information was collected when a systematic approach that relied heavily on open-ended questions was used. Furthermore, this approach was also conducive to parental expressions of emotion, since it involved less talking on the part of the interviewer and gave more time for parents to discuss their concerns. On the other hand, a noninterventionist approach resulted in the provision of less relevant information, while challenging interpretations and a confrontational style proved less effective in eliciting emotions (Cox, Holbrook, & Rutter, 1981; Cox, Hopkinson, & Rutter, 1981; Cox, Rutter, & Holbrook, 1981; Hopkinson, Cox, & Rutter, 1981; Rutter & Cox, 1981; Rutter, Cox, Egert, Holbrook, & Everitt, 1981). Thus open-ended questions can be effective in collecting information efficiently, but, of necessity, respondent-based interviews must rely on closed questions. On the other hand, closed questions are necessary to elicit information that is otherwise not forthcoming, and respondent-based interviews have been a substantial help to the developers of interviewer-based interviews in establishing well-thought-out logical structures for series of closed questions. Respondent-based interviews provide little or no opportunity for the use of open-ended questions, because each question has to be formulated to produce a response that is directly codable in that item's response format. Thus a probe like "What was it like when you were depressed?" is of no use in a respondent-based interview, because it can lead to an infinite variety of answers. Rather, a large number of specific closed questions about the possible characteristics of depressed mood have to be asked. On the other hand, when interviewers are trained to recognize and code the characteristics of symptoms, such open-ended questions can generate a large amount of information.

Redundant Questions

"Redundant" questions are ones that pose the same query more than once in different ways—that is, questions that contain two phrasings or presentations of the same item. An example of a redundant question would be "Have you been more irritable than usual?," followed by "or made angry more easily?" The adult survey literature (Cannell, Marquis, & Laurent, 1977) suggests that such redundancy is actually helpful in providing both additional time for thought and a second chance to pick up symptoms. If the answer to one question is positive and the other negative, this is no problem for an interviewer-based interview, where follow-up questions can be used to clarify the situation. However, this cannot be done in a respondent-based interview, where specific chains of questions in response to initially discrepant information are required. Collapsing the two questions into one is no help, because this generates a "multiple question," which requires the respondent to remember and process the two parts of the question simultaneously. The "recency effect" means that in many cases, only the last part of a multiple question will actually be answered.

Intensity of Training

There is no doubt that an interviewer-based interview makes greater demands on an interviewer than does a respondent-based interview. Each interviewer must make a substantial effort to understand a range of concepts, some of them difficult ones, and to apply them during a live interview. For instance, training on the full CAPA package takes a month, compared with a few days for the DISC. However, training time is a relatively small part of most clinical or research budgets, so this problem comes down to a question of whether, for each individual study, this increased effort and expense is worthwhile. That will always depend on the questions being asked. To give a purely personal example: If we were designing a study that required only the assessment of the diagnosis of conduct disorder in a general population sample, we know of no reason not to use a respondent-based interview (unless we also needed additional information that can only be collected in one of the interviewer-based interviews). On the other hand, for a study with a primary need for assessments of obsessive–compulsive disorder, we should certainly prefer an interviewer-based interview. There is also little reason not to consider "mixing and matching," though this has rarely been done. There is no evidence that there is any advantage to using material from only one interview throughout an assessment, and all of the current major interviews are more or less "modularized." Most interview studies also employ questionnaires for some purposes, so why not combine components from different interviews?

Quality Control

"Interviewer drift" occurs with respondent-based interviews, necessitating continuing quality control throughout a study. For instance, the National Comorbidity Survey, which used the respondent-based Composite International Diagnostic Interview with adults, recently reported that two separate checks on the whole of every interview were conducted. On the other hand, there is more to check with an interviewer-based interview. Not only must care be taken that the interview is being conducted and coded properly, but mechanisms must also be in place to ensure that interviewers continue to interpret the responses of interviewees correctly. Once again, whether this additional burden is worth the effort depends on the situation in which the interview is being used.

Variation in Symptom Definitions

The fact that there is no generally agreed-upon standard for symptom definitions is a real problem for the developers of interviewer-based interviews. The same problem applies to the wording of questions in respondent-based interviews. As a result, there are substantial divergences between different interviews in how they approach the definition of symptoms. Perhaps the clearest example is that the K-SADS-IVR includes the level of psychosocial impairment resulting from a symptom in the severity coding for certain symptoms (such as depressed mood), whereas the CAPA explicitly excludes such considerations from the measurement of symptom severity, including such material instead in separate ratings of "incapacity." There are advantages and disadvantages to both approaches (Angold, 1994), but the problem is that with different instruments, items with similar names may mean different things. A further problem is that, in order to specify clear coding rules for symptoms, numerous arbitrary (but, one hopes, sensible) decisions have to be made, and there may be several perfectly reasonable alternatives. All developers of interviewer-based instruments have spent many hours arguing with themselves and others over countless fine points, but so far there exists no forum for developers to come to any consensus. We know very little about the comparative functioning of different interviews, because direct comparisons have rarely been made, but there is certainly a need for such work. For instance, it would be very helpful to know to what degree differences in rates of disorders from different studies represent real population differences, and to what degree they simply reflect differences in the interviews used.

COMBINING INFORMATION FROM DIFFERENT INFORMANTS AND MAKING A DIAGNOSIS

Three basic approaches to the combination of information from multiple informants have been adopted: (1) Best estimate from a "reconciliation interview," (2) best estimate from a review of the data from separate assessments, and (3) algorithmic combination.

Best Estimate from a "Reconciliation Interview"

In both the K-SADS-P and the ADIS-C, the separate interviews with parent and child are followed by a joint interview with both, to attempt to sort out disagreements between them as to the symptom ratings. The idea here is to generate an agreed-upon *single* rating of each symptom. When disagreements result from one party's misunderstanding a question, or from a parent's having been unaware of a child's behavior or feelings, it is easy to see how such an interview would help with producing a better estimate of the symptoms in question. However, there are some problems with this approach. First, there is the possibility that a child will lie about things that he/she would like to keep secret from a parent, creating a "worst" rather than a "best" estimate. Second, there are ethical problems with such a procedure for many sorts of research studies. What right does a researcher have to reveal a child's responses to a parent in a community survey study, for instance? The usual procedure in such studies is to guarantee that the information will not be transmitted to other family members, except in cases of abuse or of suicidal or homicidal risk. Clearly, such a guarantee precludes the use of a reconciliation interview. Third, an unstructured and largely uncontrollable process is introduced into the assessment—the process by which a parent and child decide how to respond to the challenge of having to agree. Fourth, the interviewer must decide what the final answer is, even when no clear agreement emerges. Neither the K-SADS nor the ADIS-C provides clear decision rules about how this is to be done, so another unstructured step is added to the diagnostic process.

Best Estimate from a Review of the Data from Separate Assessments

In the second approach, a "best estimator" (usually a clinician) is given the results of the interviews and instructed to come up with final ratings for each child. Though guidance on how to do this is provided, clear decision rules are not specified. Given that humans do a poor job of applying decision rules consistently, this is very likely to result in extra variation in final codings.

Algorithmic Combination

Computers, on the other hand, are exceedingly good at applying utterly consistent decision rules. The trouble is that someone must write those rules quite explicitly. It is an enormous task to write a full set of diagnostic algorithms for an interview that covers a wide range of disorders, but this has now been done for most of the interviews considered here, and computer algorithms have largely supplanted best estimating except with the K-SADS and the ADIS-C. Of course, such algorithms, though completely defined, also require their developers to make numerous arbitrary decisions about cutoff points for such terms as "often," which appear so frequently in diagnostic manuals. However, in this case both interviewer-based and respondent-based interviews are in the same boat, and they share the problem of deciding exactly how to combine information from multiple informants (parents, children, and often teachers). The two commonest approaches to this problem involve either making the diagnosis separately on the basis of the parent and child interviews and then concluding that a diagnosis is present if either is positive, or combining parent and child information at the symptom level and then deciding whether diagnostic criteria are met on the basis of these combined symptoms. The latter approach now appears to be becoming the standard, as it is increasingly recognized that different informants all make a contribution, even though they do not agree very highly with one another.

RELIABILITY

Table 2.1 shows the results of studies of the *test–retest* reliabilities (kappas) of diagnoses measured by the instruments considered in this chapter. It can be seen that all do a reasonably good job, and that there is not much basis for choosing among them as far as test–retest reliability of diagnosis is concerned. These reliability coefficients are similar to those reported for the DISC and for psychiatric interviews with adults.

Studies of interrater reliability have been published for some of the instruments considered here. However, since this measure of "reliability" only shows that when different interviewers are presented with exactly the same material, they make very similar ratings, we have not presented details of these studies. A user of an interviewer-based interview is allowed to use questions that differ from another user's. Since the measurement of interrater reliability excludes this key feature (and potential source of unreliability), it is not a useful guide to an interviewer-based interview's performance. The only exception to this rule is during the development phase of an interview, when interrater reliability lower than .7–.8 indicates to test constructors that an item is too poorly specified to be of much use, or that much better training on its assessment is needed.

VALIDITY

The problem with trying to assess the validity of psychiatric interviews is that there is no noninterview test for most psychiatric disorders. The structured interview itself has become the closest approximation we have to a "gold standard." So how are we to "validate" the diagnoses obtained from such interviews? This is a version of a very old problem in psychology—one that led to the concept of "construct validity." The key idea is that the validity of an instrument for the measurement of a psychological construct inheres not in some single agreement coefficient with one external standard, but in the instrument's performance within the "nomological net" of theory and empiri-

TABLE 2.1. Test–Retest Reliabilities (Kappas) of the Instruments Considered in this Chapter

Instrument	MDD	Dysthymia/ minor depression	Any depressive disorder	GAD/ OAD	Simple phobia	Social phobia	Any anxiety disorder	PTSD	ADHD	CD	ODD	SA/D
K-SADS-P	.54	.70					.24					
K-SADS-P IIIR	.77	.89					.72		.91			.46
K-SADS-PL (current)	.90			.78			.80	.67	.63		.74	
K-SADS-PL (lifetime)	1.00			.78			.60	.60	.55	.83	.77	
CAS	1.00	.85	.83	.38			.72		.43			
DICA			.90				.76		1.00		.61	
CAPA (child only)	.90		.82	.79			.64	.64		.55		
ADIS-C (combined parent and child)				.64	.84	.73	.75					1.00

Note. MDD, major depressive disorder; GAD, generalized anxiety disorder; OAD, overanxious disorder of childhood; PTSD, posttraumatic stress disorder; ADHD, attention-deficit hyperactivity disorder; CD, conduct disorder; ODD, oppositional defiant disorder; SA/D, substance abuse/dependence.

cal data concerning the construct or constructs that the instrument purports to measure (Anastasi, 1950; Anastasi, 1986; Cronbach & Meehl, 1955; Gulliksen, 1950; Jenkins, 1946; Novick, 1985; Peak, 1953; Wallace, 1965; Weitz, 1961). As Gulliksen (1950) remarked, "at some point in the advance of psychology it would seem appropriate for the psychologist to lead the way in establishing good criterion measures, instead of just attempting to construct imperfect tests for attributes that are presumed to be assessed more accurately and more validly by the judgment of experts" (p. 511).

Structured interviews were developed because of the poor psychometric properties of unaided clinical diagnosis, so comparisons with clinical judgment are flawed tests of diagnostic interview validity. In considering the validity of any interview, we should take a construct validation approach; that is, we should describe what we currently know about it in relation to the nomological net pertaining to child and adolescent psychiatric diagnosis. So far, only the developers of the CAPA have explicitly laid out the evidence for the validity of the CAPA using this approach, but all of the interviews considered here can point to similar chains of evidence. The construct validity of the CAPA is attested to by the following findings: (1) Diagnostic rates and age and gender patterns of disorder given by the CAPA are consistent with those found when other interviews are used; (2) patterns of diagnostic comorbidity are consistent with those found by other interviews; (3) symptomatic diagnoses are associated with psychosocial impairment; (4) parent and child reports of psychopathology on the CAPA are related to parent and teacher reports of problems on well-established scales for detecting psychopathology; (5) children with CAPA-identified disorders use more mental health services than children without diagnoses of such disorders; (6) CAPA-diagnosed children tend to come from families with a history of mental illness; (7) there is genetic loading for a number of CAPA scale scores and diagnoses; (8) CAPA diagnoses show consistency over time; and (9) CAPA diagnoses predict negative life outcomes (Angold & Costello, in press).

CAS scores have been found to discriminate among inpatient, outpatient, and normal groups, and to correlate with scores on the Child Behavior Checklist and on Spielberger's (1973) State–Trait Anxiety Inventory for Children (Hodges, Kline, et al., 1982; Hodges, McKnew, et al., 1982; Verhulst, Berden, & Sanders-Woudstra, 1985). Diagnostic concordance between the CAS and the K-SADS-P, administered by lay interviewers, was found to be moderate in a study of 30 clinically referred children (kappas between .36 and .75).

The DICA has been found to discriminate between pediatric and psychiatric clinic referrals (Herjanic & Campbell, 1977), although the methods of analysis used in this study make it hard to tell just how the parent and child interviews performed as a whole. A comparison of 42 children who each had a parent with a panic disorder and 42 children from families where neither parent had a psychiatric disorder found much higher rates of disorder (especially emotional disorder) in the children of the disordered probands.

The need is for a change from concentration on single correlation coefficients describing the interview's level of agreement with "experts" as evidence of validity, to concentration on comparisons of the information collection properties of different measures. When one is deciding which interview will be best for any clinical or research application, the key question is "Which collects the information I want in the way that I want to collect it in a reasonably reliable and efficient manner?" A second useful question is "Is there any strong reason (practical or based on research on the instrument's properties) why I should *not* use this instrument?" The current evidence certainly does not support the notion that any single interview is "best" for all applications.

HOW TO SELECT AN INTERVIEW

Some General Comments on What Is Not Helpful

A brief review of Table 2.1, and of the reliability data on the DISC presented by Shaffer, Fisher, and Lucas in Chapter 1 of this book, demonstrates that reliability is not a helpful guide in interview selection. The confidence intervals around the kappas presented are sufficiently wide that no firm statement that any interview is definitely more reliable than any other in any area is possible. Rather, such reliability data as we have indicate that all the interviews considered here do a reasonably good job. That none of them does much better than any other, after so much effort at revision, probably indicates that we have pretty much reached the limits of reliability for diagnostic interview methods. However, it is perfectly possible to make reliability worse by deciding to make substantial changes to an interview that has benefited from a prolonged development process, so users should be careful before deciding to make such modifications—especially if they are not going to test the effects of those changes.

Similarly, all the instruments reviewed here (and the DISC) can make good claims to be "valid" measures of what they purport to measure, from the perspective of construct validity. So reports on validity also do not provide a useful means for choosing among instruments.

All of the diagnostic interviews take a long time to administer. Furthermore, the time they take is proportional to a child's level of symptomatology. There is no clear evidence that any is reliably shorter in practice than any other, so, once again, the reported duration of the interview does not help in choosing among them.

Question 1: What Interview Characteristics Does My Application Demand?

The upshot of our review of reliability and validity is that the question "What is the best interview?" is the wrong question. Rather, you need to ask, "What is the best interview for my particular application?" This changes the focus of the choice process very substantially, because it directs the mind to being very clear about what that application demands. This means having thought through what the ideal interview for your purposes would be like, so that the characteristics of each can be matched against your criteria. For instance, if you need an interview for a 3-month follow-up study, one with a time frame of 1 year is not going to be very helpful. It is also helpful to prioritize these demand characteristics in advance. It may not be possible to have everything you want, so it is a big help to have thought through the relative impact of different tradeoffs.

Question 2: What Assessment Time Frame Do I Need?

A key question here relates to whether a lifetime interview is required. The addition of a lifetime frame involves either compromises in the assessment of current or recent symptomatology (as with the K-SADS-PL) or combining an interview that has a short time frame with a separate lifetime interview, which results in a very long assessment. Are such compromises worth it for your study, or would you be better off just concentrating on the recent past?

A second question concerns whether you want to use a fixed time frame (like the 3 months of the CAPA) or an indeterminate "present" or "current" time frame (like that of the K-SADS-P IVR)? If the former, how long do you want the time frame to be? Versions of the DISC-IV are available for 1 year or 1 month.

Question 3: What Sort of Interviewers Will I Be Using?

In general, clinicians are not enthusiastic about using the DISC because they have to follow a fixed schedule of questions, and it provides no means of collecting more detailed information that may be relevant to a variety of treatment decisions. So it makes sense for them to use one of the interviewer-based interviews. Such interviews can also be very useful clinical training tools, since they provide excellent models for the clinical interviewing process.

If lay interviewers are to be used, then the K-SADS family of interviews may not be the best choice, because these interviews have all been developed for use by clinicians and provide less guidance for the training of lay interviewers. No reliability data on their use with lay interviewers are available.

On the other hand, the CAS, CAPA, and DICA, were all developed for use with trained lay interviewers and have been shown to have acceptable reliability in their hands. On the other hand, all of these interviews are also acceptable to clinicians.

Question 4: What Are the Ages and Developmental Levels of My Subjects?

It is clear that "adult-style" diagnostic interviews (all of the interviews considered in this chapter fall into this category) with preschool children are a waste of time, because they simply cannot provide all the information required by the diagnostic criteria of the DSM-IV or the *International Classification of Diseases*, 10th revision. Several groups are working on this problem at present, but none of the instruments reviewed here is of any use for very young children. The K-SADS and DICA are said to be suitable for face-to-face use with children down to the age of 6, but others doubt that a *full* diagnostic interview really works with children under the age of 8 or 9, unless an interviewer simply "goes off interview" to get a relatively impressionistic view of a child's symptomatology. Even parent interviews require substantial modification for preschoolers. We would not recommend the use of any of these instruments in face-to-face interviews with children under the age of 8 or 9. Special versions of the DICA and CAPA for use with younger children are currently under development, but their feasibility and reliability remain to be determined. The same problem applies to older individuals with substantial intellectual deficits. When an individual's IQ is much below 70, it becomes very difficult to complete a full diagnostic interview. Interviews with parents and teachers may still be conducted, but we know little about their performance characteristics in such circumstances.

At the other end of the "juvenile" age range (late adolescence and early adulthood), the researcher or clinician has the choice of shifting to an "adult" measure, or using an age-appropriate modification of a child interview (such as the YAPA).

Question 5: How Much Can I Afford to Spend on Training and Quality Control?

"How much can I afford to spend?" here refers to both time and money. If less than a week is available, then none of the interviewer-based interviews is suitable, because good training for them demands a greater time investment. However, DISC training can be provided in as short a time as this, because the DISC requires far less of interviewers. On the other hand, when amortized over the life of a study or clinical program, initial costs for training usually turn out to be only a small percentage of the total costs; therefore, good training on an interviewer-based interview may constitute a good investment.

For both the DICA and the CAPA, once the interview is over, it should be reviewed for appropriateness of codings. In addition, regular, continuing training sessions for interviewers (the authors of both interviews recommend weekly) are required to prevent interviewer drift. Are funds and personnel available to support such continuing quality control and training procedures? The CAS and the K-SADS interviews do not appear to include standard recommendations for quality control and continuing training, but there is no reason to suppose that data quality and consistency are any easier to maintain with these instruments. Since the DISC-IV is computerized, and the DISC interviewer's task is much less arduous than that of interviewers using any of the interviews considered in this chapter, it demands less effort to control interviewer drift.

Question 6: What Needs and Resources Do I Have for Data Entry and Manipulation?

The K-SADS family of interviews produces diagnoses through the medium of scoresheets completed by the interviewer and scored by that person to produce diagnoses. The CAS provides formal algorithms for making diagnoses, which can be implemented by either the interviewer or a computer. The CAPA offers only computerized algorithms, because its developers (like those of the DISC) believe that the process of producing a final diagnosis from a large array of symptom data is of such complexity that errors are bound to occur if humans do it unaided. These different approaches to producing a final diagnostic formulation have very different implications for data entry and manipulation. If the computer is to make the diagnoses, then all the symptom information must be entered (this task easily runs to hundreds or thousands of variables per case), and diagnostic algorithms must be available. If a clinician makes the final diagnosis, then he/she could simply enter only that information (or not computerize any data at all in a clinical setting where the interview is being used just as a clinical assessment whose results appear only in the medical record). The CAPA is probably the interviewer-based instrument that makes the most demands on data entry (because of its molecular approach to symptom severity), so it has extensive data entry, checking, and diagnostic programs. Even so, the budget must allow for setting up and training people in the use of these programs.

Action 1: Review the Available Instruments and Make a Short List

It may seem surprising that we place a review of available measures so late in the process. There are two reasons for doing this. First, the choice of measure should be dependent on the nature of the application, not the other way around; therefore, until the application has been well defined, the issue of instrumentation is moot. Second, once you have answered questions 1–6, a brief review of instruments may indicate that only one is even remotely suitable. To put it another way, it is more efficient to decide which interview to use relatively late in the process, because you may be able to save a lot of time that would otherwise have been spent in considering instruments that cannot meet the needs of the study. If you are in the happy position of seeming to have several possibilities at hand, you have at least reduced the number of instruments that need to be considered to a short list for further evaluation.

Action 2: Get Copies of the Instruments on the Short List and Conduct a Detailed Evaluation

Unfortunately, there is absolutely no substitute for getting copies of the instruments still left on the short list and reviewing them in detail. The manifold differences among instruments make it impossible to provide more than a very general sense of what an interview is like in a review chapter such as this. It is worth remembering that you will be asking the interview developers to send you several hundred pages of schedules, glossaries, instruction manuals, and the like, and that you will need to pay for these. At this stage, it should be possible to make a final choice; however, if there are still questions that have not been answered in all these materials, a phone call to someone in the relevant interview development group can be very helpful. If you have done the "homework" outlined above, it is also likely to be well received.

Action 3: Plan Training Well Ahead of Time

It is not unknown for an interview developer to get a call that runs roughly as follows: "Hello, I put the _____ in a grant proposal, and the funding has just come through. I need you to train my interviewers next month." Interview developers usually have busy research and clinical programs to run, and they cannot drop everything to provide training programs at a moment's notice. The time to be setting a tentative date for training is when the grant proposal is submitted, not after it has been reviewed and funded!

CONCLUSIONS

All in all, there has never been a better time for choosing a psychiatric diagnostic interview for use with children and adolescents. All of the well-known instruments have produced reasonable evidence of their reliability and validity. There is a substantial range of choices, which allows different users to suit the needs of their applications to the properties of an interview. Many problems remain to be solved (particularly in the area of interviewing younger children), but work in this area will shortly be producing results. Although we are often taken up with debates over the advantages and disadvantages of different interviews, it behooves us also to remember how far we have come in the last 20 years.

REFERENCES

Achenbach, T. M. (1985). *Assessment and taxonomy of child and adolescent psychopathology.* Beverly Hills, CA: Sage.

Ambrosini, P., Metz, C., Prabucki, K., & Lee, J.-C. (1990). Videotape reliability of the third revised edition of the K-SADS. *Journal of the American Academy of Child and Adolescent Psychiatry, 28,* 723–728.

Anastasi, A. (1950). The concept of validity in the interpretation of test scores. *Journal of Psychology and Educational Measures, 10,* 67–78.

Anastasi, A. (1986). Evolving concepts of test validation. *Annual Review of Psychology, 37,* 1–15.

Angold, A. (1994). Clinical interviewing with children and adolescents. In M. Rutter, E. Taylor, & L. Hersov (Eds.), *Child and adolescent psychiatry: Modern approaches.* Oxford: Blackwell Scientific.

Angold, A., & Costello, E. J. (1995). A test–retest reliability study of child-reported psychiatric symptoms and diagnoses using the Child and Adolescent Psychiatric Assessment (CAPA-C). *Psychological Medicine, 25,* 755–762.

Angold, A., & Costello, E. J. (in press). The Child and Adolescent Psychiatric Assessment (CAPA). *Journal of the American Academy of Child and Adolescent Psychiatry.*

Angold, A., Messer, S. C., Stangl, D., Farmer, E. M. Z., Costello, E. J., & Burns, B. J. (1998). Perceived parental burden and service use for child and adolescent psychiatric disorders. *American Journal of Public Health, 88,* 75–80.

Angold, A., Prendergast, M., Cox, A., Harrington, R., Simonoff, E., & Rutter, M. (1995). The Child and Adolescent Psychiatric Assessment (CAPA). *Psychological Medicine, 25,* 739–753.

Angold, A., Weissman, M. M., John, K., Merikangas, K. R., Prusoff, B. A., Wickramaratne, P., Gammon, G. D., & Warner, V. (1987). Parent and child reports of depressive symptoms in children at low and high risk of depression. *Journal of Child Psychology and Psychiatry, 28,* 901–915.

Ascher, B. H., Farmer, E. M. Z., Burns, B. J., & Angold, A. (1996). The Child and Adolescent Services Assessment (CASA): Description and psychometrics. *Journal of Emotional and Behavioral Disorders, 4,* 12–20.

Breslau, N. (1987). Inquiring about the bizarre: False positives in Diagnostic Interview Schedule for Children (DISC) ascertainment of obsessions, compulsions, and psychotic symptoms. *Journal of the American Academy of Child and Adolescent Psychiatry, 26,* 639–644.

Cannell, C. F., Marquis, K. H., & Laurent, A. (1977). *A summary of studies of interviewing methodology* (Vital and Health Statistics, Series 1, No. 2). Washington, DC: U.S. Government Printing Office.

Cantwell, D. P. (1988). DSM-III studies. In M. Rutter, A. H. Tuma, & I. S. Lann (Eds.), *Assessment and diagnosis in child psychopathology.* New York: Guilford Press.

Chaput, F., Fisher, P., Klein, R., Greenhill, L., & Shaffer, D. (1999). The Columbia

K-SADS (Schedule for Affective Disorders and Schizophrenia for School Aged Children). Child Psychiatry Intervention Research Center, New York State Psychiatric Institute, 1051 Riverside Drive, New York, NY 10032.

Costello, A. J., Edelbrock, C. S., Dulcan, M. K., Kalas, R., & Klaric, S. H. (1984). *Development and testing of the NIMH Diagnostic Interview Schedule for Children in a clinic population: Final report* (Contract No. RFP-DB–81-0027). Rockville, MD: NIMH Center for Epidemiologic Studies.

Costello, E. J., Angold, A., Burns, B. J., Stangl, D. K., Tweed, D. L., Erkanli, A., & Worthman, C. M. (1996). The Great Smoky Mountains Study of Youth: Goals, designs, methods, and the prevalence of DSM-III-R disorders. *Archives of General Psychiatry, 53,* 1129–1136.

Costello, E. J., Angold, A., March, J., & Fairbank, J. (1998). Life events and post-traumatic stress: The development of a new measure for children and adolescents. *Psychological Medicine, 28,* 1275–1288.

Cox, A., Holbrook, D., & Rutter, M. (1981). Psychiatric interviewing techniques: VI. Experimental study: Eliciting feelings. *British Journal of Psychiatry, 139,* 144–152.

Cox, A., Hopkinson, K., & Rutter, M. (1981). Psychiatric interviewing techniques: II. Naturalistic study: Eliciting factual information. *British Journal of Psychiatry, 138,* 283–291.

Cox, A., Rutter, M., & Holbrook, D. (1981). Psychiatric interviewing techniques: V. Experimental study: Eliciting factual information. *British Journal of Psychiatry, 139,* 27–37.

Cronbach, L. J., & Meehl, P. E. (1955). Construct validity in psychological tests. *Psychological Bulletin, 52,* 281–302.

di Nardo, P. A., Moras, K., Barlow, D. H., Rapee, R. M., & Brown, T. A. (1993). Reliability of DSM-III-R anxiety disorder categories: Using the Anxiety Disorders Interview Schedule—Revised (ADIS-R). *Archives of General Psychiatry, 50,* 251–256.

Edelbrock, C. & Costello, A. J. (1990). Structured psychiatric interviews for children and adolescents. In G. Goldstein & M. Hersen (Eds.), *Handbook of psychological assessment.* New York: Pergamon Press.

Ezpeleta, L., de la Osa, N., Doménech, J. M., Navarro, J. B., & Losilla, J. M. (1995). La Diagnostic Interview for Children and Adolescents—Revised (DISC-R): Acuerdo diagnostico entre ninos/adolescentes y sus padres. *Revista de ea Psiquiatria Facultad de Medicina de Barcelona, 22,* 153–163.

Ezpeleta, L., de la Osa, N., Júdez, J., Doménech, J. M., Navarro, J. B., & Losilla, J. M. (1997). Diagnostic agreement between clinician and the Diagnostic Interview for Children and Adolescents—Revised (DICA-R) in an outpatient sample. *Journal of Child Psychology and Psychiatry, 38,* 431–440.

Farmer, E. M. Z., Angold, A., Burns, B. J., & Costello, E. J. (1994). Reliability of self-reported service use: Test–retest consistency of children's responses to the Child and Adolescent Services Assessment (CASA). *Journal of Child and Family Studies, 3,* 307–325.

Geller, B., Zimerman, B., Williams, M., & Frazier, J. (1996). *WASH-U-KSADS.* St. Louis, MO: Department of Psychiatry, Washington University.

Gould, M. S., Shaffer, D., Rutter, M., & Sturge, C. (1988). UK/WHO study of ICD–9. In M. Rutter, A. H. Tuma, & I. S. Lann (Eds.), *Assessment and diagnosis in child psychopathology.* New York: Guilford Press.

Graham, P., & Rutter, M. (1968). The reliability and validity of the psychiatric assessment of the child: II. Interview with the parent. *British Journal of Psychiatry, 114,* 581–592.

Gulliksen, H. (1950). Intrinsic validity. *American Psychologist, 5,* 511–517.

Guze, S. B., Goodwin, D. W., & Crane, J. B. (1969). Criminality and psychiatric disorders. *Archives of General Psychiatry, 20,* 583–591.

Herjanic, B., & Campbell, W. (1977). Differentiating psychiatrically disturbed children on the basis of a structured interview. *Journal of Abnormal Child Psychology, 5,* 127–134.

Herjanic, B., Herjanic, M., Brown, F., & Wheatt, T. (1975). Are children reliable reporters? *Journal of Abnormal Child Psychology, 3,* 41–48.

Herjanic, B., & Reich, W. (1982a). Development of a structured psychiatric interview for children: Agreement between child and parent. *Journal of Abnormal Child Psychology, 10,* 307–324.

Herjanic, B., & Reich, W. (1982b). Development of a structured psychiatric interview for children: Agreement between child and parent on individual symptoms. *Journal of Abnormal Child Psychology, 10,* 307–324.

Hodges, K., Cools, J., & McKnew, D. (1989). Test–retest reliability of a clinical research interview for children: The Child Assessment Schedule. *Journal of Consulting and Clinical Psychology, 1,* 317–322.

Hodges, K., Kline, J., Stern, L., Cytryn, L., & McKnew, D. (1982). The development of a child assessment interview for research and clinical use. *Journal of Abnormal Child Psychology, 10*(2), 173–189.

Hodges, K., McKnew, D., Burbach, D. J., & Roebuck, L. (1987). Diagnostic concordance between the Child Assessment Schedule (CAS) and the Schedule for Affective Disorders and Schizophrenia for School-Age Children (K-SADS) in an outpatient sample using lay interviewers. *Journal of the American Academy of Child and Adolescent Psychiatry, 26,* 654–661.

Hodges, K., McKnew, D., Cytryn, L., Stern, L., & Kline, J. (1982). The Child Assessment Schedule (CAS) diagnostic interview: A report on reliability and validity. *Journal of the American Academy of Child Psychiatry, 21,* 468–473.

Hodges, K., & Saunders, W. (1989). Internal consistency of a diagnostic interview for children: The Child Assessment Schedule. *Journal of Abnormal Child Psychology, 17*(6), 691–701.

Hodges, K., Saunders, W., Kashani, J., Hamlett, K., & Thompson, R. J., Jr. (1990). Internal consistency of DSM-III diagnoses using the symptom scales of the Child Assessment Schedule. *Journal of the American Academy of Child and Adolescent Psychiatry, 29*(4), 635–641.

Hodges, K., & Wong, M. M. (1996). Psychometric characteristics of a multidimensional measure to assess impairment: The Child and Adolescent Functional Assessment Scale. *Journal of Child and Family Studies, 4,* 445–467.

Hodges, K., & Wong, M. M. (1997). Use of the Child and Adolescent Functional Assessment Scale to predict service utilization and cost. *Journal of Mental Health Administration, 24,* 278–290.

Hodges, K., Wong, M. M., & Latessa, M. (1998). Use of the Child and Adolescent Functional Assessment Scale (CAFAS) as an outcome measure in clinical settings. *Journal of Behavioral Health Services and Research, 25,* 325–336.

Hopkinson, K., Cox, A., & Rutter, M. (1981). Psychiatric interviewing techniques: III. Naturalistic study: Eliciting feelings. *British Journal of Psychiatry, 138,* 406–415.

Jenkins, J. G. (1946). Validity for what? *Journal of Consulting and Clinical Psychology, 10,* 93–98.

Kaufman, J., Birmaher, B., Brent, D., Rao, U., Flynn, C., Moreci, P., Williamson, D., & Ryan, N. (1997). Schedule for Affective Disorder and Schizophrenia for School-Age

Children—Present and Lifetime Version (K-SADS-PL): Initial reliability and validity data. *Journal of the American Academy of Child and Adolescent Psychiatry, 36,* 980–988.

Lewinsohn, P. M., Hops, H., Roberts, R. E., Seeley, J. R., & Andrews, J. A. (1993). Adolescent psychopathology: I. Prevalence and incidence of depression and other DSM-III-R disorders in high school students. *Journal of Abnormal Psychology, 102,* 133–144.

Messer, S. C., Angold, A., Costello, E. J., & Burns, B. J. (1996). The Child and Adolescent Burden Assessment (CABA): Measuring the family impact of emotional and behavioral problems. *International Journal of Methods in Psychiatric Research, 6,* 261–284.

Novick, M. R. (1985). *Standards for educational and psychological testing.* Washington, DC: American Psychological Association.

Orvaschel, H., Puig-Antich, J., Chambers, W., Tabrizi, M. A., & Johnson, R. (1982). Retrospective assessment of prepubertal major depression with the Kiddie-SADS-E. *Journal of the American Academy of Child Psychiatry, 21,* 392–397.

de la Osa, N., Ezpeleta, L., Doménech, J. M., Navarro, J. B., & Losilla, J. M. (1997). Convergent and discriminant validity of the structured Diagnostic Interview for Children and Adolescents (DICA-R). *Psychology in Spain, 1,* 37–44.

Peak, H. (1953). Problems of objective observation. In L. Festinger & D. Katz (Eds.), *Research methods in the behavioral sciences.* New York: Dryden Press.

Puig-Antich, J., & Chambers, W. (1978). *The Schedule for Affective Disorders and Schizophrenia for School-Age Children (K-SADS).* New York: New York State Psychiatric Institute.

Regier, D. A., Myers, J. K., Kramer, M., Robins, L. N., Blazer, D. G., Hough, R. L., Eaton, W. W., & Locke, B. Z. (1984). The NIMH Epidemiological Catchment Area Program: Historical context, major objectives, and study population characteristics. *Archives of General Psychiatry, 41,* 934–941.

Reich, W. (1999). *Diagnostic Interview for Children and Adolescents (DICA).* Manuscript submitted for publication.

Reich, W., Cottler, L., McCallum, K., Corwin, D., & VanEerdewegh, M. (1995). Computerized interviews as a method of assessing psychopathology in children. *Comprehensive Psychiatry, 36,* 40–45.

Reich, W., & Earls, F. (1987). Rules of making psychiatric diagnoses in children on the basis of multiple sources of information: Preliminary strategies. *Journal of Abnormal Child Psychology, 15,* 601–616.

Reich, W., Herjanic, B., Welner, Z., & Gandhy, P. R. (1982). Development of a structured psychiatric interview for children: Agreement on diagnosis comparing child and parent interviews. *Journal of Abnormal Child Psychology, 10,* 325–336.

Remschmidt, H. (1988). German study of ICD-9. In M. Rutter, A. H. Tumain, & I. S. Lann (Eds.), *Assessment and diagnosis in child psychopathology.* New York: Guilford Press.

Robins, L. N., Helzer, J., Croughan, J., Williams, J. B. W., & Spitzer, R. L. (1979). *The NIMH Diagnostic Interview Schedule (DIS): Version II.* Rockville, MD: National Institute of Mental Health.

Rutter, M., & Cox, A. (1981). Psychiatric interviewing techniques: I. Methods and measures. *British Journal of Psychiatry, 138,* 273–282.

Rutter, M., Cox, A., Egert, S., Holbrook, D., & Everitt, B. (1981). Psychiatric interviewing techniques: IV. Experimental study: Four contrasting styles. *British Journal of Psychiatry, 138,* 456–465.

Rutter, M., & Graham, P. (1968). The reliability and validity of the psychiatric assessment of the child: I. Interview with the child. *British Journal of Psychiatry, 114,* 563–579.

Shanee, N., Apter, A., & Weizman, A. (1997). Psychometric properties of the K-SADS-PL in an Israeli adolescent clinical population. *Israeli Journal of Psychiatry and Related Sciences, 34,* 179–186.

Silverman, W. K. (1991). Diagnostic reliability of anxiety disorders in children using structured interviews. *Journal of Anxiety Disorders, 5,* 105–124.

Silverman, W. K., & Eisen, A. R. (1992). Age differences in the reliability of parent and child reports of child anxious symptomatology using a structured interview. *Journal of the American Academy of Child and Adolescent Psychiatry, 31,* 117–124.

Silverman, W. K., & Nelles, W. B. (1988). The Anxiety Disorders Interview Schedule for Children. *Journal of the American Academy of Child and Adolescent Psychiatry, 27,* 772–778.

Silverman, W. K., & Rabian, B. (1995). Test–retest reliability of the DSM-III-R childhood anxiety disorders symptoms using the Anxiety Disorders Interview Schedule for Children. *Journal of Anxiety Disorders, 9,* 139–150.

Simonoff, E., Pickles, A., Meyer, J. M., Silberg, J. L., Maes, H. H., Loeber, R., Rutter, M., Hewitt, J. K., & Eaves, L. J. (1997). The Virginia Twin Study of adolescent behavioral development: Influences of age, sex and impairment on rates of disorder. *Archives of General Psychiatry, 54,* 801–808.

Spielberger, C. D. (1973). *Manual for the State–Trait Anxiety Inventory for Children.* Palo Alto, CA: Consulting Psychologists Press.

Spitzer, R. L., Endicott, J., & Robins, E. (1978). Research Diagnostic Criteria: Rationale and reliability. *Archives of General Psychiatry, 35,* 773–782.

Verhulst, F. C., Berden, G. F. M. G., & Sanders-Woudstra, J. A. R. (1985). Mental health in Dutch children: II. The prevalence of psychiatric disorder and relationship between measures. *Acta Psychiatrica Scandinavica, 72,* 1–45.

Wallace, S. R. (1965). Criteria for what? *American Psychologist, 20,* 411–417.

Weissman, M. M., Wickramaratne, P., Warner, V., John, K., Prusoff, B. A., Merikangas, K. R., Gammon, G. D., Weisz, J. R., & Cicchetti, D. (1987). Assessing psychiatric disorders in children: Discrepancies between mothers' and children's reports. *Archives of General Psychiatry, 44,* 747–753.

Weitz, J. (1961). Criteria for criteria. *American Psychologist, 16,* 228–231.

Welner, Z., Reich, W., Herjanic, B., Jung, K. G., & Amado, H. (1987). Reliability, validity, and parent–child agreement studies of the Diagnostic Interview for Children and Adolescents (DICA). *Journal of the American Academy of Child and Adolescent Psychiatry, 26,* 649–653.

Wing, J. K. (1974). *Measurement and classification of psychiatric symptoms.* Oxford: Oxford University Press.

3

General Child Behavior
Rating Scales

✧

ELIZABETH L. HART
BENJAMIN B. LAHEY

This chapter presents an overview of the qualities and uses of omnibus rating scales for assessing child behavior problems, followed by a review of some of the most widely used multidimensional scales. Scales designed to assess specific domains of childhood behavior (e.g., anxiety, disruptive behavior problems) are reviewed elsewhere in this volume.

The past two decades have seen a dramatic increase in the availability of rating scales and checklists designed for use in assessing the emotional and behavioral functioning of children and adolescents. Such assessment instruments have become a mainstay of psychological/psychiatric research and clinical practice.

In recent years there has been increasing sophistication in the development of behavior rating scales. More attention has been paid to issues of the reliability and validity of assessment instruments, as well as to developmental considerations. As a result, there are now large numbers of empirically developed, psychometrically sound rating scales appropriate for use in both clinic and research settings. In addition, although most rating scales rely on adult informants, there has been a move toward viewing older children and adolescents as reliable informants on their own behavior; thus we have seen increasing availability of parallel rating scales for different informants. This growing emphasis on multi-informant assessment is based on the assumption that each informant provides a unique, valid perspective on a young person's behavior, and thus information from all sources should be utilized in diagnostic decision making even when the informants disagree with one another

(Achenbach, McConaughy, & Howell, 1987). The use of multi-informant in-struments also allows the examination of differences in a child's or adoles-cent's behavior across settings, providing a more comprehensive picture of his/her functioning.

GENERAL CONSIDERATIONS

Dimensions of childhood dysfunction are defined by deviations in the fre-quency or duration of intercorrelated clusters of maladaptive behaviors. Rating scales provide operational rules for obtaining, combining, and inter-preting data, and typically provide a basis for determining whether a sub-ject's behavior is deviant relative to that of normative samples. Rating scales allow objective assessment of behavior, and make it possible to obtain infor-mation about the occurrence of rare behaviors that would not be captured through time-sampling observational measures.

Compared to unstructured clinical interviews, rating scales allow for data collection in a more objective and systematic fashion; this makes it possi-ble to compare data obtained for a particular child or adolescent to that of some relevant norm group, and to compare data obtained across different points in time. Similarly, rating scales allow information to be obtained from multiple informants in a time- and cost-efficient manner. Clinical interviews typically require a significantly greater investment of time and economic and professional resources.

These potential advantages over the clinical interview come at the cost of decreased flexibility and possibly a decrease in the depth and breadth of coverage, however. For example, rating scales generally do not provide infor-mation concerning how long a given behavior has been present, temporal co-occurrence of behaviors, age at onset of problem behaviors, or stressors and other factors that may play an important role in the expression of the behav-ior. Often behavior rating scales do not contain probes designed to clarify the nature of a reported behavior. This type of information is more easily ob-tained through clinical or structured diagnostic interviews.

Behavior rating scales also have several limitations that are shared by other assessment procedures. Like some observational methods, rating scales may be subject to errors related to social desirability effects, halo effects, a le-niency–severity bias, or a central tendency bias (Martin, Hooper, & Snow, 1986). In addition, responses to rating scale items may be affected by such factors as (1) characteristics of the checklist rating scale used, such as the con-tent and wording of items; (2) characteristics of the child/adolescent, such as age, gender, and presenting problem; (3) characteristic of the informant, in-cluding expectancies, familiarity with the child/adolescent, and tendency to-ward response bias (Bond & McMahon, 1984); (4) setting (i.e., home, school, clinic); and (5) purpose of the evaluation (e.g., screening, diagnosis, educational placement). Finally, rating scales typically do not provide information on specific criteria for psychiatric diagnosis, although they usually provide diagnostically relevant information.

Analyses of the factor structure of omnibus behavior rating scales have yielded varying results. Although there is considerable consistency in the identification of certain broad-band syndromes (e.g., internalizing and externalizing behaviors), there are frequently differences in the number and nature of empirically derived syndromes. This results largely from differences in the item pools, sample characteristics, and statistical analysis. In addition, comparison of the factors and syndromes identified in different rating scales is complicated by the fact that the same label maybe given to different factors in different scales. On the other hand, similar factors across rating scales may be given different labels.

RELIABILITY AND VALIDITY

In order to provide useful data for either research or clinical purposes, rating scales must have adequate reliability and validity, as well as clinical utility. There are several different indices of reliability, each reflecting a different characteristic of the instrument. The three most common indices of reliability are test–retest reliability (i.e., the likelihood of obtaining the same score on two separate occasions), interrater reliability (i.e., the likelihood that two different raters will arrive at the same score), and internal consistency (i.e., the extent to which items on the scale are all measuring the same construct). Internal consistency usually increases with the number of items on the scale (Streiner, 1993). Most parent and teacher rating scales have high internal consistency and yield high test–retest reliability (.80–.90) over 1-week to 1-month intervals. The test–retest reliability of self-ratings by children and adolescents is lower, but still moderately high (McMahon, 1984).

Findings concerning interrater reliability for various rating scales require more thoughtful consideration. Differences in ratings across raters (or settings) may mean that a child's behavior varies according to the situation, that the response tendencies of the raters differ, or that one or more of these raters are not reliable, among other factors. Studies consistently find that although behavior ratings by mothers and fathers agree fairly well, agreement between parent and teacher ratings is generally low (.30–.40), and child self-ratings do not correlate highly with the ratings made by adult informants. In general, parents report more externalizing behaviors, and children report more internalizing symptoms. These findings are consistent with the suggestion of Achenbach, McConaughy, and Howell (1987) that different informants provide unique perspectives on a child's behavior and so should be retained even in the face of discrepancy. Overall, most rating scales designed for adult informants are highly reliable. Those designed for children and adolescents are less so, but most are still acceptable for clinical and research purposes.

In addition to reliability, rating scales should also demonstrate the following types of validity:

1. *Construct validity:* The extent to which the assessment instrument measures the theoretical construct or trait it is intended to measure.
2. *Content validity:* The extent to which the scale items fully represent the content to be measured.
3. *Face validity:* The extent to which the items on a scale appear to be measuring what they purport to measure.
4. *Criterion validity:* The extent to which scores on the measure predict scores on other relevant measures or criteria. Criterion validity may be either concurrent (when the relevant criterion is measured at the same time) or predictive (when the outcome criterion is measured at a later time).

Several factors serve to increase the reliability and/or validity of rating scales. These include clearly defined anchor points, the inclusion of more than two rating points, and raters with extensive experience with the child/adolescent being rated (O'Leary & Johnson, 1979).

Another important consideration in the selection of a behavior rating scale is clinical utility. Specifically, a useful scale is one that is relevant to the questions to be addressed in the assessment, is acceptable to the rater, provides adequate coverage, is brief enough to be practical, and is sensitive to treatment effects. Typically, rating scales make use of standard instructions and response formats, are designed to minimize subjective inferences by the rater, allow the calculation of quantitative scores for each area of functioning measured, have identified clinical cutoffs for determining the deviance of scores, and are standardized on large samples. Thanks to their practicality, several rating scales have a large amount of data on the reliability and validity of their scores, allowing information on the variance of scores that can typically be expected.

CLINICAL USES

The majority of behavior rating scales are well suited to the initial assessment of children and adolescents referred for mental health services. They provide an economical means of identifying salient emotional and behavioral problems, and they pinpoint areas of behavioral deviance. Most rating scales have normative data available, allowing the determination of the statistical deviance of the ratings of behavior. In addition, they provide a means for obtaining information from significant individuals in a child's environment; they also aid in the identification of problem behaviors that, while significant, occur infrequently, and are thus unlikely to be captured by direct observational measures. When completed early in the assessment process, rating scales may serve as a natural springboard to treatment. Finally, they can provide a useful means of monitoring changes in behavior and of evaluating treatment effects.

Although most multidimensional rating scales do not assess specific diagnostic criteria per se, they typically assess relevant behaviors and/or syndromes, and can often discriminate among diagnostic groups.

RESEARCH APPLICATIONS

Many behavior rating scales are well suited to epidemiological research in particular, because they provide a simple, reliable, and efficient method for surveying large populations. Often rating scales are used in the initial stage of multistage studies as a means of obtaining information about large numbers of individuals, for the purpose of identifying subjects for more intensive assessment (Verhulst & Koot, 1992). The use of rating scales does not depend on the inferences of trained clinicians—a need that makes the cost of clinical interviews prohibitive for large-scale epidemiological studies. In addition, rating scales provide an efficient means of screening potential subjects for inclusion in or exclusion from sample groups, monitoring response to experimental treatment protocols, and assessing degree of pretest–posttest change.

A representative sample of general child behavior rating scales is reviewed here. As is the case for most rating scales, these measures are scored in terms of empirically derived scales rather than categorical syndromes. They ask the informant (parent, teacher, or child/adolescent) to rate the presence, frequency, and/or severity of the behavior problems. The rating scales reviewed all have face or content validity. Criterion-related validity is supported by their ability to discriminate between criterion groups (e.g., clinic-referred vs. nonreferred groups). Most also distinguish between diagnostic groups, although, as indicated above, rating scales generally do not provide sufficient information for determining diagnostic status.

PARENT RATING SCALES

Personality Inventory for Children

The Personality Inventory for Children (PIC; Wirt, Lachar, Klinedinst, & Seat, 1977, 1984; Wirt, Seat, Broen, & Lachar, 1989; see Table 3.1) is a parent-completed measure of affect, behavior, cognitive status, and family characteristics; it was modeled on the Minnesota Multiphasic Personality Inventory. It is appropriate for use with children aged 3–16, and, according to the authors, requires a sixth- to seventh-grade reading level to complete (Harrington & Follet, 1984). The original version of the PIC consisted of 600 items that were chosen on the basis of both rational and empirical methods. It has since undergone two revisions. In the first of these (Wirt et al., 1984), the PIC was revised to consist of four versions of varying lengths ranging from 131 to 600 items. The most recent revision (Wirt et al., 1989) eliminates the 600-item option and the associated experimental scales. It now includes 420 true–false items divided into three sections; this division allows users to choose to administer 131, 280, or 420 items. The scale may be either hand- or computer-administered and scored.

The 1989 PIC Profile contains 16 subscales, including four validity and screening scales (Lie, Frequency, Defensiveness, and Adjustment), three scales measuring cognitive status (Achievement, Development, and Intellectual Screening), and nine measuring specific types of problems (Depression, Somatic Concerns, Family Relations, Delinquency, Withdrawal, Anxiety, Psychosis, Hyperactivity, and Social Skills). In addition, there are four broadband scales derived from factor analysis of PIC protocols for 1,226 clinic-referred children (Undisciplined/Poor Self-Control, Social Incompetence, Internalization/Somatic Symptoms, and Cognitive Development). Separate profile forms are used for children aged 3–5 and 6–16, and for males and females, but the scales are the same across age and gender.

Part I of the PIC (items 1–131) includes the Lie scale and the four broad-band scales. Completion of Parts I and II (items 1–280) allows scoring of the broad-band and Lie scales plus the Development scale, shortened versions of the other 14 profile scales, and some critical items. Completion of all

TABLE 3.1. Personality Inventory for Children (PIC)

Developed by: Robert D. Wirt, David Lachar, James K. Klinedinst, and Philip D. Seat (1977, 1984)

Most recent version: Wirt, Seat, Broen, and Lachar (1989)

Ages: 3–16   **Items:** 131–420 (three versions)   **Scaling:** 0–1

Informant: Parent   **Completion time:** Approximately 20–90 minutes

Normative data: $n = 2,390$ (6–16 years); preliminary norms ages 3–5

Factors assessed: Undisciplined/Poor Self-Control, Social Incompetence, Internalization/Somatic Symptoms, and Cognitive Development

Scales: Achievement, Development, Intellectual Screening, Depression, Somatic Concerns, Family Relations, Delinquency, Withdrawal, Anxiety, Psychosis, Hyperactivity, Social Skills, Lie, Frequency, Defensiveness, and Adjustment

---

420 items of the PIC (Parts I–III) provides a measure of the four factor scales, all 16 profile scales, and the complete set of critical items.

One disadvantage of the PIC is that the scales were developed through various methodologies, including both empirical procedures and "rational" judgments. As a result, there is significant overlap in the item content of several of the scales. In addition, the full version of the PIC is quite long, making the scale impractical for research purposes. Although the short version (Part I only) may have some utility as a research tool, the longer versions of the PIC would seemed to be better suited for use as part of a clinical evaluation.

Louisville Behavior Checklist

The Louisville Behavior Checklist (LBC; Miller, 1984; see Table 3.2) is one of the most comprehensive behavior rating scales for children currently available. Designed to be completed by parents, the LBC has three separate forms (E1, E2, E3) for use with children aged 4–6 years, 7–12 years, and 13–17 years, respectively. The 164-item form for school-age children (E2) provides scores for 19 scales. It takes approximately 30–45 minutes to complete and requires a 10th-grade reading level.

The first 11 scales of the LBC (Infantile Aggression, Hyperactivity, Antisocial Behavior, Aggression, Social Withdrawal, Sensitivity, Fear, Inhibition, Academic Disability, Immaturity, Learning Disability) are factor scales, and are similar to the scales found on other omnibus rating scales. The remaining 8 scales (Severity Level, Normal Irritability, Prosocial Deficit, Rare Deviance, Neurotic Behavior, Psychotic Behavior, Somatic Behavior, Sexual Behavior)

TABLE 3.2. Louisville Behavior Checklist (LBC)

Developed by: Lovick C. Miller (1984)

Ages: 4–17	**Items:** Approx. 160 (three versions)	**Scaling:** 0–1
Informant: Parent	**Completion time:** 30–45 minutes	
Normative data: n = 425 (4–12 years)		

Factors assessed (school-age form): Aggression, Hyperactivity, Antisocial Behavior, Learning Disability, Infantile Aggression, Inhibition, Social Withdrawal, Fear, Sensitivity, Academic Disability, and Immaturity

Rationally developed scales: Severity Level, Normal Irritability, Prosocial Deficit, Rare Deviance, Neurotic Behavior, Psychotic Behavior, Somatic Behavior, and Sexual Behavior were developed through a rational strategy, similar to that used in the development of the PIC. The items and subscales contained on the E1 and E3 forms are somewhat different from those presented above. The LBC may be hand-scored with templates, or computer-scored by Western Psychological Services.

The norm sample for the LBC consisted of relatively small numbers of school children drawn from the Louisville area, although additional normative data have been reported (e.g., Tarte, Vernon, Luke, & Clark, 1982). Reliability data as reported in the manual indicate moderate to good (.60-.92) test–retest reliability over 3 months, parent–teacher agreement of .06–.57, and generally high internal consistency coefficients for subscales, with the lowest coefficient on the Sexual Behavior subscale (.60). Validity data reported in the manual include several studies supporting the ability of the LBC to distinguish clinical from nonclinical groups.

TEACHER RATING SCALES

Comprehensive Behavior Rating Scale for Children

The Comprehensive Behavior Rating Scale for Children (CBRSC; Neeper, Lahey, & Frick, 1990; see Table 3.3) is a teacher-completed rating scale designed to assess behavioral, emotional, cognitive, and social functioning in the school setting for children aged 6–14 years. The 70-item CBRSC includes nine scales derived through factor analysis: Inattention-Disorganization, Reading Problems, Cognitive Deficits, Oppositional–Conduct Disorder, Motor Hyperactivity, Anxiety, Sluggish Tempo, Daydreaming, and Social Competence. The teacher uses a 5-point Likert scale to rate how characteristic each item is of the child.

According to the authors, the scale was developed to cover content areas

---

TABLE 3.3. Comprehensive Behavior Rating Scale for Children (CBRSC)

Developed by: Ronald Neeper, Benjamin B. Lahey, and Paul J. Frick (1990)

Ages: 6–14   **Items:** 70   **Scaling:** 1–5

Informant: Teacher   **Completion time:** 10–15 minutes

Normative data: $n = 2,153$ (6–14 years)

Factors assessed: Inattention–Disorganization, Reading Problems, Cognitive Deficits, Oppositional–Conduct Disorder, Motor Hyperactivity, Anxiety, Sluggish Tempo, Daydreaming, and Social Competence

---

not included in other teacher rating scales, particularly in the area of cognitive functioning. Although three of the nine scales contain fewer than five items, all scales have high internal consistency and appear to be quite homogeneous. Scales were generated through factor analysis of data from a sample of nonreferred school children. Normative data are based on a sample of 2,153 children aged 6–14 years.

The authors have endeavored to create a rating scale that is consistent with the current diagnostic nomenclature by including items similar to those found in the third and revised third editions of the *Diagnostic and Statistical Manual of Mental Disorders* (DSM-III and DSM-III-R; American Psychiatric Association, 1980, 1987). The validity studies reported authors provide evidence for the significant correspondence between certain CBRSC subscales and the relevant DSM-III/DSM-III-R diagnostic categories in a sample of clinic-referred children. The manual is clear and comprehensive, and provides normative tables based on sex or on age and sex.

Limitations of the CBRSC include the fact that data on the test–retest reliability of the scale are based on an earlier 102-item version; thus the reliability of the 70-item version is in need of further evaluation. In addition, African American and Hispanic children are somewhat underrepresented in the normative sample, and girls are underrepresented in the clinic validation sample. The lack of a parallel parent or self-report version of this scale may also make it less than ideal, particularly for some research purposes.

School Behavior Checklist

The School Behavior Checklist (SBC; Miller, 1981; see Table 3.4) is a multidimensional scale designed for use with teachers of preschool and school-age children. The SBC consists of two forms, A–1 (104 items) and A–2 (96 items) for ages 3–6 years and 7–13 years, respectively. Form A–1 provides scores on six factors (Low Need for Achievement, Aggression, Anxiety, Cog-

---

TABLE 3.4. School Behavior Checklist (SBC)

Developed by: Lovick C. Miller (1981)

Ages: 3–13	**Items:** 104/96 (two versions)	**Scaling:** 0–1
Informant: Teacher	**Completion time:** 20 minutes	

Normative data: n = 5,912 (4–13 years)

Factors assessed (school-age form): Low Need for Achievement, Aggression, Anxiety, Academic Disability, Hostile Isolation, and Extraversion

Rationally developed subscales: School Disturbance and Normal Irritability

nitive Disability, Hostile Isolation, and Extraversion), as well as scores on two rationally developed subscales (School Disturbance and Normal Irritability). Normative data appear to be adequate, and norms are provided by age and gender.

Form A-2 provides scores on the six factors listed above (the Cognitive Disability factor is renamed Academic Disability). The normative sample for this form is quite large; norms are available by gender only. Information provided in the manual indicates that test–retest and internal consistency reliability estimates are moderate to high, and that the scale distinguishes among diagnostic groups, thus supporting its validity (Miller, 1981). Both forms utilize a true–false format and require approximately a sixth-grade reading ability.

MULTI-INFORMANT RATING SCALES AND SYSTEMS

Behavior Assessment System for Children

The Behavior Assessment System for Children (BASC) is a multidimensional system for evaluating the behavior of children and adolescents 4–18 years of age. This assessment system includes parent and teacher rating scales, as well as a self-report scale for children and adolescents aged 8–18 years. In creating this system of instruments, the emphasis was on developing measures with good content and construct validity, rather that on developing scales based primarily on factor-analytic data, because scales with good content and construct validity are more stable and more replicable than purely empirically derived scales (Reynolds & Kamphaus, 1992).

The BASC also includes a Structured Developmental History form, which contains questions pertaining to social, developmental, educational, medical, and family history, and a Student Observation System form, on which the clinician may record 15 minutes of direct observation of classroom behavior.

Both the parent and teacher rating scales have three forms with items for ages 4–5, 6–11, and 12–18 years. The frequency of each item is rated on a 4-point scale ranging from "never" to "almost always." Unlike most other child behavior rating scales, the BASC also identifies positive attributes that can be used in treatment planning. This set of measures has been shown to have high internal consistency and test–retest reliability.

The subscales of the BASC are consistent across genders, age levels, and informants (parent and teacher), allowing easy interpretation across times and settings. The BASC may be interpreted with norms based on a large, representative national sample or a clinical sample; both sets of norms are differentiated by age, gender, and clinical status. In addition, critical items that may be interpreted individually are included.

Scores for each of the three behavior rating instruments are reported as *T* scores and percentiles by gender and age for both norm samples. The BASC instruments come in either hand-scored or computer-scored formats. The hand-scored format consists of carbonless forms on which responses are automatically transferred to an easy-to-use scoring grid. Computer administration and/or scoring is also available. The computer software calculates scale and composite scores, and displays them in both tabular and profile formats. In addition, the software program generates an interpretive report, which identifies similarities between a child's profile and those of children with various diagnoses. The manual accompanying this assessment system is comprehensive, well written, and easy to use.

Advantages of the BASC are its inclusion of positive items, which may increase its acceptability to users, and the use of scales that are both clinically relevant and consistent across ages, genders, and informants. The disadvantage is that the scales may take slightly longer to complete than other multidimensional rating scales.

Teacher Rating Scale

The 130-item Teacher Rating Scale (TRS; see Table 3.5), designed to be used by teachers, teacher aides, or day care providers, measures both adaptive behaviors and problem behaviors in a school setting. It assesses three broad domains—Internalizing Problems, Externalizing Problems, and School Problems—and also measures Adaptive Skills. In addition, the TRS provides from 10 to 14 narrow-band scales (depending on the age of the child), as well as a Behavioral Symptoms Index composite score to assess the overall level of problem behavior. The TRS also includes an F ("fake bad") index to assess the validity of the teacher report. The TRS takes approximately 10–20 minutes to complete.

TABLE 3.5. Behavior Assessment System for Children (BASC): Teacher Rating Scale (TRS)

Developed by: Cecil R. Reynolds and Randy W. Kamphaus (1992)

Ages: 4–18   **Items:** Approx. 130 (three versions)   **Scaling:** 0–3
Informant: Teacher   **Completion time:** 10–20 minutes
Normative data: $n = 2,401$

Narrow-band scales (these vary with age): Aggression, Hyperactivity, Conduct Problems, Anxiety, Depression, Somatization, Attention Problems, Learning Problems, Atypicality, Withdrawal, Adaptability, Leadership, Social Skills, and Study Skills

Broad-band domains: Internalizing Problems, Externalizing Problems, and School Problems

Parent Rating Scale

The Parent Rating Scale (PRS; see Table 3.6) is designed to measure a child's adaptive and problem behaviors in home and community settings. Like the TRS, the 130-item PRS has three forms for use at three different age levels. The PRS has the same broad-domain scales as the TRS, with the exception of the School Problems composite, and does not include the Learning Problems and Study Skills subscales. Like the TRS, the PRS includes an F index and takes approximately 10–20 minutes to complete.

Self-Report of Personality

The Self-Report of Personality (SRP; see Table 3.7) consists of approximately 170 true–false items. It has two forms at two age levels (8–11 years and 12–18 years). Composite scores for both scales include School Maladjustment, Clinical Maladjustment, Personal Adjustment, and an Emotional Symptoms Index. The child form (8–11 years) consists of 12 subscales, while the adolescent form (12–18 years) has 14 subscales. Two of the subscale scores (Somatization and Self-Reliance) have been shown to have low reliability and should be interpreted with caution. The SRP also includes an L ("fake good") scale for the adolescent version, and a V (validity) index to detect invalid responding as a result of poor reading comprehension, failure to follow instructions, or poor reality testing. The SRP takes approximately 30 minutes to complete and may be interpreted with respect to age, gender, or clinical status norms. Unlike the Youth Self-Report version of the Achenbach scales (described below), the two forms of the BASC SRP allow the assessment of favorable adjustment, self-esteem, attitudes toward teachers and

TABLE 3.6. Behavior Assessment System for Children (BASC): Parent Rating Scale (PRS)

Developed by: Cecil R. Reynolds and Randy W. Kamphaus (1992)

Ages: 4–18	**Items:** Approx. 130 (three versions)	**Scaling:** 0–3
Informant: Parent	**Completion time:** 10–20 minutes	
Normative data: n = 3,483		

Narrow-band scales (these vary with age): Aggression, Hyperactivity, Conduct Problems, Anxiety, Depression, Somatization, Attention Problems, Atypicality, Withdrawal, Adaptability, Leadership, and Social Skills

Broad-band domains: Internalizing Problems, Externalizing Problems, and School Problems

TABLE 3.7. Behavior Assessment System for Children (BASC): Self-Report of Personality (SRP)

Developed by: Cecil R. Reynolds and Randy W. Kamphaus (1992)

Ages: 8–18   **Items:** Approx. 170 (two versions)   **Scaling:** T–F

Informant: Child/adolescent   **Completion time:** 30 minutes

Normative data: $n = 9,861$

Narrow-band scales (these vary with age): Anxiety, Atypicality, Locus of Control, Social Stress, Somatization, Attitude to School, Attitude to Teachers, Sensation Seeking, Depression, Sense of Inadequacy, Relations with Parents, Interpersonal Relations, Self-Esteem, and Self-Reliance

Broad-band domains: Internalizing Problems, Externalizing Problems, and School Problems

---

school, locus of control, and perceived social stress. On the other hand, these instruments provide less complete coverage of emotional and behavioral problems than does their Achenbach counterpart.

Child Behavior Checklist System

The Child Behavior Checklist (CBCL) is perhaps the most widely used general behavioral scale for assessing children and adolescents. The original CBCL (now known as the CBCL/4–18; Achenbach & Edelbrock, 1983; Achenbach, 1991b) has been translated into almost three dozen languages. Since 1983, several additional forms have been modeled on the CBCL, and all these forms together constitute a family of assessment instruments. They include the CBCL/2–3 (Achenbach, Edelbrock, & Howell, 1987; Mc-Conaughy & Achenbach, 1988), a downward extension of the CBCL, designed to be used for young children; the Teacher's Report Form (TRF; Achenbach, 1991c; Achenbach & Edelbrock, 1986) to be completed by teachers of children aged 5–18; the Youth Self-Report (YSR; Achenbach & Edelbrock, 1987; Achenbach, 1991d), for adolescents aged 11–18; and the Direct Observation Form (DOF; Achenbach, 1986), which is completed by an observer after a 10-minute observation of the classroom behavior of school-age children. Unlike the BASC instruments, these instruments were developed largely through empirical means rather than being conceptually driven. As a result, the original versions of the scales had different factors for each gender, at each age group, and for each informant. Revisions of the scoring profiles of the CBCL/4–18, TRF, and YSR, based on larger samples of clinically referred and nonreferred children, were completed in 1991

(Achenbach, 1991a, 1991b, 1991c, 1991d). These revised profiles allow for scoring of syndromes that are common to the three informants (parent, teacher, and youth), as well as additional syndromes that are specific to particular forms. Norms for the 1991 profiles are based on a single U.S. national sample. As for the BASC instruments, hand-scored profiles and computer-scoring programs are available for all of these measures.

Child Behavior Checklist/4–18

The CBCL/4–18 (Achenbach, 1991b; Achenbach & Edelbrock, 1983; see Table 3.8) is a parent-completed measure designed to assess a child's emotional and behavioral problems, as well as his/her social and academic competence. It includes 20 competence items and 112 behavior problem items, plus 2 open-ended items. The behavior problem items were originally developed through clinical case descriptions and consultation with mental health professionals (Achenbach, 1966). These items cover both internalizing and externalizing behaviors, which are rated by the parent on a scale of 0–2 for how true the item is for the child currently or within the past 6 months. The competence items pertain to the child's academic performance, participation in recreational activities, and involvement with friends and social organizations. The 1991 Profile has separate forms for each gender and for ages 4–11 and 12–18. Scores are provided for Total Competence; Activities, Social Competence, and School Competence; Internalizing and Externalizing Problems; and nine narrow-band syndrome scales. Unlike the 1983 Profile, which had different scales for each gender and each of three age groups (4–5, 6–11, 12–16), the 1991 Profile has the same scales for all groups, normed separately for each gender at each of the two age groups noted above. Scales

---

TABLE 3.8. Child Behavior Checklist/4–18 (CBCL/4–18)

Developed by: Thomas Achenbach and Craig Edelbrock (1983)
Most recent version: Achenbach (1991b)

Ages: 4–18   **Items:** 112   **Scaling:** 0–2
Informant: Parent   **Completion time:** 10–15 minutes
Normative data: n = 2,600 nonreferred children (4–18 years)

Narrow-band scales (these vary with age/gender): Delinquent Behavior, Aggressive Behavior, Withdrawn, Somatic Complaints, Anxious/Depressed, Social Problems, Thought Problems, and Attention Problems

Broad-band scales: Total Competence, Activities, Social Competence, School Competence, Internalizing Problems, and Externalizing Problems

were derived through principal-components factor analysis for 4,455 clinically referred children (McConaughy, 1992).

Child Behavior Checklist/2–3

The CBCL/2–3 (Achenbach, Edelbrock, & Howell, 1987; see Table 3.9) contains 99 problem items, 59 of which have direct counterparts on the CBCL/4–18. A parent rates how true each item is for a child within the past 2 months. The CBCL/2–3 Profile provides scores for both genders for Total Problems; Internalizing and Externalizing Problems; and six narrow-band scales, derived through factor analysis for referred, nonreferred, and low-birth-weight children.

Teacher's Report Form

The TRF (Achenbach, 1991c; Achenbach & Edelbrock, 1986; see Table 3.10) is designed for use with teachers of children and adolescents aged 5–18 years, to assess academic performance, adaptive functioning, and behavior problems. In addition to 118 behavior problem items scored 0–2, the TRF asks the teacher to rate school performance in each academic subject on a 5-point scale, and each of four areas of adaptive functioning on a 7-point scale. Ninety-three TRF items have counterparts on the CBCL/4–18; the remaining items refer to school behaviors that a teacher has more opportunity to observe.

The original 1986 version of the TRF Profile was designed for use for children aged 6–16. The 1991 TRF Profile has been expanded to cover ages 5–11 and 12–18. In addition to scores for Academic and Adaptive Functioning, Total Problems, and Externalizing and Internalizing Problems, the 1991 TRF Profile includes eight narrow-band syndrome scales normed separately for each gender/age group.

TABLE 3.9. Child Behavior Checklist/2–3 (CBCL/2–3)

Developed by: Thomas Achenbach, Craig Edelbrock, and C. T. Howell (1987)

Ages: 2–3   **Items:** 99   **Scaling:** 0–2

Informant: Parent   **Completion time:** 10–15 minutes

Normative data: n = 273 nonreferred children (2–3 years)

Narrow-band scales: Social Withdrawal, Depressed, Sleep Problems, Somatic Problems, Aggressive, and Destructive

Broad-band scales: Total Competence, Activities, Social Competence, School Competence, Internalizing Problems, Externalizing Problems

TABLE 3.10. Child Behavior Checklist (CBCL): Teacher's Report Form (TRF)

Developed by: Thomas Achenbach and Craig Edelbrock (1984)
Most recent version: Achenbach (1991c)

Ages: 5–18	**Items:** 118	**Scaling:** 0–2
Informant: Teacher	**Completion time:** 10–15 minutes	

Normative data: n = 1,391 nonreferred children (5–18 years)

Narrow-band scales (these vary with age/gender): Withdrawn, Somatic Complaints, Anxious/Depressed, Social Problems, Thought Problems, Attention Problems, Delinquent Behavior, and Aggressive Behavior

Broad-band scales: Total Competence, Activities, Social Competence, School Competence, Internalizing Problems, Externalizing Problems

Youth Self-Report

The YSR (Achenbach, 1991d; Achenbach & Edelbrock, 1987; see Table 3.11) is designed to obtain self-reports of emotional and behavioral functioning from adolescents 11–18 years of age. It contains 102 behavior problem items that correspond to CBCL/4–18 items, 16 positive items, and one open-ended item that an adolescent uses to rate himself/herself during the past six months. YSR responses are scored on the 1991 YSR Profile, which has separate forms for each gender and includes scores for Activities, Social Competence, and Total Competence; Total Problems; Internalizing and Externalizing Problems; and nine narrow-band scales, eight of which have counterparts on the CBCL/4–18 and TRF. According to the authors, the YSR requires a mental age of 10 years and a fifth-grade reading level.

There are numerous advantages of the CBCL system. The system consists of comprehensive, empirically sound scales that are easy to use and not

TABLE 3.11. Child Behavior Checklist (CBCL): Youth Self-Report (YSR)

Developed by: Thomas Achenbach and Craig Edelbrock (1987)
Most recent version: Achenbach (1991d)

Ages: 11–18	**Items:** 102	**Scaling:** 0–2
Informant: Adolescent	**Completion time:** 10–15 minutes	

Normative data: n = 1,315 nonreferred adolescents (11–18 years)

Factors assessed: Withdrawn, Somatic Complaints, Depressed, Thought Disorder, Unpopular, Aggressive, Attention Problems, Delinquent

time-consuming. A major disadvantage of the original CBCL profiles was the lack of correspondence of scales across the forms, making it difficult to compare scores across time or setting. This has changed in the revised profiles. Another disadvantage is the fact that, compared to some of the measures reviewed above, the empirically derived scales of the CBCL instruments correspond less closely to the symptom dimensions identified in the current diagnostic nomenclature.

Revised Behavior Problem Checklist

As its name indicates, the Revised Behavior Problem Checklist (RBPC; Quay & Peterson, 1983, 1984; see Table 3.12) is a revision of the Behavior Problem Checklist (Quay & Peterson, 1979). The expansion of the RBPC from the original 55-item checklist (present–absent format) to an 89-item scale (3-point severity format) has allowed for a more comprehensive assessment of the dimensions of childhood psychopathology, and has greatly improved the psychometric properties of the scale. The RBPC uses an 0–2 scale (0 = "does not constitute a problem," 1 = "mild problem," 2 = "severe problem") for rating behavior problems of children and adolescents aged 6 to 18 years. It takes approximately 5 minutes to complete. The RBPC items are grouped into six scales—four major scales (Conduct Disorder, Socialized Aggression, Attention Problems–Immaturity, and Anxiety–Withdrawal) and two additional scales (Psychotic Behavior and Motor Tension–Excess). The scales of the RBPC were constructed on the basis of factor analyses of various clinical samples. The developers made an effort to exclude items representing behaviors of high frequency in a normal population, items requiring inference on the part of the rater, items describing global aspects of pathology (e.g., "obsessions"), and items referring to somatic complaints and sexual behavior.

The manual provides normative data on parent and teacher ratings of large samples of children in kindergarten through 12th grade, as well as extensive reliability data. Means and standard deviations of scale scores are

---

TABLE 3.12. Revised Behavior Problem Checklist

Developed by: Herbert C. Quay and Donald Peterson (1983, 1984)

Ages: 5–17	**Items:** 89	**Scaling:** 0–2
Informant: Parent or teacher	**Completion time:** 15–20 minutes	

Normative data: $n = 1,315$ nonreferred children and adolescents (kindergarten–12th grade)

Factors assessed: Conduct Disorder, Socialized Aggression, Attention Problems–Immaturity, Anxiety–Withdrawal, Psychotic Behavior, and Motor Tension–Excess

provided from diverse clinical and nonclinical samples, and from both parent and teacher ratings. Internal consistency coefficients for the six scales range from .70 to .95. This represents a significant improvement in internal consistency for the shorter scales in the original 55-item version, due to an increase in the length of these scales. Interrater reliability for teachers ranges from .52 to . 85, depending on the subscale. No data on parent–teacher agreement are provided. Test–retest reliability of the RBPC appears to be adequate. In addition, the RBPC has been shown to discriminate between clinic-referred and nonreferred children (Aman & Werry, 1984), and between children with attention deficit disorder with and without hyperactivity as defined by DSM-III (Lahey, Schaughency, Strauss, & Frame, 1984).

Although it is designed to be used by both parents and teachers, one disadvantage of the RBPC is the relative absence of items that are specifically relevant to the school setting. This makes the RPBC more useful for obtaining information from parents than from teachers.

Revised Conners Rating Scales

Revised Conners Parent Rating Scale

The Revised Conners Parent Rating Scale (CPRS-R; Conners, Sitarenios, Parker, & Epstein, 1998a; see Table 3.13) is a revision and restandardization of the Conners Parent Rating Scale, originally published in 1970. The original scale was designed as a comprehensive measure for obtaining parent reports of behavior problems in children seen in an outpatient mental health setting. It assessed problems in areas such as eating, sleep, social relationships, and school functioning, in rationally derived groups. Another scale was later added that covered symptoms of inattention, hyperactivity, and impulsivity. Factor-analytic studies (Blouin, Conners, Seidel, & Blouin, 1989) later identified eight empirically derived factors constituting the 93-item scale: Conduct Disorder, Anxious–Shy, Learning Problems, Restless–Disorganized, Obsessive Compulsive, Antisocial, Psychosomatic, and Hyper-

---

TABLE 3.13. Revised Conners Parent Rating Scale (CPRS-R)

Developed by: C. Keith Conners, Gill Sitarenios, James Parker, and Jeffery Epstein (1998)

Ages: 3–17   **Items:** 57   **Scaling:** 0–3

Informant: Parent   **Completion time:** 10–15 minutes

Normative data: $n = 2,200$ nonreferred children (3–17 years)

Factors assessed: Oppositional, Cognitive Problems, Hyperactivity–Impulsivity, Anxious/Shy, Perfectionism, Social Problems, and Psychosomatic

active–Immature. The various versions of the original scale have perhaps been most widely used as methods of assessing treatment outcomes in children presenting with disruptive behavior problems. Some of these versions included a 48-item restandardized subset of the original item set (Goyette, Conners, & Ulrich, 1978), as well as an abbreviated 10-item version (Conners, 1994). Although the original scale demonstrated good test–retest and interrater reliability, as well as good validity, it suffered from some significant limitations. Most importantly, the norms were based upon a small, nonrepresentative sample.

The CPRS-R was constructed and validated on a sample of 2,200 children 3 to 17 years of age, obtained from schools across Canada and the United States. The resulting scale includes 57 items, which are measured on a 4-point Likert scale (0 = "not at all true," 3 = "very much true"). The scale takes approximately 5–10 minutes to complete. Factor analysis of the CPRS-R identified seven factors: Oppositional, Cognitive Problems, Hyperactivity–Impulsivity, Anxious/Shy, Perfectionism, Social Problems, and Psychosomatic. The scales have excellent internal reliability, with coefficient alphas ranging from .75 to .94. The CPRS-R scales also have excellent test–retest reliability, with the exception of the Social Problems scale, which has a correlation of .13 over 6 weeks. Good discriminative validity is evident as well.

In comparison to the original scale, the CPRS-R provides a briefer format, with better coverage of symptoms and behaviors related to attention deficit disorders. The factor structure is more consistent with the DSM-IV conceptualization of attention-deficit/hyperactivity disorder. In addition to the Hyperactivity–Impulsivity factor, the Cognitive Problems factor includes symptoms of inattention, which were not fully assessed in the original scale. Like most rating scales, the CPRS-R is most useful as a screening tool or as an adjunct to a comprehensive assessment. In addition, it may be useful as a measure of treatment outcome. The existence of a corresponding teacher version of the scale further enhances its utility in the assessment of childhood behavior problems.

Revised Conners Teacher Rating Scale

The original Conners Teacher Rating Scale was designed as a tool for assessing the effectiveness of stimulant medication in treating children with disruptive behavior disorders. The original version contained 39 items, and several abbreviated versions have also been developed and used in both clinical and research settings. Like the original parent scale, the original teacher scale lacked a representative norm group and a consistent, empirically derived factor structure. The Revised Conners Teacher Rating Scale (CTRS-R; Conners, Sitarenios, Parker, & Epstein, 1998b; see Table 3.14) was normed on a nationwide U.S. and Canadian sample of more than 1,700 children ranging in age from 3 to 17 years. The resulting scale contains 38

TABLE 3.14. Revised Conners Teacher Rating Scale (CTRS-R)

Developed by: C. Keith Conners, Gill Sitarenios, James Parker, and Jeffery Epstein (1998)

Ages: 3–17	**Items:** 38	**Scaling:** 0–3
Informant: Teacher	**Completion time:** 5–10 minutes	

Normative data: n = 1,702 non-referred children (3–17 years)

Factors assessed: Oppositionality, Inattention/Cognitive Problems, Hyperactivity–Impulsivity, Anxious/Shy, Perfectionism, and Social Problems

---

items rated on a 4-point Likert scale (0 = "not at all true," 3 = "very much true," as well as temporal descriptions for each point). It takes approximately 5 minutes to complete. Factor-analytic studies have revealed a consistent six-factor solution. These six factors correspond directly to the CPRS-R scales, with the exception of the Psychosomatic factor, which is not present on the CTRS-R. Assessment of the scale's psychometric properties indicates very good internal and test–retest reliability overall, as well as solid discriminant validity. Of note, however, is the somewhat lower test–retest reliability of the Inattentive/Cognitive Problems factor (r = .47). In addition, a significant decrease in Hyperactivity–Impulsivity scores was observed with repeated administrations. The authors suggest obtaining multiple-baseline ratings of children, particularly when the scale is being used to assess treatment effects.

DISCUSSION

A number of well-developed rating scales provide clinically relevant information from multiple sources, serving a significant role in the comprehensive assessment of the behavior problems of children and adolescents. The use of rating scales has numerous advantages. Compared to other assessment modalities, such as clinical interviews and direct observation, rating scales represent an easy and inexpensive means of obtaining data from multiple informants in a standardized fashion. Because most behavior problems are more likely to occur in natural settings (e.g., home, school) than in the clinic, information from parents and teachers is crucial for the assessment of children; rating scales provide an efficient way of obtaining this information. In addition, they yield quantitative indices that are useful for determining changes in behavior over time and in response to treatment.

Of course, rating scales, as well as other types of assessment measures, should not be used in isolation to make decisions concerning diagnostic, treatment, or educational placement. The comprehensive assessment of child and adolescent functioning necessitates the use of various assessment modalities. Information should be obtained through interviews, direct observation, and other methods, as well as through rating scales. Moreover, like other assessment instruments, rating scales should not be used by untrained personnel. Finally, the use of rating scales both in clinical and research contexts should conform to guidelines for ethical and professional conduct.

REFERENCES

Achenbach, T. M. (1966). The classification of children's psychiatric symptoms: A factor-analytic study. *Psychological Monographs, 80*, (7, Whole No. 615).

Achenbach, T. M. (1986). *The Direct Observation Form of the Child Behavior Checklist* (rev. ed.). Burlington: University of Vermont, Department of Psychiatry.

Achenbach, T. M. (1991a). *Integrative Guide to the 1991 CBCL, YSR, and TRF Profiles*. Burlington: University of Vermont, Department of Psychiatry.

Achenbach, T. M. (1991b). *Manual for the Child Behavior Checklist/4–18 and 1991 Profile*. Burlington: University of Vermont, Department of Psychiatry.

Achenbach, T. M. (1991c). *Manual for the Teacher's Report Form and 1991 Profile*. Burlington: University of Vermont, Department of Psychiatry.

Achenbach, T. M. (1991d). *Manual for the Youth Self-Report and 1991 Profile*. Burlington: University of Vermont, Department of Psychiatry.

Achenbach, T. M., & Edelbrock, C. (1983). *Manual for the Child Behavior Checklist and Revised Child Behavior Profile*. Burlington: University of Vermont, Department of Psychiatry.

Achenbach, T. M., & Edelbrock, C. (1986). *Manual for the Teacher's Report Form and Teacher Version of the Child Behavior Profile*. Burlington: University of Vermont, Department of Psychiatry.

Achenbach, T. M., & Edelbrock, C. (1987). *Manual for the Youth Self-Report and Profile*. Burlington: University of Vermont, Department of Psychiatry.

Achenbach, T. M., Edelbrock, C., & Howell, C. (1987). Empirically based assessment of the behavioral/emotional problems of 2–3 year old children. *Journal of Abnormal Child Psychology, 15*, 629–650.

Achenbach, T. M., McConaughy, S. H., & Howell, C. (1987). Child/adolescent behavioral and emotional problems: Implications of cross-informant correlations for situational specificity. *Psychological Bulletin, 101*, 213–232.

Aman, M. G., & Werry, J. S. (1984). The Revised Behavior Problem Checklist in clinic attenders and nonattenders: Age and sex effects. *Journal of Clinical Child Psychology, 13*, 237–242.

American Psychiatric Association. (1980). *Diagnostic and statistical manual of mental disorders* (3rd ed.). Washington, DC: Author.

American Psychiatric Association. (1987). *Diagnostic and statistical manual of mental disorders* (3rd ed., rev.). Washington, DC: Author.

Barkley, R. A. (1988). Child behavior rating scales and checklists. In M. Rutter, A. H. Tuma, & I. S. Lann (Eds.), *Assessment and diagnosis in child psychopathology* (pp. 113–155). New York: Guilford Press.

Blouin, A. G., Conners, C. K., Seidel, W. T., & Blouin, J. (1989). The independence of hyperactivity from Conduct Disorder: Methodological considerations. *Canadian Journal of Psychiatry, 34,* 279–282.

Bond, C. R., & McMahon, R. J. (1984). Relationships between marital distress and child behavior problems, maternal personal adjustment, maternal personality, and maternal parenting behavior. *Journal of Abnormal Psychology 93,* 348–351.

Conners, C. K. (1994). The Conners Rating Scales: Use in clinical or assessment treatment planning and research. In M. Maruish (Ed.), *Use of psychological testing for treatment planning and outcome assessment.* Hillsdale, NJ: Erlbaum.

Conners, C. K., Sitarenios, G., Parker, J. D. A., & Epstein, J. N. (1998a). The Revised Conners Parent Rating Scale (CPRS-R): Factor structure, reliability, and criterion validity. *Journal of Abnormal Child Psychology, 26,* 257–268.

Conners, C. K., Sitarenios, G., Parker, J. D. A., & Epstein, J. N. (1998b). Revision and restandardization of the Conners Teacher Rating Scale (CTRS-R): Factor structure, reliability, and criterion validity. *Journal of Abnormal Child Psychology, 26,* 279–291.

Edelbrock, C., & Achenbach, T. A. (1984). The teacher version of the child behavior profile: I. Boys ages 6–11. *Journal of Consulting and Clinical Psychology, 52,* 207–217.

Goyotte, C. H., Conners, C. K., & Ulrich, R. F. (1978). Normative data on Revised Conners Parent and Teacher Rating Scales. *Journal of Abnormal Child Psychology, 6,* 221–236.

Harrington, R. G., & Follet, G. M. (1984). The readability of child personality assessment instruments. *Journal of Psychoeducational Assessment, 2,* 37–48.

Lahey, B. B., Schaughency, E. A., Strauss, C. C., & Frame, C. L. (1984). Are attention deficit disorders with and without hyperactivity similar or dissimilar disorders? *Journal of the American Academy of Child Psychiatry, 48,* 566–574.

Martin, R. P., Hooper, S., & Snow, J. (1986). Behavior rating scale approaches to personality assessment in children and adolescents. In H. M. Knoff (Ed.), *The assessment of child and adolescent personality* (pp. 309–351). New York: Guilford Press.

McConaughy, S. (1992). Objective assessment of children's emotional and behavioral problems. In C. E. Walker & M. C. Roberts (Eds.), *Handbook of clinical child psychology* (2nd ed., pp. 163–180). New York: Wiley.

McConaughy, S., & Achenbach, T. (1988). *Practical guide for the Child Behavior Checklist and related materials.* Burlington: University of Vermont, Department of Psychiatry.

McMahon, R. J. (1984). Self-report instruments. In T. H. Ollendick & M. Hersen (Eds.), *Child behavioral assessment: Principles and procedures* (pp. 80–105). New York: Pergamon Press.

Miller, L. C. (1981). *School Behavior Checklist manual.* Los Angeles: Western Psychological Services.

Miller, L. C. (1984). *Louisville Behavior Checklist manual.* Los Angeles: Western Psychological Services.

Neeper, R., Lahey, B. B., & Frick, P. J. (1990). *Manual for the Comprehensive Behavior Rating Scale for Children.* San Antonio, TX: Psychological Corporation.

O'Leary, D. K., & Johnson, S. B. (1979). Psychological assessment. In H. C. Quay & J. S. Werry (Eds.), *Psychological disorders in childhood* (pp. 210–246). New York: Wiley.

Quay, H. C., & Peterson, D. R. (1979). *Manual for the Behavior Problem Checklist.* New Brunswick, NJ: Rutgers University.

Quay, H. C., & Peterson, D. R. (1983). *Interim manual for the Revised Behavior Problem Checklist.* Unpublished manuscript, University of Miami.

Quay, H. C., & Peterson, D. R. (1984). *Appendix I to the interim manual for the Revised Behavior Problem Checklist.* Unpublished manuscript, University of Miami.

Reynolds, C. R., & Kamphaus, R. W. (1992). *Manual for the Behavior Assessment System for Children.* Circle Pines, MN: American Guidance Service.

Streiner, D. L. (1993). A checklist for evaluating the usefulness of rating scales. *Canadian Journal of Psychiatry, 38,* 140–148.

Tarte, R. D., Vernon, C. R., Luke, D. E., & Clark, H. B. (1982). Comparison of responses by normal and deviant populations to the Louisville Behavior Checklist. *Psychological Reports, 50,* 99–106.

Verhulst, F. C., & Koot, H. M. (1992). *Child psychiatric epidemiology: Concepts, methods, and findings.* London: Sage.

Wirt, R. D., Lachar, D., Klinedinst, J. K., & Seat, P. D. (1977). *Multidimensional description of child personality: A manual for the Personality Inventory for Children.* Los Angeles: Western Psychological Services.

Wirt, R. D., Lachar, D., Klinedinst, J. K., & Seat, P. D. (1984). *Multidimensional description of child personality: A manual for the Personality Inventory for Children* (rev. ed.). Los Angeles: Western Psychological Services.

Wirt, R. D., Seat, P. D., Broen, W. E., & Lachar, D. (1989). *Personality Inventory for Children: Revised format administration booklet.* Los Angeles: Western Psychological Services.

Witt, J. C., Heffer, R. W., & Pfeifer, J. (1990). Structured rating scales: A review of self-report and informant rating processes, procedures, and issues. In C. R. Reynolds & R. W. Kamphaus (Eds.), *Handbook of psychological and educational assessment of children: Personality, behavior, and context* (pp. 364–394). New York: Guilford Press.

II

MEASURES FOR ASSESSING SPECIFIC SYNDROMES

✦

4

Behavior Rating Scales in the Assessment of Disruptive Behavior Problems in Childhood

✧

STEPHEN P. HINSHAW
JOEL T. NIGG

Behavior rating scales—also known as checklists or questionnaires—have undoubtedly become the most widely used instruments for the assessment of externalizing or disruptive behavior problems of childhood. Their ability to tap the impressions of key adult informants about child behavior, their ease of use and flexibility, and (in some cases) their broad normative base have all fostered this surge in popularity. Our goals in this chapter are (1) to highlight key conceptual issues pertaining to the use of behavior rating scales as assessment devices; (2) to discuss advantages and disadvantages of these tools; and (3) to present pertinent psychometric information on selected rating scales for attention-deficit/hyperactivity disorder (ADHD), oppositional defiant disorder (ODD), and conduct disorder (CD). Throughout, we feature discussion of the relative advantages and disadvantages of checklists in relation to other evaluation strategies, and we debate the merits of "narrow" rating scales of externalizing problems versus "broad" scales that capture wider domains of behavioral and emotional functioning (see Hart & Lahey, Chapter 3, this volume).

At the outset, we should state that several of the practical advantages of rating scales—namely, their utility and ease of administration—may also be disadvantages for some critical purposes, such as obtaining formal diagnoses. For instance, data regarding onset of symptomatology are crucial for ascertaining a diagnosis, but rating scales typically fail to yield sufficiently sensitive information regarding precise problem onset. In addition, because of halo effects (see extended discussion below), ratings also tend to yield higher inter-correlations between subdomains than do objective observations, limiting the construct validity of the information yielded (e.g., Hinshaw, Simmel, & Heller, 1995). Furthermore, reliance on the behavioral ratings of any one informant may present a skewed picture of a child's functioning. In short, questionnaires have an established niche in the evaluation of disruptive behavior problems, but they are rarely if ever sufficient as assessment or diagnostic tools. Our goal is for the reader to take from this chapter a deeper appreciation of the proper roles for the use of behavior rating scales in the appraisal of disruptive behavior problems in children.

BACKGROUND ISSUES

Disruptive Behavior Problems

First, what constitutes the domain under consideration—the disruptive behavior problems of childhood? Importantly, it was the early use of rating scales in the field that helped to differentiate such disruptive or acting-out behaviors from other types of child dysfunction (Quay, 1986). In parsing the domain of maladaptive behavior in children, the field has made a fundamental distinction between (1) disruptive or externalizing behavior problems,[1] which include aggressive, antisocial, hyperactive, impulsive, and sometimes inattentive behaviors, and (2) internalizing problems (formerly termed emotional or overcontrolled problems), which include somatic complaints, social withdrawal, dysphoric affect, anxiety, and thought disturbance (Achenbach & Edelbrock, 1978; Achenbach, 1991a, 1991b). These two "broad-band" domains, which have been documented from the early days of empirical research in the field (e.g., Jenkins & Glickman, 1947; Peterson, 1961), yield orthogonal dimensions in factor-analytic studies and form the basis for much current conceptualization about child psychopathology (e.g., Quay, 1986).

It has become quite clear, however, that marked overlap exists between disruptive and internalizing problems (e.g., Achenbach, 1991a, 1991b; Biederman, Newcorn, & Sprich, 1991; Capaldi, 1991; Jensen, Martin, & Cantwell, 1997). Furthermore, diagnostic comorbidity is of extreme importance with respect to research on underlying mechanisms, long-term course, and (potentially) treatment response. Overall, whereas internal coherence and substantial temporal stability pertain to the disruptive behavior problems of childhood—and whereas the nature of such impulsive, aggressive, and assaultive problems renders them quite salient to adults—their interrelationships with internalizing symptomatology cannot be neglected. Thus, in considering rating scales for disruptive problems, assessors must be appropriately cautious about using only narrow checklists of "aggression" or "hyperactivity," given the frequent overlap of these domains with internalizing dysfunction and the clinical and theoretical implications of such comorbidity (Caron & Rutter, 1991). Indeed, evaluators who rely solely on narrow checklists or questionnaires may well overlook such crucial comorbidity, with disastrous consequences for both clinical and research endeavors (for discussion, see Loney & Milich, 1982).

Considerable empirical and theoretical attention has been paid in recent years to the viability of subdistinctions within the disruptive class of behaviors. First, it is increasingly recognized that a dimension of inattention/hyperactivity is separable from interpersonal aggression/conduct problems (see Hinshaw, 1987, for a review). In addition, inattention is distinct from impulsivity and motoric overactivity: The latter two dimensions typically load together in factor-analytic investigations, separately from inattention/disorganization (Lahey et al., 1988; Healey et al., 1993). Furthermore, overt aggression (fighting, assaults, defiance) is distinguishable from such clandestine or covert activities as lying, stealing, truancy, and substance abuse (Hinshaw et al., 1995; Loeber & Schmaling, 1985).[2] The essential consideration regarding any such subcategorizations is not simply whether separate factors or clusters emerge, but whether such distinctions show empirical separability with respect to external criteria (e.g., family history, biological markers, course, or treatment response). Although validation of narrow syndromes in child psychopathology is not as clear-cut as might be supposed (Werry, Elkind, & Reeves, 1987), increasing evidence points to the validity of these key syndromal distinctions (Hinshaw, 1987; Lahey et al., 1988; Loeber & Schmaling, 1985), with the implication that users of rating scales must consider instruments that can distinguish inattention, impulsivity/hyperactivity, overt aggression, and covert antisocial behavior. Even finer distinctions are emphasized in some existing scales—for example, distinguishing predatory, intentional aggression from affective, reactive aggression (Vitiello, Behar, Hunt, Stoff, & Ricciuti, 1990).

Some narrow rating scales in the field focus on only one such subdimension (consider the plethora of "hyperactivity" or "ADHD" checklists). A key question centers on the utility of (1) such highly focused scales, (2) those concentrating on more complete coverage of the disruptive domains, and (3) those extremely broad scales spanning both disruptive and internalizing problems (see Hart & Lahey, Chapter 3). The decision to use a given instrument often hinges on key tradeoffs—for instance, the scale's thoroughness versus its repeatability. Although longer instruments yield more comprehensive data across a number of aspects of psychopathology, the more specific scales contained within these broad checklists may be relatively undifferentiated. For example, the Attention Problems scale of the Child Behavior Checklist (Achenbach, 1991a, 1991b) combines items pertaining to inattention, impulsivity, and motoric hyperactivity. Thus, without further subanalysis of this scale, teasing apart the constituent problems related to ADHD is problematic. Furthermore, broad scales are typically too unwieldy for daily or weekly use in the monitoring of treatment response. Investigators and clinicians must therefore be knowledgeable about both (1) the purposes of the assessment situation at hand and (2) the important psychometric properties of the scales under consideration, if they are to make informed decisions about particular instruments (see Hinshaw & Zupan, 1997).

Issues Pertinent to Ratings from Adult Informants

Although a comprehensive review of the conceptual issues that pertain to the use of behavior ratings is far beyond the scope of this chapter, we discuss several key points. Our intention is to provide an appropriate framework for decision making about checklists for appraising disruptive behavior problems.

Ratings versus Observations

The first point is definitional: What constitutes a "rating," as opposed to an alternative means of assessment—for example, a "behavior observation"? For our purposes, "ratings" are defined as quantified appraisals of behavioral items or domains, made over relatively lengthy time periods—sometimes as brief as a day, but often periods of several months. Although self-report ratings clearly fall under this category, as do peer sociometric ratings, our focus herein is on reports from adult informants (e.g., parents, teachers, staff members of treatment facilities).[3] "Behavior observations," on the other hand, are exemplified by repeated assessments of far shorter periods of behavior—typically no more than a few seconds—with rigorously operationalized codes to define discrete behavioral events (see Reid, Patterson, Baldwin, & Dishion, 1988). Thus, although ratings obviously require observation of a child, behavior ratings are distinguishable from formal behavior observations, in which well-trained, "objective" adults make precise counts of the frequency, duration, and/or intensity of discrete behavioral acts.

Which are preferable—behavior ratings or formal behavior observations? The answer, of course, depends upon the purpose of the assessment. If the goal is to appraise response to treatment in an unbiased fashion, behavior observation methodology appears preferable, despite its greater cost. In the classic investigation of Kent, O'Leary, Diament, and Dietz (1974), behavior ratings and behavior observations were contrasted in an analogue study. Adult observers of videotaped disruptive behaviors in children were also asked to complete global ratings of their impressions. For the randomly assigned group of these raters/observers who were led to believe that the children had improved as a result of treatment (in actuality, levels of behavior were distributed randomly across tapes), ratings likely to indicate such "improvement," but objective observations did not yield spurious treatment gains. Presumably, the discreteness and objectivity of the observational methodology insulated the observations (but not the ratings) from bias. A related point is that in psychosocial intervention studies with children, parents and teachers are (in most cases) actively involved in the delivery of treatment; their ratings therefore cannot serve as so-called "blind" outcome measures. Because of these points, objective observations should supplement adult ratings for formal treatment outcome studies (e.g., Gittelman et al., 1980; Hinshaw et al., 1997).

Yet it would be a mistake to assume that behavior observation strategies are the unbiased, entirely valid criterion measures against which all other assessment techniques (including ratings) should be appraised. For one thing, the selection of discrete observational categories is often arbitrary; for another, the observation of extremely brief units of behavior may distort the context or flow of the interchange. In addition, when discrete behavioral units are summed, it is unclear that a high frequency of mildly aggressive acts should outweigh the display of one infrequently occurring but intense action (e.g., an assault). The apparent objectivity of observation strategies may thus be more apparent than real, and there may be advantages to the higher levels of inference used by raters as opposed to objective behavioral observers (see Kenrick & Funder, 1988).

Furthermore, ratings can definitely be of assistance in monitoring treatment outcome. With the use of brief rating scales in which an informant appraises behavior over relatively short time intervals (a classroom period, a day's behavior), ongoing treatment-related change *can* be monitored with sensitivity (see examples in Conners, 1994; see also McBurnett, Swanson, Pfiffner, Tamm, & Phan, 1995). Indeed, intervention effects that are gleaned from ratings correspond reasonably well with those from observational methodology in studies of medication and behavioral interventions (Gittelman et al., 1980; Whalen et al., 1978). A key problem, however, is that when ratings are made, supposedly distinct domains of outcome may be difficult to differentiate, given the tendency for rater halo effects (Abikoff & Gittelman, 1985). As an example, Hinshaw et al. (1995) found that whereas discrete observations of overt aggression versus covert antisocial actions (stealing, property destruction) were modestly associated ($r = .28$), global staff ratings of the same constructs were virtually collinear ($r = .91$). In research investigations with sufficient resources, the dual use of rating scales and objective observation methodologies may be the ideal solution (Hinshaw et al., 1997).

From another perspective—that of the literature on appraising personality traits—it appears that ratings yield extremely valid portrayals of an individual's dispositions. Indeed, as argued by Kenrick and Funder (1988), when multiple raters who know a subject well quantify their impressions of observable behaviors over long periods, they can capture, with high validity, important traits of the observed individual.[4] The features of ratings—recall and amalgamation of memories of behavior over time—that tend to bias discrete description may well serve to enhance the appraisal of enduring, cross-situational aspects of personality.

Bias and Distortion

The foregoing discussion has implicitly raised a number of conceptual issues pertinent to ratings; several of these are noted explicitly. (For a far more comprehensive perspective on validity issues regarding assessment tools, see Foster & Cone, 1995.) In a heuristic review, Saal, Downey, and Lahey (1980) pointed to the traditional critiques of ratings as potentially subjective and biased. More specifically, ratings may yield data subject to (1) "halo" effects, wherein all of the attributes being rated for a given subject are high or low on the scale; (2) "leniency" or "severity" effects, in which the rater consistently uses one or the other side of the scale across subjects (e.g., all subjects are rated as aggressive); (3) range restriction, wherein the full metric of the scale is not employed; and (4) logical errors, in which the rater's implicit personality theory (and not the "real" interrelation between domains of behavior) shapes the patterns of association across different items. Schweder's (1982) discussion of the systematic distortion hypothesis is a thorough exposition of the latter point. Overall, key concerns regarding ratings are that items may be defined idiosyncratically by different informants, that nonexistent relationships between behavioral constructs will be inferred by raters, and that raters' perceptions of behavior are distorted in memory. Any of these can lead to biased appraisal.

How real are such concerns for the domain of disruptive behavior problems? Investigations by Schachar, Sandberg, and Rutter (1986) and by Abikoff, Courtney, Pelham, and Koplewicz (1993) are quite pertinent in this regard. In both investigations, raters inappropriately inferred the presence of inattentive/hyperactive behaviors when only conduct-disordered or oppositional behaviors were displayed by a target child. For example, Abikoff et al. (1993) used child actors who were trained to portray solely inattentive/hyperactive or solely oppositional/aggressive behavioral patterns; objective observations confirmed the fidelity of the actors to their scripts. When teachers viewed the tapes and completed behavior rating scales, however, the group observing the oppositional/aggressive model inferred a significant presence of inattentive/hyperactive behaviors. The converse, however, was not true: Raters of the inattentive/hyperactive child did not infer aggression. Thus comorbidity between CD and the spectrum of behaviors pertinent to ADHD may be inflated in samples of CD youth when ratings are used as the primary assessment tool. Recently, Stevens, Quittner, and Abikoff (1998) found that this unidirectional bias was attenuated when rating scales containing behaviorally precise rather than ambiguous items were utilized. This unidirectional bias underscores the subjectivity of the rating process and has implications for the accurate separation of these two important externalizing subdomains in studies that utilize rating scales.

Interinformant Agreement

How well do parents and teachers—the two primary groups of informants for child behavior problems—agree when they complete similar or identical rating scales with respect to the same children? As systematically reviewed in an influential meta-analytic report by Achenbach, McConaughy, and Howell (1987), the initial answer is rather pessimistic. Across numerous investigations, similar informants (e.g., two parents; a teacher and a teacher's aide) showed an average correlation of .60 for ratings of problem behavior. Yet the average parent–teacher association was .27.[5] Although this coefficient was statistically significant across the large number of investigations reviewed, it is obviously not of strong magnitude. We hasten to point out that parent–teacher correspondence was somewhat stronger for the externalizing domain ($r = .41$) than for internalizing aspects of children's functioning (which is closer to $r = .2$) (Achenbach et al., 1987). Interinformant agreement thus appears stronger for more readily observable aspects of a child's behavioral repertoire. Yet within the externalizing domain, it is important to note that some types of covert antisocial behavior may be far more difficult to observe than overt aggression.

Given these rather low levels of correspondence, an initial assumption is that parents and teachers are inherently unreliable informants when they rate child problem behavior. Achenbach et al. (1987), however, contend that the levels of disagreement may reflect true differences in children's behavior across situations, rather than unreliability of the ratings; in fact, the temporal stability and internal consistency of adult ratings are of acceptable magnitude. Indeed, Achenbach (1990) has developed the argument that a multiaxial system of diagnoses for children should include the different sources of assessment data on the various axes, reflecting the importance of obtaining diverse sources of information about a child's functioning. Certainly, if parents and teachers agree regarding (for example) severe levels of inattentive, impulsive, and hyperactive behavior, such cross-situationality predicts considerable impairment in a child (Schachar, 1991).

Yet how is *disparate* information to be amalgamated to yield a coherent picture of a child? Indeed, the optimal weighting of different information sources is an area in need of empirical attention. A healthy heuristic in this regard has been established by Piacentini, Cohen, and Cohen (1992). These authorities contend that in the absence of clear decision rules as to the primacy of one or another source, relatively "simple" means of combining data (e.g., counting a symptom as present if *either* informant has scored it so) will always be psychometrically superior to complex algorithms for amalgamating disparate sources. For now, it should suffice to realize that multiple perspectives on child problem behavior are essential for careful assessment and diagnosis, but that the field currently lacks the database to make fully informed decisions regarding the primacy of different sources of information.

Summary

The focus of this chapter is on the disruptive (or externalizing) problems of childhood, which include the spectrum of inattentive/impulsive/hyperactive difficulties, as well as interpersonal aggression and other forms of antisocial behavior. Although this broad domain is often contrasted with so-called internalizing problems, the overlap between these domains is usually substantial in clinical populations. Because of the partial independence of inattention, impulsivity/hyperactivity, overt aggression, and covert antisocial behavior within the disruptive spectrum of behaviors, checklists that can differentiate or separate such domains should be sought when fine-grained analysis is necessary.

Behavior ratings can be distinguished from objective observational strategies with respect to the discreteness of the events to be recorded and the length of time that behavior is sampled. Whereas observations may be less subject to bias, ratings have a clear place in the identification of relevant dimensions of problem behavior. Furthermore, brief scales have been validated for monitoring treatment response, and global ratings are essential for inferring trait-like entities (i.e., complex patterns of behavior). Several types of distortion and bias inherent in rating methodologies have been identified, and empirical evidence as to the inaccurate inference of inattentive/hyperactive behaviors from children displaying pure aggression has been discussed. Even for the rather visible behaviors of the disruptive domain, parent–teacher correspondence is modest with respect to rating data; the field is grappling with the problem of how to amalgamate disparate sources of information for accurate identification of problematic functioning.

ADVANTAGES AND DISADVANTAGES OF RATING SCALES

As discussed earlier, any consideration of the validity of an assessment device must pertain to the goals of the evaluation. Thus the advantages and disadvantages of rating scales must be considered in explicit relation to the underlying purpose of the assessment. Establishing a formal diagnosis is a different endeavor from periodically monitoring a child's response to treatment; appraising the number of problematic symptoms or behaviors is not the same as establishing the levels of impairment that such problems create. Our discussion of "pros" and "cons" must therefore be contextualized with respect to the objectives of the assessment procedures in which rating scales may be used.

Advantages

Several of the advantages of rating scales have been highlighted already. First and foremost, they are quite easy to use: Parents and teachers simply read the items and appraise each problem on the metric of the particular scale in use (e.g., yes vs. no; the 4-point Conners scale metric of the extent to which the item is a problem, labeled "not at all," "just a little," "pretty much," and "very much"). No special training is necessary, and the time required to complete even the longest scales for disruptive behavior is rarely over 20 minutes. (Indeed, brief scales designed for repeated use in treatment monitoring may require only a minute or two.)

Second, most such scales are designed not for the clinician in the office, but for the parent who deals with the child at home and/or the teacher who observes the child daily at school. It is increasingly clear that the problems of disruptive children, particularly those with inattentive/hyperactive behaviors, are not readily apparent during a clinic visit (Sleator & Ullmann, 1981). Those persons who observe day-to-day disruptive behaviors in the natural environment are the best equipped to provide meaningful information. Thus the types of assessment data that are necessary to evaluate the classroom, home, and peer-related behavior of children with disruptive problems are readily accessible from rating scale formats (Hinshaw, 1994).

Third, for the most part the checklists reviewed herein show good to excellent reliability, in terms of both test–retest stability and internal consistency, with factor structures that yield acceptable alpha reliabilities for the various subdomains. Some aspects of validity are also strong: Most of the scales differentiate clinical from comparison samples ("known groups" validity), and the briefer scales designed for repeated use have been shown to be responsive to active pharmacological or psychosocial intervention. A more difficult criterion is to establish the scale's ability to discriminate different clinical groups from one another. Some positive evidence has accumulated for selected scales (see Loney & Milich, 1982, regarding the IOWA Conners Scale; see also various investigations with the Child Behavior Checklist), but the diagnostic specificity of most rating scales remains to be established.

Fourth, rating scales exemplify the dimensional approach to classification (Eysenck, 1986), in which problem behaviors are considered on a quantified scale of frequency, duration, or severity. Indeed, rated information retains the full range of scores along the domain(s) of interest, in keeping with such a dimensional approach. Although debate as to the relative value of quantitative/dimensional versus categorical/diagnostic conceptions of child psychopathology is still active (e.g., Hinshaw, Lahey, & Hart, 1993; Jensen et al., 1996), evidence exists (for example) that dimensional assessment outperforms categorical (threshold) evaluation with regard to the predictability of adult substance use patterns from earlier aggression and conduct problems (Robins & McEvoy, 1990). Cutoff scores can be also applied to rating scale data to yield subgroups, attesting to the flexibility of checklist data. In short, feasibility, reliability, ecological validity, and compatibility with dimensional assessment are key advantages of behavior checklists and rating scales.

Disadvantages

One class of disadvantage has been discussed earlier—namely, the potential for subjective, biased information to emerge from rating scales. As highlighted, there are various types of such bias; several are reiterated or discussed anew here. First, untrained parents or teachers may variously interpret items on rating instruments. Does, for example, the item "nervous" refer to inner sensations of anxiety or to jittery, overactive behavior? Differing interpretations of the items on a scale can compromise the quality and validity of information reported on checklists. Second, it is conceivable that adults' ratings reflect their own inner states—or, more specifically, their attitudes toward a child—as opposed to the "actual" behaviors displayed by the youngster. Indeed, most clinicians can recall the inflated ratings made by a distressed parent in comparison with the relatively mild problem behaviors reported by a teacher or observed in a clinic playgroup.

A sizable literature, in fact, has developed around the contention that parental (and particularly maternal) depression induces inflated ratings of child misbehavior, particularly in the disruptive domain. Although an extensive discussion of this literature is not possible here, the incisive review of Richters (1992) makes it clear that definitive tests of this depression-distortion hypothesis are difficult to execute and that no fully satisfactory investigation has yet been performed. The best evidence to date, however, suggests that distress and depression in mothers are associated with independently corroborated elevations of children's disruptive behaviors. Thus, rather than evidencing distortion, mothers' ratings may well be accurately reflecting disruptive tendencies in their children. As work in the field continues to substantiate this conclusion, the viability of ratings of the disruptive/externalizing domain is bolstered.

A related issue is that despite the extraction of orthogonal dimensions of disruptive behavior during the derivation of rating scales, in most samples the factors or subscales pertinent to such behavior are rather substantially intercorrelated. Indeed, such associations are typically far higher than those of comparable domains yielded from objective behavior observations (Abikoff & Gittelman, 1985; Hinshaw et al., 1995). Such factors as the subjectivity of the rating process, raters' implicit personality theories, and halo effects may conspire to inflate associations across domains that are believed (or hoped) to be relatively independent. This collinearity is a decided disadvantage, particularly for research investigations that aim to appraise partially independent behavioral domains or for clinicians desiring differential diagnosis.

Another potential disadvantage pertains to the norms for most extant rating scales. Unfortunately, the normative base for the vast majority of "narrow" rating scales for disruptive behavior problems is thin and unrepresentative. Furthermore, as discussed below, it is rare that normative samples contain sufficient numbers of ethnic minority groups.[6] Certainly, obtaining a large and truly representative sample of children is a costly enterprise—one that only the best-funded psychological tests or rating scales can afford. With poor norms, any standardized score (e.g., T or z score) used to appraise the deviance of a given youngster is suspect. Potential users of rating scales would be well advised to scrutinize the normative base of instruments they are considering, particularly if a score in a particular checklist's deviant range could lead to diagnostic labeling. In this regard, there are clear advantages to using broad scales, which are more likely to have been extensively normed. On the other hand, if the purpose of the rating is to perform repeated monitoring of a child and not to make normative comparisons for diagnostic purposes, the thin normative base of selected narrow scales may not be as problematic.

Yet another issue pertains to evidence that scores from rating scales for the disruptive behavior problems show a drop in magnitude from the initial rating to the second rating provided by parents or teachers. This so-called "regression" or "practice" effect may be an issue if single ratings are utilized to ascertain diagnostic status. Evidence, however, from Diamond and Deane (1990) reveals that with further repetition of questionnaire administration, subsequent scores increase to levels near or above those from the initial rating. Further research on untreated populations is needed to clarify the viability of such within-subject fluctuations in rating scale scores.

Crucially, questionnaires are not adequate when the goal is formal diagnosis. Despite the utility and validity of rating scales for many purposes, ascertaining a diagnosis is not performed optimally or even well through use of ratings. The chief issue here is that cross-sectional symptom patterns are diagnostically nonspecific. For example, a host of situational factors may precipitate inattention, poor impulse control, and motoric restlessness—as indicated by a high score on a hyperactivity rating scale—but ADHD per se is marked by impairing levels of such problems over long time periods (American Psychiatric Association, 1994). With structured interviews, precise appraisal of symptom onset and offset can be determined with far more accuracy than with checklists, and impairment indicators are typically omitted from questionnaire formats. In addition, the meticulous reading of items by a structured interviewer facilitates uniformity in a parent's or teacher's response to the questions; rating scale items, as suggested earlier, may be interpreted ambiguously. Furthermore, the often utilized procedure of applying a simple cutoff score to a dimension of behavior on a rating scale is bound to yield arbitrary groupings unless extensive validation of a particular cutoff is performed.[7] In optimal assessment paradigms, rating scales constitute the initial step of case identification. If scores approach or exceed the clinical range, the assessor will need to gather developmental histories, structured interviews, and psychological testing to facilitate formal differential diagnosis.

Summary

Advantages of rating scale methodology include ease of use, ecological validity, respectable to excellent psychometric properties, and consonance with a dimensional approach to child psychopathology. Key disadvantages involve the potential for subjectivity and bias, the relatively poor norms for most narrow scales, and the invalidity of rating scales for determining formal diagnoses. Such disadvantages may be mitigated by embedding the use of rating scales in a broader assessment strategy that includes (1) a thorough developmental history, (2) objective observations when feasible, (3) structured diagnostic interviews, and (4) psychological testing.

BROAD VERSUS NARROW SCALES

We have highlighted the difference between narrow scales, which pertain solely to disruptive problems or syndromes, and broader instruments, which more comprehensively span internalizing and externalizing symptomatology (see also Hart & Lahey, Chapter 3). Briefly, which class of rating instrument should an investigator or clinician select? As we have repeatedly emphasized, the answer depends on the referral or research questions to be addressed and the time and resources available.

If the goal is comprehensive evaluation of a child's functioning and if time allows, broader scales must be considered, at least for the initial evaluation. Indeed, given the strong likelihood of symptom overlap or diagnostic comorbidity in the field (e.g., Biederman et al., 1991; Caron & Rutter, 1991), the sole use of narrow scales may severely restrict the available database and result in neglect of important associated symptomatology. If the broad instrument reveals deviance in ADHD-related domains, narrower scales that afford differentiation of inattention from hyperactivity and impulsivity may then be useful. We also point out that with respect to internalizing problems, adult informants may lack the sensitivity of children themselves in revealing key problem domains; again, assessment tools beyond rating scales (e.g., structured interviews) are important to consider.

Regarding the superiority of broad-based assessment instruments, Mc-Conaughy, Achenbach, and Kent (1988) demonstrated that children with identical scores on given narrow behavioral dimensions (e.g., aggression, inattention) may differ markedly, depending on their profile of scores on additional scales. Indeed, configurational or profile approaches have been profitably utilized for decades with adult instruments such as the Minnesota Multiphasic Personality Inventory. A comparable situation exists in the field of learning disabilities, wherein children with the same absolute scores in reading skill may differ markedly with respect to neuropsychological profiles—and potentially in response to intervention—depending on their levels of performance in other academic areas (for extensive examples, see Rourke, 1985; Lyon, 1996).

We should note also that the psychometric properties of the specific ADHD- or aggression-related externalizing scales from comprehensive checklists are comparable or superior to those from syndrome-specific questionnaires. Indeed, the Attention Problems, Aggressive Behavior, and Delinquent Behavior scales from the Child Behavior Checklist (Achenbach, 1991a, 1991b) show reliability and validity data at least as good as those of the narrower scales reviewed below. Furthermore, as noted earlier, the broader scales are more likely to have a sounder normative base—a crucial characteristic if subject selection or potential diagnosis is the goal.

On the other hand, disruptive-behavior-related scales from broad checklists typically lack the specific item content in a particular domain to yield full differentiation of important constructs. As discussed earlier, the Attention Problems scale from the various forms of the Child Behavior Checklist (e.g., Achenbach, 1991a, 1991b) spans inattention and disorganization as well as impulsivity and hyperactivity in one omnibus scale. Many of the narrower scales we review below, however, are specifically designed to differentiate such subdomains. Similarly, if there is a need to cover relatively rare but important domains of acting-out behavior, broad scales may be insufficiently detailed. And, as noted earlier, if the aim is to perform repeated monitoring of response to ongoing intervention, the broad scales are typically too unwieldy, placing undue burden on informants for daily or weekly completion. In all, the needs of the particular assessment situation, the resources of the clinician or investigator, the time available from the respondents, and the scale's psychometric properties all influence the decision regarding choice of instrument.

ETHNICITY AND CULTURE

Given the rapidly developing diversity of the U.S. population of children and adolescents, a growing problem in the field of assessment is the lack of research on and development of instruments appropriately sensitive to variations in culture or ethnicity (e.g., Vargas & Willis, 1994). Adequate explication of the many facets of this topic is beyond the scope of our brief coverage (for reviews, see Neighbors, Jackson, Campbell, & Williams, 1989; Prinz

& Miller, 1991; Schweder & Sullivan, 1993; Snowden & Todman, 1982), which is necessarily selective (please see Cohen & Kasen, Chapter 11, this volume, for a thorough discussion). First, the limited data available suggest modest prevalence differences in some cases (see, e.g., Lambert, Knight, Taylor, & Achenbach, 1994) as well as cultural bias in severity ratings of disruptive behavior problems (e.g., Bauermeister, Berrios, Jimenez, Acevedo, & Gordon, 1990; Mann et al., 1992). Evaluation of such effects within U.S. subcultures is understudied. On the other hand, studies of potential bias in major rating instruments have supported the validity and utility of some of the rating scales in question (e.g., Kline & Lachar, 1992). Examination of bias issues is needed for instruments in use in the field.

Second, many scales fail to report the ethnic composition of their norming samples. Even if proportional representation of ethnic minorities is attained and reported, separate subgroup norms are nearly always lacking. Moreover, the levels of acculturation of subgroup members (admittedly difficult to define) are rarely assessed or reported. In addition, the potential for differential predictive validity of scores across cultural groups is rarely appraised. As a result, nearly all scales must be used with caution when one is assessing nonmainstream clients who are not well represented in the norming sample.

Several alternative approaches do exist. For one thing, with some instruments a "correction" formula is used to adjust scores according to both ethnicity and empirically established psychosocial risk factors (see Mercer & Lewis, 1978, regarding the System of Multicultural Pluralistic Assessment). This approach has been applied primarily to cognitive test data rather than to behavior ratings; it remains controversial (e.g., Figueroa, 1979; Snowden & Todman, 1982). Second, there is a precedent for translation of major scales into other languages (e.g., the Spanish translation of the Revised Behavior Problem Checklist; Rio, Quay, Santisteban, & Szapocznik, 1989). Third, some scales have been standardized in minority populations (see Bauermeister et al., 1990).

Swanson (1992) raises several pertinent issues about cultural and ethnic factors in the school-based assessment of disruptive behavior problems. For one thing, whereas epidemiological data do not reveal effects of socioeconomic status (SES) or ethnicity on attention deficits/hyperactivity per se (e.g., Szatmari, Offord, & Boyle, 1989), concurrent aggression and antisocial behavior are found preponderantly in lower SES strata and are therefore overrepresented in ethnic minority populations. Rating instruments that can disentangle these two key subdomains of disruptive symptomatology are therefore crucial. Second, Swanson (1992) recommends that sensitive questioning of parents who disagree with teachers regarding the presence of ADHD symptoms in children may help to clarify the situational and contextual factors that "pull" for the display of problematic behaviors in one setting but not another. In all, we urge interested readers to pursue such issues in the cited literature.

REVIEW OF SPECIFIC SCALES

Because of the presence of the Hart and Lahey chapter in this volume (see Chapter 3), and because of Barkley's (1988) earlier book chapter,[8] we restrict our coverage to "narrow" scales that emphasize externalizing or disruptive symptomatology and that have not been covered in these two chapters. The sheer number of rating scales that specifically cover disruptive behavior problems renders exhaustive coverage impossible. Indeed, in a review from the earlier part of this decade, Dykman, Raney, and Ackerman (1993) uncovered 42 different checklists that deal with the domain of ADHD alone. That number has grown substantially since 1993. We make no claim whatsoever for the thoroughness of our treatment of the large number of extant instruments in the material below; the coverage is of necessity selective and illustrative. Table 4.1 provides an overview of the scales that we review herein. In addition, interested readers should consult the Appendix to this chapter, which provides addresses for further information about these (and related) questionnaires.

Conners Scales

The Conners Rating Scales merit specific attention. These widely used scales have undergone several revisions since their initial publication in the late

TABLE 4.1. Selected "Narrow" Rating Scales for Disruptive Behavior Problems

Scale	Informant	Normative n	Age range	No. of items	Factors
CASQ	P, T	2,345 (P) 1,736 (T)	3–17 years	10	1. Restless/Impulsive 2. Emotional Lability
IOWA Conners	T	608	K–5th grade	10	1. Inattention/Overactivity 2. Aggression or Oppositional/Defiant
CLAM	P, T	[a]	[a]	16	(This scale contains the CASQ plus the two IOWA Conners factors; see above)

(continued)

TABLE 4.1 (continued)

Scale	Informant	Normative n	Age range	No. of items	Factors
SNAP-IV	P, T	[b]	[b]	41	[c]
SKAMP	T	109	2nd–5th grades	10	1. Attention 2. Deportment
ACTeRS-R	T	2,362	5–13 years	24	1. Attention 2. Hyperactivity 3. Social Skills 4. Oppositional Behavior
CAAS-S	T	3,674	5–13 years	31	1. Inattention 2. Impulsivity 3. Hyperactivity 4. Conduct Problems
CAAS-H	P	183	5–13 years	31	1. Inattention 2. Impulsivity 3. Hyperactivity 4. Conduct Problems
ADDES-H	P	1,754	4–20 years	46	1. Inattention 2. Impulsivity 3. Hyperactivity
ADDES-S	T	4,876	4–20 years	60	1. Inattention 2. Impulsivity 3. Hyperactivity
YCI	T	260	8–14 years	62	1. Behavior 2. Cognitive[d]
NYTRS	T	1,264	1st–10th grade	48	1. Defiance 2. Physical Aggression 3. Delinquent Behaviors 4. Peer Problems

Note. CASQ, Conners Abbreviated Symptom Questionnaire; CLAM, Conners, Loney, and Milich Scale; SNAP-IV, Swanson, Nolan, and Pelham Rating Scale, fourth edition; SKAMP, Swanson, Kotkin, Agler, M-Flynn, and Pelham Rating Scale; ACTeRS-R, ADD-H Comprehensive Teacher Rating Scale—Revised; CAAS, Children's Attention and Adjustment Survey (H, home, and S, school); ADDES, Attention Deficit Disorders Evaluation Scale (H, home, and S, school); YCI, Yale Children's Inventory; NYTRS, New York Teacher Rating Scale.

[a]See separate norms for CASQ and IOWA Conners.

[b]For the DSM-III items, Swanson (1981) provides norms for the original SNAP; for teacher-rated DSM-III-R items, see Pelham et al. (1992) regarding normative and psychometric data.

[c]This scale contains (1) the DSM-III criteria for attention deficit disorder with and without hyperactivity as well as for Oppositional Disorder; (2) the DSM-III-R criteria for ADHD and ODD; (3) the ADHD and attention deficit disorder without hyperactivity symptoms from the DSM-IV field trial; and (4) the final 18 ADHD symptoms and the final 8 ODD symptoms from the DSM-IV criteria.

[d]From these two major factors, 11 smaller factors emerged; see text.

1960s and early 1970s (Conners, 1969, 1970). In the comprehensive manual of 1990, Conners has helped to clarify some of the confusion that surrounds these scales, which emanates in part from the two different forms of the Conners Parent Rating Scale (93-item and 39-item) and the two different forms of the Conners Teacher Rating Scale (48-item and 28-item) that have been in use. It is noteworthy that these different forms have different factor structures and different norming samples.

Moreover, the Conners scales were revised again in 1997, with new and extensive normative data (Conners, 1997). Because current assessors are likely to be utilizing this version of the Conners Scales, we next describe the revised scales. Although not selected in stratified, random fashion, the new normative sample (aged 3–17) is reasonably representative of the United States and Canada regarding region, ethnicity, sex, and SES. In the 1997 revision, the "long" parent version contains 80 items, and the "long" teacher version has 59. Each version has scales for Oppositional, Conduct, Hyperactivity, Anxious–Shy, Perfectionism, and Social Problems. Each also contains a Conners Global Index, parallel to the former versions' Hyperactivity Index (HI) or Conners Abbreviated Symptom Questionnaire (CASQ); a specific ADHD Index intended to discriminate ADHD from non-ADHD children; and the 18 ADHD items from the DSM-IV. National norms are thus available for these items. Psychometric properties of these scales are quite acceptable, except in some instances for late adolescence.

In addition, the 1997 revision contains "short forms" (27 items for parents, 28 for teachers), each of which yields Oppositional, Cognitive Problems, and Hyperactivity factors, as well as the ADHD Index and the Global Index. We focus here on the briefer versions of these instruments that specifically address hyperactivity and oppositional/aggressive behavior: the CASQ, the IOWA Conners Scale, and the Conners, Loney, and Milich (CLAM) Scale.

Conners Abbreviated Symptom Questionnaire, Hyperactivity Index, and ADHD Index

From each of the earlier versions of the Conners scales, 10 of the most medication-sensitive items (as well as those loading highest on externalizing factors) have been selected as the Conners HI. Note that these scales differ slightly, depending on whether (1) the longer or shorter version or (2) the parent or teacher scale serves as the basis. Published separately have been two versions of the HI known as the CASQ: a 10-item parent CASQ and a similar 10-item teacher CASQ. Scores on each scale range from 0 to 30, given the 0–3 metric for the component 10 items. Their internal consistency and test–retest reliabilities are excellent, in the neighborhood of .9; Conners (1994) lists numerous investigations attesting to the concurrent and predictive validity of the HI/CASQ with external criterion measures. These brief scales have received perhaps their most widespread use to monitor children's response to pharmacological (and psychosocial) intervention: Their historical precedent, extremely brief format, and amenability to repeated administration have been key factors in such use.

Furthermore, for many years these abbreviated scales set a standard for the field with regard to the selection of "hyperactive" samples of children. With a national mean of approximately 5 and a standard deviation of approximately 5 (Goyette, Conners, & Ulrich, 1978), the cutoff score of 15 (or sometimes 18) from the possible 30 was often invoked as a screen for this diagnostic category. Over and above the general problems involved in use of brief rating instruments to yield diagnostic categories (see earlier discussion), the main critique of these scales has been that they confound the domains of inattention, hyperactivity, and defiance/negative emotionality (e.g., Furlong & Fortman, 1984). Thus their exclusive use as screening devices for ADHD may exclude youngsters with primary problems of inattention and may limit inclusion to children with comorbid hyperactivity and aggression (Ullmann, Sprague, & Sleator, 1985).[9] In fact, a recent confirmatory factor analysis (Parker, Sitarenios, & Conners, 1996) demonstrates that both the teacher and parent HIs comprise two factors, one pertinent to restless/impulsive behavior and the other dealing with emotional lability. In part because of this dual nature of the index, the brief Conners scales have also been used as screening tools for preliminary identification of youth at risk for the development of CD (August, Realmuto, Crosby, & MacDonald, 1995). Related to such concerns, alternative means have been utilized to derive brief scales from the original Conners items that show greater divergent validity and diagnostic specificity (see below).

New to the 1997 revision is the ADHD Index, consisting of 12 items empirically selected for their ability to discriminate ADHD from non-ADHD children. The scale appears to exhibit solid sensitivity and specificity (Conners, 1997), with actual psychiatric diagnosis as the criterion and with a matched control group. Sensitivity ranges from .91 to 1.00, and specificity from .77 to .93. With a 50% base rate of ADHD, these figures yield positive and negative predictive powers above .85; however, when the base rate of ADHD is considerably lower (as would be the case in a general community screen), false positives predominate, substantially lowering the positive predictive power.

Although the sensitivity and specificity data are impressive, limitations are that recent publications (e.g., Conners, Sitarenios, Parker, & Epstein, 1998) do not yield information on (1) the discrimination of ADHD from other disorders or (2) the utility of alternate cutoff scores regarding predictive validity (Conners et al., 1998, used discriminant-function analysis incorporating information from all items and scales). It is one thing to discriminate a case from a control; it is another, more difficult endeavor to make a differential diagnosis (e.g., of ADHD from ODD) based on a rating scale. Furthermore, cutoff scores for individual Conners scales and factors would enhance utility. In all, however, the most recent revision of the Conners scales has made a leap forward with respect to psychometric properties.

IOWA Conners Scale

Loney and Milich (1982) reported on their derivation of a two-factor, brief Conners scale for use in screening and treatment evaluation. In short, they selected only those items from the Conners Teacher Rating Scale that (1) correlated exclusively with chart-derived, independently appraised inattention/overactivity but not with the domain of oppositionality/aggression, or (2) the converse (i.e., items converging with the aggression construct but diverging from inattention/overactivity). Their analyses yielded a 5-item Inattention/Overactivity scale (IO) and a 5-item Aggression scale (later named Oppositional/Defiant, or OD); together, the 10 items constitute the IOWA (Inattention/Overactivity with Aggression) Conners Scale. It must be pointed out that the IO and OD scales do, in clinical samples, correlate moderately (on the order of .6), attesting to the actual overlap between these two domains of disruptive behavior. Yet the two subscales show excellent psychometric properties (e.g., test–retest reliabilities of .86 to .89 and alpha coefficients of .89 to .92; Loney & Milich, 1982), and their construct validity is ascertained by their differential prediction of key correlates and outcomes (Atkins, Pelham, & Licht, 1989; Loney & Milich, 1982).

Pelham, Milich, Murphy, and Murphy (1989) summarize validational evidence for the IOWA Conners Scale and provide norms for teacher administration based on a sample of 608 elementary-school-age children in Florida. They recommend research screening scores for each scale, arguing for different cutoffs according to a child's age but identical scores for boys and girls. Given its brevity, built-in construct validity, and excellent psychometric properties, the IOWA Conners Scale should clearly be considered as a brief device for initial school-based screening or for treatment monitoring in work with disruptive youngsters. The lack of parental norms limits its use to school settings at this time, however.

Conners, Loney, and Milich Scale

In order to retain, on a brief checklist, the widely used CASQ as well as the two IOWA Conners factors, a 16-item scale known as the CLAM Scale is available (Swanson, 1992). This scale allows scoring of the IO and OD factors of the IOWA Conners Scale, as well as the total score from the CASQ. The scale is brief enough to be usable in repeated treatment outcome studies while maintaining the divergently valid scales from the IOWA Conners. Norms for parents are in the process of being gathered; teacher norms are available for the CASQ and the two IOWA factors (see Table 4.1).

Swanson, Nolan, and Pelham Rating Scale, Fourth Edition

The Swanson, Nolan, and Pelham Rating Scale, fourth edition (SNAP-IV) is the latest version of a rating instrument that corresponds to diagnostic criteria for attention deficits and hyperactivity from the recent editions of the DSM. The SNAP instruments utilize a 4-point, Conners-style metric to dimensionalize these criteria. To provide historical continuity, the SNAP-IV contains (1) the DSM-III criteria for attention deficit disorder (with and without hyperactivity) and oppositional disorder (American Psychiatric Association, 1980); (2) the DSM-III-R criteria for ADHD and ODD (American Psychiatric Association, 1987); and (3) the DSM-IV criteria for the Inattentive and Hyperactive–Impulsive (and therefore Combined) subtypes of ADHD, as well as for ODD (American Psychiatric Association, 1994). Because of item overlap across these changing diagnostic criteria, the total item set is 41. The SNAP-IV has the advantage of normative data for the DSM-III and DSM-III-R criteria, as well as the ability to generate norms for the new DSM-IV criterion set. In addition, one can readily ascertain whether a given child would meet diagnostic cutoffs according to each of the recent operational definitions of attention deficits/hyperactivity.

As has been highlighted throughout this chapter, however, potential users must maintain extreme caution in assuming that the surpassing of rating scale cutoffs is tantamount to a clinical diagnosis. Indeed, as is true of nearly all other rating instruments, criteria for symptom duration and impairment are not included in the SNAP-IV.[10] Parent and teacher completion of the SNAP-IV could well serve as an initial screen comprising a stimulus for subsequent unstructured and structured interviews designed to generate data on developmental history, symptom onset and offset, patterns of impairment, and contextual factors.

Other ADHD Symptom Checklists

The past several years have witnessed the development of a flurry of brief ADHD symptom checklists based on the DSM-IV ADHD criteria: the ADHD Rating Scale (DuPaul et al., 1998), which includes the DSM-IV ADHD items; the Vanderbilt AD/HD Diagnostic Teacher Rating Scale (Wolraich, Feurer, Hannah, Baumgaertel, & Pinnock, 1998), which includes symptoms of ADHD and ODD as well as a screen for CD; and the ADHD Symptom Checklist—4 (Gadow & Sprafkin, 1997). These scales demonstrate solid reliability, some factor-analytic support, attempts at norms, and varying degrees of predictive validity. The most impressive data pertain to the ADHD Rating Scale, for which tables demonstrate the performance of various parent and teacher cutoff scores for distinguishing children with ADHD from control children (and, more tentatively, ADHD subtypes from one another). Because negative predictive power figures are above .8, clinicians may be in the advantageous position of being able to rule out ADHD with a brief symptom checklist. Because these scales include the DSM-IV items of ADHD, they are not listed in Table 4.1.

Swanson, Kotkin, Agler, M-Flynn, and Pelham Rating Scale

Swanson (1992) and McBurnett et al. (1995) present preliminary data on a brief, 10-item scale called the Swanson, Kotkin, Agler, M-Flynn, and Pelham Rating Scale (SKAMP), designed specifically to monitor a child's response to psychosocial interventions in classroom settings. Item selection was based not on diagnostic criteria for psychopathology, but rather on the types of classroom target behaviors typically utilized in behavioral treatment strategies. The SKAMP items divide evenly into an Attention factor and a Deportment factor, both of which have been found to display construct validity with respect to important school criterion variables (McBurnett et al., 1995). Whereas the small normative database should caution assessors about using this instrument for identification of cases, its use as a brief, repeated assessment of treatment outcome appears promising. (Note that a more recent version of this device, the McBurnett, Swanson, Kotkin, Agler, M-Flynn, and Pelham Rating Scale [McSKAMP], also includes room for individually assigned target behaviors and can thus be tailored to a particular child's school-based problems.)

ADD-H Comprehensive Teacher Rating Scale—Revised

The first edition of the ADD-H Comprehensive Teacher Rating Scale (ACTeRS) was reviewed by Barkley (1988), who pointed out the problems of sparse validity data and norming on a community sample with uncertain applicability to clinical populations. The revised edition of the ACTeRS (ACTeRS-R) partially addresses those concerns. The primary accomplishments of the newer edition are (1) to extend the age range from kindergarten through fifth grade to kindergarten through eighth grade, and (2) to provide cross-validation of the factor structure.

The theoretical conceptualization underlying both versions of the ACTeRS, developed by Rina Ullmann and colleagues at Illinois, is that inattention is the core feature of ADHD. The original version's subscales, derived by factor analysis, are Attention, Hyperactivity, Social Skills, and Oppositional Behavior. For the ACTeRS-R, a new sample was gathered for cross-validation and restandardization. The factors were again validated, and efforts were made to create relatively "factor-pure" item lists, so that each item loads above .68 on its primary factor and below .25 and on any other factor. Factor intercorrelations range from .38 to .78. Additional validity data are not provided, however, and differential external validation of the discrete subscales is not offered. For example, all scales show positive response to stimulant medication treatment, but the Oppositional Behavior scale's sensitivity to such intervention was lower than that of other factors. Because lenient cutoffs are recommended for the scale, so that the upper 10% of the distribution would be diagnosed as having ADHD, the potential for overdiagnosis appears to be a concern (cf. recent epidemiological prevalence estimates for ADHD ranging from approximately 1% to 7% of the school-age population; Hinshaw, 1994). Gender and age means are provided, but normative data (standard score conversions) are possible only by gender. Information regarding ethnicity or SES of the norming sample is not provided. In all, more extensive validity data would be welcome for this promising scale.

Children's Attention and Adjustment Survey

School Version

The school version of the Children's Attention and Adjustment Survey (CAAS) is a substantive addition to the teacher inventories available to researchers and clinicians (Lambert, Hartsough, & Sandoval, 1990). Targeted at externalizing problems in the ADHD-to-CD spectrum, it explicitly attempts to capture the DSM-III diagnoses of attention deficit disorder with and without hyperactivity and the DSM-III-R ADHD diagnosis, as well as the aggression dimension. The scales were developed out of programmatic research into hyperactivity in school settings carried out over nearly two decades. In their research, Lambert et al. (1990) have adopted an explicit social-interactional model of ADHD, seeking from the outset to incorporate school and home sources into their formation of the instrument. Many items were originally selected on a rational basis after literature searches for items believed to display discriminant validity and sensitivity to medication response; the source of each item is provided in the manual.

Follow-up factor analysis of these items was conducted on large, randomly sampled groups of first- through fifth-grade children representing a wide ethnic and sociodemographic cross-section, yielding three basic factors (Conduct Problems, Hyperactivity, and Inattention). An additional factor analysis with Conduct Problems items removed resulted in three factors corresponding to the core list for ADHD—Hyperactivity, Impulsivity, and Inattention. These results were used to form the clinical scales, with elimination of items loading highly on more than one factor. The manual reports scale properties in detail, including extensive reliability and validity data, although the latter are primarily in the form of correlations with other teacher rating scales. Scale alphas range from .78 to .91; test–retest stability ranges from .32

to .44 over 3 years. The scale intercorrelations range from .67 to .74, demonstrating the clear overlap of these domains of externalizing behavior in rating data.

Although brief, the school version consists of well-researched items and is accompanied by age norms based on a diverse community sample. Furthermore, data on the predictive validity of the scales in a longitudinal sample are presented. The major limitation is that the normative sample was primarily a community sample (only 1.19% met "social system criteria" for hyperactivity), raising questions about how the scale performs within a referred population; the manual also does not provide ethnicity or gender norms. Overall, this is a solid instrument for use in epidemiological research, initial diagnostic screening, and school-based investigations.

Home Version

To generate a home version of the CAAS, Lambert et al. (1990) performed factor analyses for parent administration of a small subset of the project's large norming sample (see above), generating subscales of Inattention, Impulsivity, Hyperactivity, and Conduct Problems. The subscales can be combined to yield scores for the DSM-III-R ADHD diagnosis, as well as for inattention with and without hyperactivity. Scale alphas range from .75 to .81, and test–retest stabilities are .44–.61. The subscales appear to be partially independent, with intercorrelations from .36 to .56.

In keeping with meta-analytic reviews (Achenbach et al., 1987), correlations between the home and school versions of the CAAS are modest. A crucial limitation is the small community sample, rendering unclear the scale's potential performance with clinic populations. Furthermore, exemplifying a ubiquitous problem for the field, the normative sample is too small to detect any but the largest age, gender, or ethnic differences; in fact, none were revealed. The primary utility of the CAAS home version would seem to be as an adjunct to assessments in schools using the more extensively normed school version.

Attention Deficit Disorders Evaluation Scale

Home Version

The Attention Deficit Disorders Evaluation Scale (ADDES) was developed by Stephen B. McCarney with the explicit goal of evaluating the DSM-III-R ADHD construct. It contains scales for Inattention, Impulsivity, and Hyperactivity. Test–retest reliability (30 days) ranges from .90 to .92, and interrater agreement between parents is in the range of .80–.94. However, external validity data for the distinct subscales are lacking; one validity study is reported, in which all three scales correlated with the Conners HI and were able to discriminate ADHD from non-ADHD children. Although item response distributions are commendably reported, the relatively narrow item ranges lead to substantial floor effects.

Items are worded in behavioral terms. Items were generated rationally, by polling "parents and clinicians," although the number and identity of these sources is not reported; the final item total is 46. A strength of this scale is that an ambitious, nationwide norming effort was carried out; the scale is unique for "narrow" instruments in that samples were drawn from all regions of the United States. The normative sample was 48% male and 84% European American. Although ethnic or cultural group results are not reported, age and gender norms are provided.

As might be expected, the three factors may not be distinct; their intercorrelations are typically above .7, and all three correlate over .80 with the Conners HI. As noted earlier, there is general empirical support for the proposition that across clinic and community samples, inattention may be distinguished from hyperactivity/impulsivity, but the latter may not yield separable dimensions (Lahey et al., 1988; Healey et al., 1993). Furthermore, the shortage of items explicitly assessing aggression or conduct problems limits the utility of this scale for separating ADHD-related symptomatology from associated antisocial behavior.

School Version

The school version of the ADDES has many of the same strengths and shortcomings as the home version. The method of scale development was nearly identical, and behavioral descriptors are emphasized within the three dimensions of Inattention, Impulsivity, and Hyperactivity. It contains 60 items, scaled 0–4. Like the home version, the school version of the ADDES boasts a unique normative sample, representatively drawn from 19 states throughout the United States. Gender-specific norms are provided, and there is a partial breakdown by age groups. Scale internal reliabilities are excellent, and test–retest reliabilities (30-day) for the scales are .89–.97. Interrater agreement (by 237 pairs of educators rating a random selection of students from the norming sample) ranged from .81 to .90 (uncorrected product–moment correlations). The properties of this instrument in clinic samples are unknown.

The three subscales of the school version are substantially intercorrelated (.77, .79, .95), calling into question their differential validity. The shortage of items to assess aggression, conduct problems, or covert antisocial behavior further limits the utility of the instrument for general research or clinical practice with disruptive behavior problems. However, the ADDES may have merit when screening or additional assessment of ADHD symptoms is needed. The impressive normative sample makes scores on both versions of this instrument of interest for local epidemiological studies of ADHD.

Yale Children's Inventory

The Yale Children's Inventory (YCI; Shaywitz, Schnell, Shaywitz, & Towle, 1986) is a parent-based rating scale. The scale is of primary interest in the differential assessment of children with learning disabilities and ADHD. Norming samples were drawn from the community, along with a sample of learning-disabled children from both schools and an outpatient clinic. Ethnicity of the sample is not reported, and all subjects were combined for all analyses, so that separate age and gender norms are not available. Factor-analytic procedures emphasized retention of simple, factor-pure items. The final item pool comprises 11 short subscales (Attention, Hyperactivity, Impulsivity, Tractability, Habituation, Conduct Disorder Socialized, Conduct Disorder Aggressive, Negative Affect, Academics, Language, Fine Motor), with four to seven items per scale. Interscale correlations were not reported, but the scales load on two general factors named Behavior and Cognitive; the authors do provide some evidence for discriminant validity of the Hyperactivity, Attention, and Impulsivity scales. With further development and a broader norm sample, the YCI may have promise in the differential assessment of children with learning problems and disruptive behavior problems.

New York Teacher Rating Scale

A new scale has been developed by Miller et al. (1995) to cover with greater representation the domain of conduct problems and aggression. As has been pointed out, many of the narrow scales currently in use fail to provide sufficient coverage of aggressive, assaultive, or covert antisocial behaviors. A key issue is that many such difficulties occur at low base rates; questionnaires may become quite lengthy if comprehensive coverage of this domain is attempted. The New York Teacher Rating Scale (NYTRS) was derived specifically to address the problem of insufficient coverage of the aggression/conduct domain. Although utilized in the initial construction of the scale, items pertinent to ADHD were not included in the final version, affording a scale with the factors of Defiance, Physical Aggression, Delinquent Aggression, and Peer Problems. Psychometric properties, in the initial report, appear promising: Scale alphas range from .73 to .96, and 6-week test–retest reliabilities range from .62 to .70. The most important attribute, according to the authors, is that the full range of oppositional defiant behavior, overt aggression, and covert conduct problems is represented in the scale.

The initial investigation of the NYTRS utilized a small clinical sample and a normative group of 1,258 (Miller et al., 1995). In a subsequent study, the instrument showed incremental validity, over and above the Child Behavior Checklist Teacher's Report Form, in predicting criterion measures of antisocial behavior (Freeman, Miller, & Wasserman, 1995). A parent version of the NYTRS is under development. The scale appears quite promising for appraising the key domain of aggression and antisocial behavior.[11]

Because of space limitations, we refer the interested reader to Hinshaw and Zupan (1997), who focus more generally on assessment and evaluation strategies related to antisocial behavior in children and adolescents.[12]

CONCLUDING ISSUES

We have reviewed only several of the most prominent narrow scales for disruptive behavior problems that are currently in use, but the astute reader should be able to detect some fundamental similarities across our descriptions. A number of scales tap, with adequacy, the domains of inattention, impulsivity, and motoric overactivity; indeed, only a finite number of items pertain to this domain, and psychometric properties of these dimensions across different scales are (not surprisingly) similar. Fewer scales pertain exclusively to the many types of aggressive and antisocial behaviors; the NYTRS is a new instrument that appears to span this domain without attempting the broad coverage of general psychopathology of a scale like the Child Behavior Checklist. Nearly all of the disruptive behavior disorder scales lack truly broad and representative norms. Specifically, whereas separate norms for various age groups (or sometimes for gender) are found, insufficient sample sizes for detecting effects of ethnicity are the rule.[13] In short, a large number of briefer rating scales for disruptive problems (particularly ADHD) share similar strengths and limitations.

It must not be assumed, however, that factors from different scales entitled "Attention Problem," "Hyperactivity," or "Aggression" are all measuring the same construct. The reification of factor names is a common problem when the results of factor-analytic strategies are used (Hinshaw, 1987), and even slight differences in item composition may alter the clinical meaning of a given dimension of disruptive behavior. The best antidote to misleading data is the careful perusal of the normative, psychometric, and validational information regarding a particular scale.

Given the superior norms and comorbidity data that are available from broad rating instruments, why would the clinician or investigator consider the use of briefer, narrow scales? As has been emphasized throughout, the purpose of the assessment always guides the choice of instrument. For ongoing monitoring of treatment response, extremely brief scales are typically in order. Furthermore, in many instances there is simply not the time available to have adult informants complete scales that take 15–20 minutes or more, even for initial evaluations. As highlighted earlier, however, we strongly advise the use of broader scales during preliminary workups, given the frequent overlap of disruptive behavior problems with internalizing features and the importance of ascertaining comorbid symptom patterns. Narrower scales may then be employed for more fine-grained analyses of externalizing problems, in the context of the types of data (developmental histories, structured interviews, and psychological/cognitive testing) necessary for accurate differential diagnosis. Overall, there are no substitutes for (1) precise specification of the research or clinical question at hand, and (2) careful scrutiny of the properties of questionnaires under consideration.

Perhaps the most important message of this chapter is a point made several times herein: Although rating scales are an important, if not essential, aspect of the beginning stages of thorough child assessment or treatment monitoring, they are rarely if ever sufficient; ratings must always be considered in light of additional developmental, psychological, medical, and diagnostic information. Their ease of use can lead to overly zealous identification of "cases" unless seasoned, well-trained evaluators learn to incorporate rating scale scores with the additional information that is necessary to diagnose and appraise disruptive behavior problems.

APPENDIX: WHERE TO OBTAIN ADDITIONAL INFORMATION ON RATING SCALES REVIEWED HEREIN

ADD-H Comprehensive Teacher Rating Scale—Revised (ACTeRS-R). MetriTech, Inc., 111 North Market Street, Champaign, IL 61820 (1-800-747-4868).

Attention Deficit Disorders Evaluation Scale (ADDES). Hawthorne Educational Services Incorporated, 800 Gray Oak Drive, Columbia, MO 65201 (1-800-542-1673).

ADHD Rating Scale. The Guilford Press, 72 Spring St., New York, NY 10012 (1-800-365-7006).

ADHD Symptom Checklist—4. Checkmate Plus Ltd., P.O. Box 696, Stony Brook, NY 11790-0696 (1-800-779-4292).

Child Behavior Checklist. Thomas Achenbach, PhD, University Associates in Psychiatry, Department of Psychiatry, University of Vermont, Burlington, VT 05401.

Children's Attention and Adjustment Survey (CAAS). Consulting Psychologists Press, Inc., 577 College Ave., Palo Alto, CA 94306.

Conners Abbreviated Symptom Questionnaire (CASQ), Revised Conners Teacher Rating Scale, Revised Conners Parent Rating Scale, Conners Hyperactivity Index (HI). Multi-Health Systems, Inc., 908 Niagara Falls Blvd., North Tonawanda, NY 14120-2060 (1-800-456-3003).

Conners, Loney, and Milich (CLAM) Scale. James Swanson, PhD, Child Development Center, 19262 Jamboree Blvd., University of California, Irvine, CA 92717.

IOWA Conners Scale. Jan Loney, PhD, Department of Psychiatry, SUNY–Stony Brook, Stony Brook, NY 11794-8790.

New York Teacher Rating Scale (NYTRS). Laurie Miller, PhD, New York State Psychiatric Institute, 722 W. 168th St., New York, NY 10032.

Self-Report Delinquency (SRD) Measure. David Huizinga, PhD, University of Colorado, Campus Box 442, Boulder, CO 80309.

Swanson, Kotkin, Agler, M-Flynn, and Pelham Rating Scale (SKAMP). James Swanson, PhD,

Child Development Center, 19262 Jamboree Blvd., University of California, Irvine, CA 92717.

Swanson, Nolan, and Pelham Rating Scale, fourth edition (SNAP-IV). James Swanson, PhD, Child Development Center, 19262 Jamboree Blvd., University of California, Irvine, CA 92717.

Vanderbilt AD/HD Diagnostic Teacher Rating Scale. Mark Wolraich, MD, Department of Pediatrics, Vanderbilt University, Nashville, TN 37204.

Yale Children's Inventory (YCI). Sally E. Shaywitz, MD, Learning Disorders Unit, Department of Pediatrics, Yale University School of Medicine, P.O. Box 3333, New Haven, CT 06510.

NOTES

1. The early terms "aggressive" or "acting out" for this domain of problem behaviors were supplanted for many years by the labels "undercontrolled" or "externalizing" (Achenbach & Edelbrock, 1978). Yet because of contentions that the term "undercontrol" is not synonymous with disruptive behavioral manifestations (Block & Gjerde, 1986), and that the label "externalizing" carries implicit etiological connotations (i.e., that underlying intrapsychic conflict is "externalized" through acting-out behavior), the recent editions of the *Diagnostic and Statistical Manual of Mental Disorders* (DSM; American Psychiatric Association, 1987, 1994) have advocated use of the more theoretically neutral term "disruptive." Indeed, DSM-IV now categorizes ADHD, ODD, and CD as "attention-deficit and disruptive behavior disorders"; for the sake of brevity, however, we refer to these in this chapter as "disruptive behavior problems."

2. The latter distinction has a long psychometric history with respect to the differentiation between undersocialized and socialized aggression (see Quay, 1986).

3. Although a thorough discussion of self-report and peer sociometric procedures is beyond the scope of this chapter, several points are in order. First, for the domains of attention deficits, hyperactivity, and oppositional defiant behavior, children are likely to underreport their own problems quite markedly and are not considered valid informants for assessment or diagnostic purposes (Loeber, Green, Lahey, & Stouthamer-Loeber, 1991). On the other hand, children appear to be crucially important sources of information regarding not only internalizing features but also interpersonal aggression and conduct problems, particularly the subdomain of covert antisocial behavior (Loeber, Stouthamer-Loeber, Van Kammen, & Farrington, 1989). Scales such as Elliott, Huizinga, and Morse's (1986) Self-Report Delinquency (SRD) measure are important in this regard (see also the Self Report of Antisocial Behavior [Loeber et al., 1989], an adaptation of the SRD for 7- to 10-year-olds). Second, given (a) the strong interrelation between externalizing behavior and peer rejection and (b) the power of negative peer status to predict long-term outcome (Parker & Asher, 1987), peer rating or peer nomination data are markedly underutilized in typical assessment procedures. Although logistic constraints curtail their routine use, peer sociometric data are not redundant with adult appraisals of peer status (Hinshaw & Melnick, 1995); evaluators are encouraged to consider obtaining peer-related data when feasible. Importantly, some teacher estimates of peer status show good validity (Dishion, 1990).

4. It should not be assumed, however, that a single rating of a child by one informant comes close to approximating this ideal.

5. Additional data from the Achenbach et al. (1987) meta-analytic review point to similarly low levels of association between (a) either parents or teachers and (b) mental health workers. Furthermore, the average correlation between parent/teacher ratings and those from child self-reports was in the low .2 range. Modest levels of interinformant correspondence (although statistically significant in the aggregate) are apparently the norm.

6. Also, without extremely large n's in the normative database, insufficient numbers of children within narrow age ranges will be available to form norms for that age group. This developmental insensitivity may be important: Across normal development in grade-school-age youngsters, inattention/hyperactivity decreases in frequency, whereas antisocial behaviors tend to increase through adolescence (e.g., Pelham, Evans, Gnagy, & Greenslade, 1992). Thus, the use of a single "hyperactivity" cutoff score for all ages may tend to overidentify younger children but to underidentify older youngsters, with the reverse pattern for serious aggression.

7. Of course, the same critique can be applied to the "official" diagnostic thresholds utilized in most structured interviews: Unless meaningful validation research has been performed, the choice of cutoff score will be arbitrary.

8. Barkley (1988) reviewed the Conners Parent Rating Scale, the Conners Teacher Rating Scale, the Child Behavior Checklist, the Personality Inventory for Children, the Louisville Behavior Checklist, the Eyberg Child Behavior Inventory, the Werry–Weiss–Peters Activity Rating Scale, the School Behavior Checklist, and the original version of the ADD-H Comprehensive Teacher Rating Scale. Because of the thoroughness of this review, because some of these instruments can be considered broad scales (Hart & Lahey, Chapter 3), and because of space limitations herein, we focus on other instruments—chiefly those that are newer. Also, despite their relevance to disruptive behavior problems, we do not cover such other broad instruments as the ACQ Behavior Checklist, the Revised Behavior Problem Checklist, or the Behavior Assessment System for Children (again, see Hart & Lahey, Chapter 3).

9. Conners (1990), in fact, considers the CASQ/HI to be a general indicator of externalizing psychopathology and not a specific tool for hyperactivity/ADHD.

10. A related scale for which space does not permit a separate review is the Disruptive Behavior Disorders Checklist for Teachers (see Pelham et al., 1992). For this scale, the DSM-III-R criteria for ADHD, ODD, and CD were randomized and scaled on a 4-point, Conners-style metric. Pelham et al. (1992) provide psychometric properties for this instrument in a special education population. The scale is dated, of course, by the advent of the DSM-IV criterion set, but it provides important information on the dimensionalized criteria for disruptive behavior disorders from the previous version of the official nomenclature in the United States.

11. Two other scales focusing specifically on the domain of acting-out/aggressive behavior are noteworthy. First, Kazdin, Rodger, Colbus, and Siegel (1987) describe the Children's Hostility Inventory, a scale based on the Buss–Durkee Hostility Inventory for adults. The chief purpose of this questionnaire is to differentiate children's hostile cognitions and perceptions from their aggressive actions per se. Separate factors for these two domains emerged in quantitative analyses; the scale differentiated youth with CD from those with other psychiatric disorders. Although extensive normative data have not been obtained, this theoretically derived scale may play a role in research programs dealing

with mechanisms of aggressive behavior. Contact Alan Kazdin, PhD, Department of Psychology, Yale University, P.O. Box 11A Yale Station, New Haven, CT 06520-7447.

Second, the recent Child Aggression Scale, with parent and teacher versions available, focuses on the display of discrete acts of physical and verbal aggression, with considerably more detail than the usual "Conduct Problem" or "Aggression" factors in extant scales. Also noteworthy is the explicit frequency-based response metric, which asks respondents to note specifically the number of actions in recent days or weeks. Psychometric data on this promising scale are forthcoming; contact Jeffrey Halperin, PhD, Department of Psychology, Queens College, CUNY, 65-30 Kissena Blvd., Flushing, NY 11367-0904.

12. We briefly note that dimensional symptom checklists are available from structured interviews such as the Diagnostic Interview Schedule for Children (DISC; see Rubio-Stipec et al., 1996). In addition to the categorical, yes–no diagnoses derived from such instruments, counts of pertinent symptoms within specific domains are available. Indeed, Rubio-Stipec et al. (1996) provide information on the excellent internal consistency and test–retest reliability of symptom scales for the domains of ADHD, ODD, and CD (as well as depression) from the DISC-2.3. Further work with respect to external validation is needed, however, and newer versions of such interviews as the DISC will require additional scale construction.

13. Furthermore, even if effects of ethnicity were to be found, it would be quite difficult to tease these apart from the effects of associated SES differences unless extensive demographic information were also obtained.

REFERENCES

Abikoff, H., Courtney, M., Pelham, W. E., & Koplewicz, H. S. (1993). Teachers' ratings of disruptive behaviors: The influence of halo effects. *Journal of Abnormal Child Psychology, 17*, 519–533.

Abikoff, H., & Gittelman, R. (1985). The normalizing effects of methylphenidate on the classroom behavior of ADDH children. *Journal of Abnormal Child Psychology, 13*, 33–44.

Achenbach, T. M. (1990). Conceptualization of developmental psychopathology. In M. Lewis & S. M. Miller (Eds.), *Handbook of developmental psychopathology* (pp. 3–14). New York: Plenum Press.

Achenbach, T. M. (1991a). *Manual for the Child Behavior Checklist/4–18 and 1991 Profile.* Burlington: University of Vermont Department of Psychiatry.

Achenbach, T. M. (1991b). *Manual for the Teacher's Report Form and 1991 Profile.* Burlington: University of Vermont Department of Psychiatry.

Achenbach, T. M., & Edelbrock, C. S. (1978). The classification of child psychopathology: A review and analysis of empirical efforts. *Psychological Bulletin, 85*, 1275–1301.

Achenbach, T. M., McConaughy, S. H., & Howell, C. T. (1987). Child/adolescent behavioral and emotional problems: Implications of cross-informant correlations for situational specificity. *Psychological Bulletin, 101*, 213–232.

American Psychiatric Association. (1980). *Diagnostic and statistical manual of mental disorders* (3rd ed.). Washington, DC: Author.

American Psychiatric Association. (1987). *Diagnostic and statistical manual of mental disorders* (3rd ed., rev.). Washington, DC: Author.

American Psychiatric Association. (1994). *Diagnostic and statistical manual of mental disorders* (4th ed.). Washington, DC: Author.

Atkins, M. S., Pelham, W. E., & Licht, M. H. (1989). The differential validity of teacher ratings of inattention/overactivity and aggression. *Journal of Abnormal Child Psychology, 17,* 423–435.

August, G. J., Realmuto, G. M., Crosby, R. D., & MacDonald, A. W. (1995). Community-based multiple-gate screening of children at risk for conduct disorder. *Journal of Abnormal Child Psychology, 23,* 521–544.

Barkley, R. A. (1988). Child behavior rating scales and checklists. In M. Rutter, A. H. Tuma, & I. S. Lann (Eds.), *Assessment and diagnosis in child psychopathology* (pp. 113–155). New York: Guilford Press.

Bauermeister, J. J., Berrios, V., Jimenez, A. L., Acevedo, L., & Gordon, M. (1990). Some issues and instruments for the assessment of attention-deficit hyperactivity disorder in Puerto-Rican children. *Journal of Clinical Child Psychology, 19,* 9–16.

Biederman, J., Newcorn, J., & Sprich, S. (1991). Comorbidity of attention deficit hyperactivity disorder with conduct, depressive, anxiety, and other disorders. *American Journal of Psychiatry, 148,* 564–577.

Block, J., & Gjerde, P. (1986). Distinguishing antisocial behavior and undercontrol. In D. Olweus, J. Block, & M. Radke-Yarrow (Eds.), *Development of antisocial and prosocial behavior: Research, theories, and issues* (pp. 177–206). Orlando, FL: Academic Press.

Capaldi, D. M. (1991). Co-occurrence of conduct problems and depressive symptoms in early adolescent boys: I. Familial factors and general adjustment at grade 6. *Development and Psychopathology, 3,* 277–300.

Caron, C., & Rutter, M. (1991). Comorbidity in child psychopathology: Concepts, issues, and research strategies. *Journal of Child Psychology and Psychiatry, 32,* 1063–1080.

Conners, C. K. (1969). A teacher rating scale for use in drug studies with children. *American Journal of Psychiatry, 126,* 884–888.

Conners, C. K. (1970). Symptom patterns in hyperkinetic, neurotic, and normal children. *Child Development, 41,* 667–682.

Conners, C. K. (1990). *Manual for Conners' Rating Scales.* North Tonawanda, NY: Multi-Health Systems.

Conners, C. K. (1994). Conners Rating Scales. In M. E. Maruish (Ed.), *The use of psychological testing for treatment planning and outcome assessment* (pp. 550–578). Hillsdale, NJ: Erlbaum.

Conners, C. K. (1997). *Conners Rating Scales Revised—Technical manual.* North Tonawanda, NY: Multi-Health Systems.

Conners, C. K., Sitarenios, G., Parker, J. D. A., & Epstein, J. N. (1998). The Revised Conners Parent Rating Scale (CPRS-R): Factor structure, reliability, and criterion validity. *Journal of Abnormal Child Psychology, 26,* 257–268.

Diamond, J. M., & Deane, F. P. (1990). Conners Teachers' Questionnaire: Effects and implications of frequent administration. *Journal of Clinical Child Psychology, 19,* 202–204.

Dishion, T. (1990). The peer context of troublesome child and adolescent behavior. In P. E. Leone (Ed.), *Understanding troubled and troubling youth* (pp. 128–153). Newbury Park, CA: Sage.

DuPaul, G. J., Anastopoulos, A. D., Power, T. J., Reid, R., Ikeda, M. J., & McGooey, K. E. (1998). Parent ratings of attention-deficit/hyperactivity disorder symptoms: Factor structure and normative data. *Journal of Psychopathology and Behavioral Assessment, 20,* 83–102.

Dykman, R., Raney, T. J., & Ackerman, P. T. (1993). Assessing children with attention deficit disorder for identification and classification. In *Proceedings of the Forum on Education of Children with Attention Deficit Disorder* (pp. 17–26). Washington, DC: Chesapeake Institute.

Elliott, D. S., Huizinga, D., & Morse, B. (1986). Self-reported violent offending: A descriptive analysis of juvenile violent offenders and their offending careers. *Journal of Interpersonal Violence, 1,* 472–514.

Eysenck, H. J. (1986). A critique of classification and diagnosis. In T. Millon & G. L. Klerman (Eds.), *Contemporary directions in psychopathology: Toward the DSM-IV* (pp. 73–98). New York: Guilford Press.

Figueroa, R. A. (1979). The system of multicultural pluralistic assessment. *School Psychology Digest, 8,* 28–78.

Foster, S. L., & Cone, J. D. (1995). Validity issues in clinical assessment. *Psychological Assessment, 7,* 248–260.

Freeman, L. N., Miller, L. S., & Wasserman, G. (1995). *Assessing children's antisocial behavior: Utility of the New York Teacher Rating Scale.* Unpublished manuscript, Columbia University School of Social Work.

Furlong, M. J., & Fortman, J. B. (1984). Factor analysis of the abbreviated Conners Teacher Rating Scale: Implications for the assessment of hyperactivity. *Psychology in the Schools, 21,* 289–293.

Gadow, K. D., & Sprafkin, J. (1997). *ADHD Symptom Checklist–4: Manual.* Stony Brook, NY: Checkmate Press.

Gittelman, R., Abikoff, H., Pollack, E., Klein, D. F., Katz, S., & Mattes, J. (1980). A controlled trial of behavior modification and methylphenidate in hyperactive children. In C. K. Whalen & B. Henker (Eds.), *Hyperactive children: The social ecology of identification and treatment* (pp. 221–243). New York: Academic Press.

Goyette, C. H., Conners, C. K., & Ulrich, R. F. (1978). Normative data on revised Conners Parent and Teacher Rating Scales. *Journal of Abnormal Child Psychology, 6,* 221–236.

Healey, J. M., Newcorn, J. H., Halperin, J. M., Wolf, L. E., Pascualvaca, D. M., Shmeidler, J., & O'Brian, J. D. (1993). The factor structure of ADHD items in DSM-III-R: Internal consistency and external validation. *Journal of Abnormal Child Psychology, 21,* 441–453.

Hinshaw, S. P. (1987). On the distinction between attentional deficits/hyperactivity and conduct problems/aggression in child psychopathology. *Psychological Bulletin, 101,* 443–463.

Hinshaw, S. P. (1994). *Attention deficits and hyperactivity in children.* Thousand Oaks, CA: Sage.

Hinshaw, S. P., Lahey, B. B., & Hart, E. L. (1993). Issues of taxonomy and comorbidity in the development of conduct disorder. *Development and Psychopathology, 5,* 31–49.

Hinshaw, S. P., March, J. S., Abikoff, H., Arnold, L. E., Cantwell, D. P., Conners, C. K., Elliott, G. R., Halperin, J., Greenhill, L. L., Hechtman, L. T., Hoza, B., Jensen, P. S., Newcorn, J. H., McBurnett, K., Pelham, W. E., Richters, J. E., Severe, J. B., Schiller, E., Swanson, J. M., Vereen, D., Wells, K., & Wigal, T. (1997). Comprehensive assessment of childhood attention-deficit hyperactivity disorder in the context of a multisite, multimodal clinical trial. *Journal of Attention Disorders, 1,* 217–234.

Hinshaw, S. P., & Melnick, S. M. (1995). Peer relationships in children with attention-deficit hyperactivity disorder with and without comorbid aggression. *Development and Psychopathology, 7,* 627–647.

Hinshaw, S. P., Simmel, C., & Heller, T. (1995). Multimethod assessment of covert antisocial behavior in children: Laboratory observations, adult ratings, and child self-report. *Psychological Assessment, 7,* 209–219.

Hinshaw, S. P., & Zupan, B. (1997). Assessment of antisocial behavior in children and adolescents. In D. M. Stoff, J. Breiling, & J. D. Maser (Eds.), *Handbook of antisocial behavior* (pp. 36–50). New York: Wiley.

Jenkins, R. L., & Glickman, S. (1947). Patterns of personality organization among delinquents. *Nervous Children, 6,* 329–339.

Jensen, P. S., Martin, D., & Cantwell, D. P. (1997). Comorbidity in ADHD: Implications for research, practice, and DSM-V. *Journal of the American Academy of Child and Adolescent Psychiatry, 36,* 1065–1079.

Jensen, P. S., Watanabe, H. K., Richters, J. E., Roper, M., Hibbs, E. D., Salzberg, A. D., & Liu, S. (1996). Scales, diagnoses, and child psychopathology: II. Comparing the CBCL and DISC against external validators. *Journal of Abnormal Child Psychology, 24,* 151–168.

Kazdin, A. E., Rodgers, A., Colbus, D., & Siegel, T. (1987). Children's Hostility Inventory: Measurement of aggression and hostility in psychiatric inpatient children. *Journal of Clinical Child Psychology, 16,* 320–328.

Kenrick, D. T., & Funder, D. C. (1988). Profiting from controversy: Lessons from the person–situation debate. *American Psychologist, 43,* 23–34.

Kent, R. N., O'Leary, K. D., Diament, C., & Dietz, A. (1974). Expectation biases in observational evaluation of therapeutic change. *Journal of Consulting and Clinical Psychology, 42,* 774–780.

Kline, R. B., & Lachar, D. (1992). Evaluation of age, sex, and race bias in the Personality Inventory for Children (PIC). *Psychological Assessment, 4,* 333–339.

Lahey, B. B., Pelham, W. E., Schaughency, E. A., Atkins, M. S., Murphy, H. A., Hynd, G., Russo, M., Hartdagen, S., & Lorys-Vernon, A. (1988). Dimensions and types of attention deficit disorder. *Journal of the American Academy of Child and Adolescent Psychiatry, 27,* 330–335.

Lambert, M. C., Knight, F., Taylor, R., & Achenbach, T. M. (1994). Epidemiology of behavioral and emotional problems among children of Jamaica and the United States. *Journal of Abnormal Child Psychology, 22,* 113–128.

Lambert, N., Hartsough, C., & Sandoval, J. (1990). *Manual for the Children's Attention and Adjustment Survey.* Palo Alto, CA: Consulting Psychologists Press.

Loeber, R., Green, S. M., Lahey, B. B., & Stouthamer-Loeber, M. (1991). Differences and similarities between children, mothers, and teachers as informants on disruptive behavior disorders. *Journal of Abnormal Child Psychology, 19,* 75–95.

Loeber, R., & Schmaling, K. B. (1985). Empirical evidence for overt and covert patterns of antisocial conduct problems: A meta-analysis. *Journal of Abnormal Child Psychology, 13,* 337–352.

Loeber, R., Stouthamer-Loeber, M., Van Kammen, W. B., & Farrington, D. P. (1989). Development of a new measure of self-reported antisocial behavior for young children: Prevalence and reliability. In M. W. Klein (Ed.), *Cross-national research in self-reported crime and delinquency* (pp. 203–225). Dordrecht, The Netherlands: Kluwer-Nijhoff.

Loney, J., & Milich, R. (1982). Hyperactivity, inattention, and aggression in clinical practice. In M. Wolraich & D. K. Routh (Eds.), *Advances in developmental and behavioral pediatrics* (Vol. 2, pp. 113–147). Greenwich, CT: JAI Press.

Lyon, G. R. (1996). Learning disabilities. In E. J. Mash & R. A. Barkley (Eds.), *Child psychopathology* (pp. 390–435). New York: Guilford Press.

Mann, E. M., Ikeda, Y., Mueller, C. W., Takahashi, A., Tao, K. T., Humris, E., Li, B. L., & Chen, D. (1992). Cross-cultural differences in rating hyperactive–disruptive behavior in children. *American Journal of Psychiatry, 149,* 1539–1542.

McBurnett, K., Swanson, J. M., Pfiffner, L. J., Tamm, L., & Phan, D. (1995). *A measure of ADHD-related classroom impairment based on targets for behavioral intervention.* Unpublished manuscript, University of California at Irvine.

McConaughy, S. H., Achenbach, T. M., & Kent, C. L. (1988). Multiaxial empirically based assessment: Parent, teacher, observational, cognitive, and personality correlates of child behavior profiles in 6- to 11-year-old boys. *Journal of Abnormal Child Psychology, 16,* 485–509.

Mercer, J., & Lewis, J. (1978). *System of Multicultural Pluralistic Assessment.* New York: Psychological Corporation.

Miller, L. S., Klein, R. G., Piacentini, J., Abikoff, H., Shah, M. R., Samoilov, A., & Guardino, M. (1995). The New York Teacher Rating Scale for disruptive and antisocial behavior. *Journal of the American Academy of Child and Adolescent Psychiatry, 34,* 359–370.

Neighbors, H. W., Jackson, J. S., Campbell, L., & Williams, D. (1989). The influence of racial factors on psychiatric diagnosis: A review and suggestions for research. *Community Mental Health Journal, 25,* 301–311.

Parker, J. D. A., Sitarenios, G., & Conners, C. K. (1996). Abbreviated Conners Rating Scales revisited: A confirmatory factor analytic study. *Journal of Attention Disorders, 1,* 55–62.

Parker, J. G., & Asher, S. R. (1987). Peer relations and later personal adjustment: Are low-accepted children at risk? *Psychological Bulletin, 102,* 357–389.

Pelham, W. E., Evans, S. W., Gnagy, E. M., & Greenslade, K. E. (1992). Teacher ratings of DSM-III-R symptoms for the disruptive behavior disorders: Prevalence, factor analyses, and conditional probabilities in a special education sample. *School Psychology Review, 21,* 285–299.

Pelham, W. E., Milich, R., Murphy, D. A., & Murphy, H. A. (1989). Normative data on the IOWA Conners Teacher Rating Scale. *Journal of Clinical Child Psychology, 18,* 259–262.

Peterson, D. R. (1961). Behavior problems of middle childhood. *Journal of Consulting Psychology, 25,* 205–209.

Piacentini, J. C., Cohen, P., & Cohen, J. (1992). Combining discrepant information from multiple sources: Are complex algorithms better than simple ones? *Journal of Abnormal Child Psychology, 20,* 51–63.

Power, T. J., Andrews, T. J., Eiraldi, R. B., Doherty, B. J., Ikeda, M. J., DuPaul, G. J., & Landau, S. (1998). Evaluating attention deficit hyperactivity disorder using multiple informants: The incremental utility of combining teacher with parent reports. *Psychological Assessment, 10,* 250–260.

Prinz, R. J., & Miller, G. E. (1991). Issues in understanding and treating childhood conduct problems in disadvantaged populations. *Journal of Clinical Child Psychology, 20,* 379–385.

Quay, H. C. (1986). Classification. In H. C. Quay & J. S. Werry (Eds.), *Psychopathological disorders of childhood* (3rd ed., pp. 1–34). New York: Wiley.

Reid, J. B., Patterson, G. R., Baldwin, D. V., & Dishion, T. J. (1988). Observations in the assessment of childhood disorders. In M. Rutter, A. H. Tuma, & I. S. Lann (Eds.), *Assessment and diagnosis in child psychopathology* (pp. 156–195). New York: Guilford Press.

Richters, J. E. (1992). Depressed mothers as informants about their children: A critical review of the evidence for distortion. *Psychological Bulletin, 112*, 485–499.

Rio, A. T., Quay, H. C., Santisteban, D. A., & Szapocznik, J. (1989). Factor-analytic study of a Spanish translation of the Revised Behavior Problem Checklist. *Journal of Clinical Child Psychology, 18*, 343–350.

Robins, L. N., & McEvoy, L. (1990). Conduct problems as predictors of substance abuse. In L. N. Robins & M. Rutter (Eds.), *Straight and devious pathways from childhood to adulthood* (pp. 182–204). Cambridge, UK: Cambridge University Press.

Rourke, B. P. (Ed.). (1985). *Neuropsychology of learning disabilities: Essentials of subtype analysis.* New York: Guilford Press.

Rubio-Stipec, M., Shrout, P. E., Canino, G., Bird, H. R., Jensen, P., Dulcan, M., & Schwab-Stone, M. (1996). Empirically defined symptom scales from the DISC 2.3. *Journal of Abnormal Child Psychology, 24*, 67–83.

Saal, F. E., Downey, R. G., & Lahey, M. A. (1980). Rating the ratings: Assessing the psychometric quality of rating data. *Psychological Bulletin, 88*, 413–428.

Schachar, R. (1991). Childhood hyperactivity. *Journal of Child Psychology and Psychiatry, 32*, 155–191.

Schachar, R., Sandberg, S., & Rutter, M. (1986). Agreement between teachers' ratings and observations of hyperactivity, inattentiveness, and defiance. *Journal of Abnormal Child Psychology, 14*, 331–345.

Schweder, R. A. (1982). Fact and artifact in trait perception: The systematic distortion hypothesis. In *Progress in experimental personality research* (pp. 65–100). New York: Academic Press.

Schweder, R. A., & Sullivan, M. A. (1993). Cultural psychology: Who needs it? *Annual Review of Psychology, 44*, 497–523.

Shaywitz, S. E., Schnell, C., Shaywitz, B. A., & Towle, V. R. (1986). Yale Children's Inventory (YCI): An instrument to assess children with attentional deficits and learning disabilities. I. Scale development and psychometric properties. *Journal of Abnormal Child Psychology, 14*, 347–364.

Sleator, E. K., & Ullmann, R. K. (1981). Can the physician diagnose hyperactivity in the doctor's office? *Pediatrics, 67*, 13–17.

Snowden, L., & Todman, P. (1982). The psychological assessment of blacks: New and needed developments. In E. Jones & S. Korchin (Eds.), *Minority mental health* (pp. 193–226). New York: Praeger.

Stevens, J., Quittner, A. L., & Abikoff, H. (1998, October). *Factors influencing elementary school teachers' ratings of ADHD and ODD behaviors.* Paper presented at the Kansas Conference on Clinical Child Psychology, Lawrence.

Swanson, J. M. (1981, August). Teacher norms for the SNAP rating scale. In W. Pelham (Chair), *DSM-III category of attention deficit disorders: Rationale, operationalization, and correlates.* Symposium conducted at the annual meeting of the American Psychological Association, Los Angeles.

Swanson, J. M. (1992). *School-based assessments and interventions for ADD students.* Irvine, CA: K. C.

Szatmari, P., Offord, D. R., & Boyle, M. H. (1989). Ontario Child Health Study: Prevalence of attention deficit disorder with hyperactivity. *Journal of Child Psychology and Psychiatry, 30*, 219–230.

Ullmann, R. K., Sleator, E. K., & Sprague, R. L. (1985). A change of mind: The Conners Abbreviated Rating Scales reconsidered. *Journal of Abnormal Child Psychology, 13,* 553–565.

Vargas, L. A., & Willis, D. J. (1994). New directions in the treatment and assessment of ethnic minority children. *Journal of Clinical Child Psychology, 23,* 2–4.

Vitiello, B., Behar, D., Hunt, J., Stoff, D., & Ricciuti, A. (1990). Subtyping aggression in children and adolescents. *Journal of Neuropsychiatry and Clinical Neurosciences, 2,* 189–192.

Werry, J. S., Elkind, G. S., & Reeves, J. C. (1987). Attention deficit, conduct, oppositional, and anxiety disorders in children: III. Laboratory differences. *Journal of Abnormal Child Psychology, 15,* 409–428.

Whalen, C. K., Collins, B. E., Henker, B., Alkus, S. R., Adams, D., & Stapp, J. (1978). Behavior observations of hyperactive children and methylphenidate (Ritalin) effects in systematically structured classroom environments: Now you see them, now you don't. *Journal of Pediatric Psychology, 3,* 177–187.

Wolraich, M. L., Feurer, I. D., Hannah, J. N., Baumgaertel, A., & Pinnock, T. Y. (1998). Obtaining systematic teacher reports of disruptive behavior disorders utilizing DSM-IV. *Journal of Abnormal Psychology, 26,* 141–152.

5

Rating Scales for Anxiety and Mood Disorders

❖

WENDY K. SILVERMAN
BRIAN RABIAN

Rating scales play an important role in the assessment of youth and are now ubiquitous in child and adolescent psychiatric clinical and research settings. A perusal of articles published in recent child psychiatry and clinical child psychology journals (e.g., *Journal of the American Academy of Child and Adolescent Psychiatry*, *Journal of Clinical Child Psychology*) reveals that a rating scale of one sort or another has been used in almost every study as a means of assessing young people's emotional and behavioral functioning. The extensive coverage given to rating scales in the present volume is testimony to just how much work has been conducted during recent years in developing, testing, and refining rating scales. As a result, there are now numerous rating scales specifically designed to assess an array of childhood emotional and behavioral states, including general behavioral disorders (Hart & Lahey, Chapter 3, this volume), disruptive behavior problems (Hinshaw & Nigg, Chapter 4), pervasive developmental and communication disorders (Volkmar & Marans, Chapter 6), and anxiety and mood disorders (this chapter).

In this chapter, the focus is on rating scales that obtain subjective self-ratings or self-reports from children and adolescents about their anxious and depressed moods. Plentiful work has been conducted in recent years on developing these types of scales. Work on developing parent, teacher, or peer rating scales for assessing children's anxious and depressed moods in youth has lagged far behind. Part of the reason for the lag in this area is that children and adolescents are considered to be more accurate reporters of their own internal subjective states, including those of anxious and depressed moods, than are other reporters (e.g., parents, teachers) (Loeber, Green, & Lahey, 1990). As a result, a minimal assessment in child psychopathology of anxiety and mood disorders customarily involves the use of youth as primary informants via self-rating scales.

This chapter has two major objectives. The first objective is to introduce the reader to a way of thinking about assessment that is pragmatic in orientation (Silverman & Kurtines, 1996). Guided by this pragmatic orientation, the reader will come to see how self-rating scales for childhood anxiety and mood disorders in youth should (and can) be used to meet specific research and clinical goals, or to solve specific problems in certain contexts. The reader also will come to see how for certain goals or problems, other methods of assessment may be more useful than self-rating scales. The second objective of the chapter is to present evaluative descriptions of the most commonly used child and adolescent self-rating scales for anxiety and depression. The chapter concludes with recommendations for future research directions.

Before we proceed, a brief description of the anxiety and mood disorders as manifested by children and adolescents (from here on, referred to as children, for the sake of brevity) is presented. In presenting this description, we rely on the fourth edition of the *Diagnostic and Statistical Manual of Mental Disorders* (DSM-IV; American Psychiatric Association, 1994).

DEFINING THE ANXIETY AND MOOD DISORDERS IN CHILDREN

Both "anxiety" and "depression" have three common referents in the literature—as symptoms, as syndromes/disorders, and as nosological entities (e.g., Beck, 1967; Lehmann, 1959). As symptoms, "anxiety" and "depression" usually refer to the layperson's denotations of these (e.g., depression is reported sad affect) (Carson, 1986). As syndromes or disorders, "depression" and "anxiety" usually refer to groups of symptoms that cluster together (e.g., depression is negative affect, loss of interest in activities, feelings of worthlessness, changes in appetite). As nosological entities, "depression" and "anxiety" usually refer not only to specific syndromes but also to sets of symptoms that should display a certain time course, prognosis, and probable treatment response (Kazdin, 1990a).

The most widely used classification system of nosological entities is the DSM. DSM-III and DSM-III-R contained a broad category called "anxiety disorders of childhood and adolescence," which consisted of three subcategories (separation anxiety disorder, overanxious disorder, and avoidant disorder; see Silverman, 1992, for a review). DSM-IV, however, no longer contains this broad category. In addition, one of the subcategories (avoidant disorder) was eliminated in DSM-IV, and another (overanxious disorder) was subsumed under the "adult" anxiety subcategory of generalized anxiety disorder. Generalized anxiety disorder is characterized by excessive anxiety and worry in areas such as future events and past behavior, as well as physiological complaints. The only anxiety disorder specific to children in DSM-IV is separation anxiety disorder, which is classified under the broader category "other disorders of infancy, childhood, or adolescence." Separation anxiety disorder is characterized by excessive anxiety concerning separation from attachment figures, evidenced by such symptoms as unrealistic/persistent worry about possible harm to attachment figures, persistent avoidance of being alone, somatic complaints when anticipating separation, and so on.

In DSM-IV (as in DSM-III and DSM-III-R), children also may receive, as appropriate, diagnoses of the "adult" anxiety disorders. In addition to generalized anxiety disorder, these disorders include panic disorder without agoraphobia, panic disorder with agoraphobia, agoraphobia without history of panic disorder, specific phobia, social phobia (social anxiety disorder), obsessive–compulsive disorder, posttraumatic stress disorder, acute stress disorder, anxiety disorder due to a general medical condition, and substance-induced anxiety disorder.

The descriptions of mood disorders found in DSM-IV are, for the most part, similar to the descriptions in DSM-III-R. The major and broader patterns (i.e., diagnostic subcategories) include major depressive disorder, dysthymic disorder, depressive disorder not otherwise specified, bipolar I and II disorders, cyclothymic disorder, bipolar disorder not otherwise specified, mood disorder due to a general medical condition, and substance-induced mood disorder.

Most child self-rating mood scales were designed for assessing major depressive episode (the primary constituent of major depressive disorder, and a component of bipolar I and II disorders) and dysthymic disorder, or their symptoms. These scales are the focus of this chapter. According to DSM-IV, a major depressive episode is characterized by five of the following symptoms, causing clinically meaningful impairment or distress: (1) depressed mood (or irritable mood in youth), (2) notably decreased pleasure or interest in most activities, (3) marked weight loss or gain, (4) insomnia or hypersomnia, (5) slowed or speeded psychomotor activity, (6) fatigue or energy loss, (7) feelings of guilt or worthlessness, (8) difficulties in concentration, and (9) recurring thoughts about death. In dysthymic disorder, many of these same symptoms are apparent but in less severe form. Specifically, the symptoms may be chronic, lasting for at least 1 year in youth (during which there has been depressed mood most of the day more days than not).

Now that the anxiety and mood disorders have been described, we discuss how these disorders (or their symptoms) can be assessed through the use of child self-rating scales. In doing so, we first provide an overview of our "pragmatic orientation." We do so because we have found this orientation to be a useful frame for guiding our clinical and research activities, including assessing anxiety and mood disorders in children. (See Silverman & Kurtines, 1996, 1997, for more comprehensive coverage of the pragmatic tradition and our pragmatic orientation.)

A PRAGMATIC ORIENTATION

"Pragmatic" sometimes means being simple and expedient; it can, however, mean much more. The pragmatic tradition in modern thought has played a key role in shaping the way we think about many issues, including complex philosophical as well as theoretical and conceptual subjects. American in origin,[1] pragmatism encompasses a long and distinguished tradition that contains some of the most prominent thinkers in American philosophy, including Peirce, James, and Dewey, as well as more contemporary thinkers (e.g., Rorty, 1979). The concept of "pragmatic" that defines our orientation draws on this tradition.

Our pragmatic orientation is not an approach, a theory, or a philosophy/metatheory. Rather, it is *a way of thinking about* all of these things and more. William James (1907/1981) said it best when he described being pragmatic as "an attitude of orientation. . . . The attitude of looking away from first things, principles, 'categories', supposed necessities; and of looking toward last things, fruits, consequences, facts" (p. 29). Hence we think of being pragmatic as an attitude of orientation toward all of human experience, and we bring this attitude to all of our work, including assessment. Moreover, this attitude has two identifiable characteristics. One is an emphasis on problem solving; the second is an emphasis on context. These two characteristics are briefly described next.

Problem Solving and Contextualism

Rather than beginning with principles or basic assumptions, a pragmatic attitude begins with concretely experienced human problems. In other words, the pragmatist adopts a *problem-solving* orientation. Specifically, it adopts a practical approach to problem solving, in that it does not believe that solving problems can be separated from the practical effects or consequences of solving problems. To borrow (and paraphrase) another expression from James, the practical meaning and significance of any problem can always be brought down to some particular consequence in future practical experience. For the pragmatist, this "pragmatic" orientation provides a practical test of the significance of a problem.

The pragmatist, for example, thinks that the solution to problems cannot be separated from the practical effects or consequences of the solutions on particular human beings in specific contexts, because what is a successful solution in one context may be a more or less successful solution in another context. The pragmatist thus considers knowledge to be contextual in significance.

Traditionally, concepts and constructs derive their meaning and significance from the theoretical frameworks in which they are embedded. A pragmatic attitude, on the other hand, holds that concepts derive their meaning and significance from the "contexts" in which they are *used*. What this means is that the utility and validity of concepts is to be found in their success in contributing to the solution to problems.

In sum, our pragmatic orientation is an attitude—an "attitude of orientation"—that includes an emphasis on the practical solving of concretely experienced problems in specific contexts. What this boils down to is relatively simple: It boils down to doing *what is useful and what works*. Although simple, such a perspective does involve a reorientation in the ways that many of us are used to thinking about many things, including assessment.

A Pragmatic Orientation to Assessment

The pragmatic attitude that we tend to use in making our assessment choices serves to remind us not to let our assumptions about assessment get in the way of choosing and using the most effective methods. Rather, our pragmatic attitude guides us to use what works with the particular problems that we are trying to solve. It also guides us to stay focused on particular problems in specific contexts.

The emphasis on context dictates that in deciding on what assessment method to use, we first identify the setting and the goal. For our purposes, by "setting" we mean the specific situation wherein the assessment takes place (e.g., private practice, clinic, school). By "goal" we mean the purpose or function of the assessment (i.e., the "problem" that we are seeking to solve). The concept of pragmatism dictates that in deciding on what assessment method to use, we choose the method that is "most useful" in a particular setting. Finally, being pragmatic, we are guided to choose the "best" assessment method that will help us to accomplish the specific goal or solve a particular problem in that particular setting.

A PRAGMATIC ORIENTATION TO USING
CHILD SELF-RATING SCALES

Now that we have presented an overview of our pragmatic orientation and its application to assessment in general, in this section of the chapter we show how a pragmatic orientation specifically guides our thinking with respect to using child self-rating scales for assessing anxiety and depression in children. We first indicate the contexts in which self-rating scales can be used, and then we discuss the problems that self-rating scales can solve or the goals they can achieve. Woven through this discussion are evaluative summaries regarding how well (or poorly) self-rating scales can solve these problems or achieve these goals. When necessary, alternative assessment methods that can solve these problems "better" than self-rating scales are suggested.

The Contexts

The concept of context dictates that in deciding on an assessment method to use, we first identify the setting. As noted, by "setting" we mean the specific situation wherein an assessment takes place. There are many different types of settings or situations where children's emotional and behavioral functioning can be assessed. These include a private practice, a busy outpatient clinic, an inpatient clinic, or a school. Although this may seem simple enough, it is important to begin with context, because some assessment methods are more feasible than others for use in particular settings.

Consider, for example, the characteristics of the school setting. Most school settings do not have the luxury of expending a great deal of staff time, student time, or funds on tasks that are nonacademic. Consequently, in school settings it is necessary to choose a method that is low in cost, and that requires minimal time and effort on the part of both staff and students.

Typically, once the setting and the characteristics of the setting have been identified, we can quickly move on and focus on the goal or the problem that we are being asked to solve. This is not the case in the school setting, however. That is, if our knowledge about the various methods of assessment is solid, we realize that the number of feasible methods for use in the school setting is limited, and that child self-rating scales are clearly the most feasible. This is because no other assessment method costs as little and is as easy to administer and score as child self-rating scales. We also know that rating scales, because of their objective scoring procedure, minimize the role of clinical inference and interpretation. As a result, there is no need to use highly trained staff members for administration and scoring. In addition, child self-rating scales contain questions that are of clear concern to members of the school district; that is, the scales possess "face validity."

These advantages of child self-rating scales hold not only for their use in school settings, but also for their use in almost every other setting (e.g., a private practice, an outpatient clinic). It is for this reason that child self-rating scales have become the most widely used method of assessment for child anxiety and mood disorders (and symptoms) in both clinical and research contexts.

The Problems or Goals

Child self-rating scales are useful for solving or achieving many different problems or goals. Jensen and Haynes (1986) have provided an outline of some of these, and their outline has been adapted in this chapter. Specifically, the problems that can be solved by using self-rating scales include (1) screening and diagnosing, (2) identifying/quantifying symptoms and behaviors, (3) identifying/quantifying alternative behaviors, (4) identifying/quantifying controlling variables, (5) evaluating treatment outcome, and (6) evaluating the role of mediators and moderators. Each of these is discussed below.

Screening and Diagnosing

A rating scale that is useful for "screening" is one that can differentiate a group of symptomatic children from the rest of the community; in other words, it is capable of "diagnosing cases." The degree to which a scale can screen cases is an aspect of its criterion-related validity (Costello & Angold, 1988). Ideally, one would like this aspect of a self-rating scale to be nearly perfect: It would be most useful to administer a brief questionnaire to a child, to score it, and then to be able to characterize the child as either a "case" or a "noncase." Unfortunately, screening and diagnosing are not that simple.

First, in an attempt to present themselves in a positive light to adult testers, children may respond to the demand characteristics of the assessment situation by responding in socially desirable ways on these measures (La Greca, 1990). Evidence for this was provided in a study that examined the relation between scores on the Revised Children's Manifest Anxiety Scale (RCMAS; described later) and scores on the Marlowe–Crowne Social Desirability Scale in a sample of 78 nonclinical high school students (Hagborg, 1991). Results indicated that with boys (but not girls), lower levels of self-reported anxiety were significantly related to higher levels of social desirability.

Because of the potential for children to present themselves in a positive light or in a socially desirable way, steps should be taken to limit the occurrence of this. One important step is to use carefully worded instructions, such as "All children have different feelings," "We are interested in how you feel about things" and "There are no right or wrong answers." Such instructions are frequently included in the directions of child self-rating scales.

If we assume that appropriate steps have been taken to reduce the potential of social desirability effects in children's self-reports, are the child self-rating scales useful for screening? As noted at the beginning of this chapter, there is now a general consensus that it is more useful to elicit information from parents and teachers than from children about observable or objective child behaviors (Loeber et al., 1990). On the other hand, it is more useful to elicit information from children themselves about subjective child behaviors, such as anxiety and mood problems.

Although child self-rating scales are more useful than parent or teacher rating scales for screening for anxiety and depression, how much criterion-related validity can be expected of childhood anxiety and depression self-rating scales? In answering this question, it is helpful to review the meaning of "sensitivity" and "specificity." "Sensitivity" is the percentage of individuals who receive the diagnosis who were positively identified by the rating scale (true positives); "specificity" is the percentage of individuals who do not receive the diagnosis and who are not identified by the rating scale as anxious or depressed (true negatives) (Vecchio, 1966). Receiver operating characteristic curves (Hanley & McNeil, 1982) are helpful and efficient ways of presenting data on a rating scale's sensitivity and specificity (see Rey & Morris-Yates, 1991, for further information on the use of such curves for scales measuring adolescent depression).

In terms of screening for child anxiety and mood disorders, the currently available self-rating scales are likely to select more false positives than true positives (Costello & Angold, 1988). Thus children identified as anxious or depressed at an initial screen are likely *not* to be anxious or depressed at the second stage of an investigation. For example, Asarnow and Carlson (1985) found sensitivity to be 54% with inpatient children (aged 8 to 13) who completed a self-report measure of depression; this indicated that 46% of the children were misclassified as depressed or nondepressed. Kazdin, Colbus, and Rodgers (1988), in a comparison of the relative sensitivity and specificity of four child completed (and parent-completed) depression rating scales with inpatient children aged 7 to 13, found that individual depression scale scores yielded a sensitivity rate of 61%. Mattison, Bagnato, and Brubaker (1988), examining the sensitivity and specificity of a childhood anxiety self-rating scale with outpatient children aged 8 to 12, found the sensitivity rates to be 41%, 36%, and 48%, depending on the cutoff technique employed. Similarly, Hodges (1990) found that self-ratings of anxiety and depression by inpatient children aged 6 to 13 were better at correctly identifying children without anxiety or depression than at identifying children with these disorders.

Although research findings on the sensitivity and specificity of the child self-rating scales are not encouraging, the findings should not be surprising, given that only a small proportion of these scales' items operationalize DSM criteria. In addition, with the exception of Kazdin et al. (1988), all of the studies relied on a single measure obtained from a single source. A multimeasure, multisource approach would be likely to perform better. Evidence for this view also comes from Kazdin et al. (1988). Specifically, when multiple measures were combined in discriminant analyses, sensitivity, specificity and overall classification accuracy improved substantially (>80%). Unfortunately, though, administering a large assessment battery combined through an empirically derived algorithm does not provide the same degree of efficiency and ease as the administration and scoring of a single self-report measure (Kazdin et al., 1988).

The acute comments of Costello and Angold (1988) nicely sum up the situation with respect to the utility of child self-rating scales as screening instruments for anxiety and mood disorders:

It would therefore seem more appropriate to regard most psychiatric screening instruments as serving to increase the concentration of true cases in the second stage population, rather than expecting them to select only the true cases. If it were really possible to identify all true cases and true noncases using a brief self-report questionnaire, large areas of diagnostic psychiatry would be redundant. It is unrealistic to expect this level of accuracy. . . . Perhaps the term "screen" is unhelpful . . . ; the process is more like trawling through a population with a net; one will catch some of the fish one wants, miss others, and pick up all sorts of other species that will have to be selected out later. Despite the poor sensitivity and specificity of the fishing net, however, it will prove efficient and cost effective for most purposes when compared with a single fishing pole. (pp. 729–730)

One implication of Costello and Angold's (1988) comments is that a useful, cost-efficient research approach would employ a multistage sampling design (e.g., Ialongo, Edelsohn, Werthamer-Larsson, Crockett, & Kellam, 1993; Kendall, Cantwell, & Kazdin, 1989; Roberts, Lewinsohn, & Seeley, 1991). At the first stage, a child self-rating scale would be administered to all participants. This would identify those cases that should undergo more precise and comprehensive assessments (e.g., structured diagnostic interviews) at the second or third stage of the research.

In most research and clinical settings it is not useful to have to rely on a detailed procedure for screening, as screening should be a quick and efficient process. A detailed procedure is more acceptable for attaining careful diagnoses. Of all assessment instruments, the structured diagnostic interview is best suited for diagnosis. Thus, once diagnoses are derived via the structured interview, self-rating scales can be administered to quantify severity of symptoms (as discussed in the next section).

Identifying and Quantifying Symptoms and Behaviors

Most of the rating scales were specifically designed for identifying symptoms and behaviors and for quantifying their severity. The summary score obtained from the scales is assumed to be a quantitative index of the degree to which a particular problem area (e.g., anxiety or depression) is relevant to a child, or the probability that the child will emit one of a class of behaviors (e.g., eating little, eating a lot) (Jensen & Haynes, 1986). Departures from the "norm" can usually be determined, based on standard deviation units that define a particular percentile of the sample (e.g., Beidel & Turner, 1988; Silverman, La Greca, & Wasserstein, 1995). As noted above, however, groups that are defined in this way are not necessarily defined as "anxious" or "depressed" via diagnoses; studies comparing diagnoses with presentation on rating scales demonstrate that optimal cutoff scores (i.e., scores that maximize classification accuracy) have a high rate of false positives and false negatives (e.g., Hodges, 1990; Kazdin et al., 1988; Mattison et al., 1988).

In this connection, Costello and Angold (1988) have pointed out how a rating scale that is optimal as a measure of symptoms (i.e., one that has satisfactory content validity) will not necessarily perform well as a screen or criterion measure (i.e., one that has satisfactory criterion validity). The reason for this is that for a measure to have criterion validity, its items must correlate strongly with the criterion. Thus, if items that correlate poorly with the criterion are dropped (thereby improving criterion validity), content validity may be reduced, as the scale's representativeness of the construct being studied is reduced as well (Cronbach, 1970).

In addition, evidence is accumulating for the lack of distinctiveness of respondents' self-ratings of anxiety and depression. Several excellent reviews of the research evidence for both children (e.g., Finch, Lipovsky, & Casat, 1989; King, Ollendick, & Gullone, 1991; Seligman & Ollendick, 1998) and adults (e.g., Feldman, 1993) have appeared, and so will not be detailed here. In essence, much of the evidence rests on the large number of studies (both monomethod and multimethod) that have found large correlations between self-report measures of anxiety and depression, such that no meaningful discrimination between self-reported anxiety and depression can be identified (e.g., Norvell, Brophy, & Finch, 1985; Saylor, Finch, Spirito, & Bennett, 1984; Treiber & Mabe, 1987).

In the adult area, most exploratory factor analyses of self-rated anxiety and depression have produced a general negative mood or dysphoria factor, rather than distinct anxiety and depression factors (e.g., Gotlib, 1984; Gotlib & Meyer, 1986). Feldman (1993) presented further support for this notion by conducting a confirmatory factor analysis on data from adult nonclinical and clinical samples, and showing that the anxiety and depression self-rating scales were not measuring distinctive mood constructs. Feldman (1993) concluded that these scales are better thought of as measures of general negative mood than of anxiety and depression.

Crowley and Emerson (1996) attempted to replicate these results with children. Specifically, these investigators administered two widely used anxiety self-rating scales (the RCMAS and the State–Trait Anxiety Inventory for Children, or STAIC) and two widely used depression self-rating scales (the Children's Depression Inventory, or CDI, and the Reynolds Child Depression Scale; all four scales are described later) to nonreferred school-age children, and investigated whether a one-factor or a two-factor model best fit the data. Unlike the findings of Feldman (1993) with adults, Crowley and Emerson identified a two-factor model as the better model, based on chi-square and goodness-of-fit indices. According to the authors, these findings suggest that the distinction between anxiety and depression should be maintained.

This study awaits replication, particularly with clinical samples of children. Nevertheless, there appears to be growing consensus that whereas anxiety and depression show overlap with respect to negative affectivity, they also have distinguishing features (e.g., Lonigan, Carey, & Finch, 1994). For example, in the study conducted by Lonigan et al. (1994), 233 inpatient children with either a pure anxiety or a pure depressive clinical diagnosis completed the RCMAS and the CDI. Results indicated that the two groups showed overlap in negative affectivity: Both groups reported similar degrees of depressed affect in terms of being sad, lethargic, bothered by things, or feeling alone and isolated. Important differences between the two groups were also found, however. Specifically, children with a depressive disorder reported more problems related to a loss of interest and low motivation, and they had a more negative view of themselves. Children with an anxiety disorder reported more worry about the future, their well-being, and the reactions of others. Moreover, one general factor that appeared to distinguish between the depressed children and the anxious children was positive affectivity, in that there was an absence of positive affect reported by depressed children. These findings suggest that to improve the distinctiveness of anxiety and depression self-rating scales, it is important to assess the degree to which respondents report high positive affective states, and to infer depression from the relative absence of such experiences. In other words, a greater number of items contained in self-rating scales need to be reflective of positive affectivity, not negative affectivity (Watson & Kendall, 1989).

In addition to using child self-rating scales to identify and quantify symptoms and behaviors, another alternative "quick" method for accomplishing this goal is to use specific sections of a child structured interview schedule as a series of minimodules. For example, to assess a particular anxiety or mood disorder, the interview questions covering that diagnostic category may be asked of a child, and a "symptom summary score" may be derived (e.g., Silverman & Eisen, 1992). When interview schedules are used in this way, questions can be asked that are in line with DSM criteria.

Identifying and Quantifying Alternative Behaviors

Another frequent goal of self-rating scales is to identify positive alternatives to undesirable problem behaviors (e.g., Jensen & Haynes, 1986; Mash & Terdal, 1997). The child anxiety and depression self-rating scales are not very successful in meeting this goal. As noted above, the items contained on these rating scales largely reflect negative affectivity, not positive affectivity; thus most scales focus on identifying problem (negative) behaviors, not on positive alternatives to these behaviors. Although there are a few exceptions (e.g., the Children's Depression Scale; Lang & Tisher, 1978), most children's rating scales for anxiety and depression do not contain items that assess children's positive symptoms or adaptive ways in which children could handle their negative affective states. To assess these issues, another questionnaire specifically designed for this purpose, or another type of assessment measure, would need to be administered.

Identifying and Quantifying Controlling Variables

Once specific symptoms and alternative symptoms or behaviors have been identified and quantified, it is also helpful to identify and quantify the controlling variables (Jensen & Haynes, 1986). The assessment of controlling variables provides an important interface between assessment and treatment (Hayes, Nelson, & Jarrett, 1987). Such assessment is critical, given that childhood behavior problems, including those of anxiety and mood, vary in frequency and/or intensity as a function of the situation (e.g., Goldfried & Kent, 1972; Silverman, 1992).

In principle, the optimal way to identify and quantify controlling variables is to conduct behavioral observations in a child's natural setting. For example, in determining the variables that "control" a child's anxious behaviors (e.g., avoidance) in the school setting, the child could be observed in his/her classroom on a number of occasions, and the specific antecedents and consequences that elicit or control such behaviors could then be identified. However, observational methods are fraught with problems and difficulties of their own, and are usually impractical to implement in clinical contexts. As a result, their use is typically restricted to specific research contexts. In light of this, can child rating scales be used to identify and quantify controlling variables? Although the majority do not, there is no reason why rating scales cannot be designed for this purpose. An example of such a scale is the School Refusal Assessment Scale (Kearney & Silverman, 1993)—a scale designed to assess a behavior frequently associated with anxious and depressed mood in children.

The School Refusal Assessment Scale is based on a functional classification model of school refusal (Kearney & Silverman, 1996). According to this model, "refusal" to attend school is classified as being maintained by at least one of the following four controlling variables: (1) avoidance of stimuli provoking specific fearfulness or general anxiousness, (2) escape from aversive social or evaluative situations, (3) attention-getting behavior, and (4) positive tangible reinforcement. The School Refusal Assessment Scale determines the functional class that a particular child's school refusal may fit, and a specific, individualized treatment is then prescribed (e.g., contingency contracting for children who refuse because of condition 4).

Preliminary support for this functional model was demonstrated when seven children with difficulties attending school were successfully treated via prescriptive treatments (Kearney & Silverman, 1990). Kearney and Silverman (in press) recently provided further evidence for the efficacy of this model by employing a multiple-baseline design and by showing that "prescriptive treatment" (i.e., assigning treatment based on a child's highest functional condition on the scale) was more efficacious than "nonprescriptive treatment" (i.e., assigning treatment based on a child's lowest functional condition on the scale). It would be worthwhile to develop other children's self-rating scales that are based on a functional approach to assessment, as such scales can enhance our explanatory and predictive powers with respect to children's anxiety and mood disorders (Kearney & Silverman, 1996).

Evaluating Treatment Outcome

Self-rating scales are also useful for evaluating the effects of treatment on targeted symptoms or behaviors. According to a tripartite model (Lang, 1977) of internalizing disorders, self-rating scales serve as one of the three sets of measures administered in outcome studies of childhood anxiety and depression. In this model, self-rating scales are used to assess the subjective channel, behavioral observations are used to assess the behavioral or motoric channel, and psychophysiological measures are used to assess the physiological channel. Change observed from pre- to posttreatment is likely to vary across the three channels, both within and between subjects (e.g., Lang, 1977; Rachman & Hodgson, 1974). Although the use of a tripartite assessment battery is a luxury in most clinical settings because of its time, cost, and effort, the assessment of the subjective channel via self-rating measures is the part of the battery that is most time- and cost-efficient and should thus be used.

In using self-rating scales to assess treatment outcome, however, it is important to bear in mind that numerous complexities are involved in the evaluation of treatment outcome. In this section, we highlight two reasons most pertinent to childhood anxiety and depression. One reason has been alluded to above: Emotional responding across the three channels is generally desynchronous, both within and between subjects. Consequently, change may be observed from pre- to posttreatment in one of the channels but not in the others (e.g., Lang, 1977; Rachman & Hodgson, 1974). The implication is that for some participants, the subjective channel assessed via self-rating scales is not necessarily the channel in which change or improvement will be observed. (This is why the complete tripartite battery is preferable.)

Another reason for exercising caution when interpreting self-rating scale scores in the evaluation of treatment outcome is that fluctuations occur with these scores, regardless of treatment. For example, in a study on the stability of "normal" children's depression self-rating scores, Finch, Saylor, Edwards, and McIntosh (1987) found significant declines in the scores between the first and subsequent administrations (2, 4, and 6 weeks later). Similarly, Nelson and Politano (1990) found significant decrements in 6- to 15-year-old inpatient children's depression self-rating scale scores from the time of the first administration to the time of the second and third administration (10 and 30 days later, respectively).

In the context of treatment evaluation, therefore, it is not clear how to interpret an observed decrease in a self-rating score. On the one hand, it may be interpreted as children's subjective reporting of reduced symptoms, and thus as a reflection of treatment efficacy. On the other hand, it may reflect an artifact of the rating scale, related in part to the heterogeneity of anxious or depressed samples' actual fluctuations in these states (Nelson & Politano, 1990). In light of the ambiguities involved in interpreting self-rating scale scores' fluctuations, Finch et al. (1987) suggested that when child self-rating scales are being used in the evaluation of treatment outcome, the scales should be administered at least twice prior to the actual intervention—once at the initial screening or assessment, and a second time immediately prior to treatment. This could help prevent the drawing of erroneous conclusions that "treatment worked," based on observed decreases in self-rating scale scores (decreases that might be observed even before the initiation of treatment). It is rare, however, for Finch et al.'s (1987) suggestion to be implemented in research or clinical contexts.

Attenuation in children's responding is not unique to self-rating scales. Symptom scale scores of interview schedules also show decrements in respondents' reporting of symptoms over time (Silverman & Eisen, 1992). Thus, as with rating scales, caution is warranted when one is interpreting observed declines in interview schedules' symptom scale scores. These declines may be due to factors extraneous to the intervention itself, and need to be carefully considered.

Evaluating the Role of Mediators and Moderators

Investigators are frequently interested not only in evaluating of treatment effects on targeted symptoms or behaviors, but also in determining the variables that may mediate or moderate treatment outcome. Many different variables can mediate or moderate intervention outcome, including anxiety and depression. For example, La Greca, Dandes, Wick, Shaw, and Stone (1988) have suggested that social anxiety may serve as an important moderator in children's peer relations. In an intervention aimed at improving children's peer relations, therefore, it might be useful to administer the Social Anxiety Scale for Children—Revised (La Greca & Stone, 1993) and to examine children's scores on the scale as a moderator of outcome. This might also be done using an adolescent version of the scale, the Social Anxiety Scale for Adolescents, if one is working to improve adolescents' peer relations (La Greca & Lopez, 1998).

Variables that are related to anxiety and depression may also serve as mediators or moderators of treatment outcome. Such variables may include feelings of hopelessness or fear. Self-rating scales have been designed specifically to assess some of these related variables. Of all available assessment procedures, self-rating scales are best suited to assess the role that anxiety and depression or other related variables play as potential mediators or moderators of intervention outcome.

EVALUATIVE DESCRIPTIONS OF ANXIETY AND DEPRESSION SELF-RATING SCALES FOR CHILDREN

It should be apparent from the preceding discussion that from a pragmatic perspective, to say that an assessment method is "best" means to be useful or clinically feasible in a specific context. It also means choosing the method that ultimately is most useful for accomplishing a specific goal or solving a specific problem in a particular context. "Best" or "most useful" is thus a concept to be evaluated in relation to a particular problem and the actual (and foreseeable) alternatives for solving that problem.

In this part of the chapter, we present evaluative descriptions of child anxiety and depression self-rating scales. Guided by our pragmatic orientation, we focus in these descriptions on those normative concepts that are most significant for the contexts in which most researchers and clinicians work—namely, scientific evidence of utility (i.e., reliability and validity). This section is not exhaustive in scope; it mainly illustrates the types of research studies that have been conducted and highlights areas that require further research. In addition, emphasis is placed on rating scales that are most widely used and that have an established research literature. Because of this emphasis, we do not review two recently developed measures: the Multidimensional Anxiety Scale for Children (March, Parker, Sullivan, Stallings, & Conners, 1997) and the Screen for Child Anxiety Related Emotional Disorders (Birmaher et al., 1997). We note, however, that the articles describing the development and initial psychometrics of these two measures (Birmaher et al., 1997; March et al., 1997) suggest that both of these measures show promise in assessing anxiety in children. Finally, in light of the proliferation of child self-rating scales in recent years, emphasis is also placed in this chapter on scales that assess the general constructs of anxiety and depression, not specific facets of these constructs (e.g., test anxiety, social anxiety) or related constructs (e.g., fear, hopelessness).

Self-Rating Scales for Anxiety

Revised Children's Manifest Anxiety Scale

The RCMAS (Reynolds & Richmond, 1978, 1985), a downward extension of the Manifest Anxiety Scale for adults (Taylor, 1953), is the most widely used self-rating scale for childhood anxiety. Developed for use with school-age children, this 37-item measure is a revision of Castaneda, McCandless, and Palermo's (1956) Children's Manifest Anxiety Scale. In addition to yielding a total anxiety score, the RCMAS yields three factor scale scores (i.e., Physiological Anxiety, Worry/Oversensitivity, and Social Concerns/Concentration), as well as a Lie scale score (e.g., "I am always nice to everyone," "I never lie").

The internal consistency of the RCMAS total scale score has been extensively studied (Reynolds & Richmond, 1978). In an initial report of internal consistency obtained during the development phase of the RCMAS, an alpha coefficient of .83 was found for the total score, based on a sample of 329 children aged 5 to 17 (Reynolds & Richmond, 1978). Reynolds and Paget (1981) reported a similar alpha coefficient (.82) for the total score during the standardization phase, based on a sample of 4,972 children (aged 6 to 19). The alpha coefficients were also found to be high for the different ethnic (primarily European American, African American, and Hispanic), grade, and gender subsample total scores, with the one exception being the alpha coefficients found for African American girls who were younger than 12 years old (alpha = .69). Alpha coefficients greater than .80 have been found for the RCMAS total score in other diverse samples, including children in kindergarten (Reynolds, Bradley, & Steele, 1980), children with learning disabilities (Paget & Reynolds, 1984), and English-speaking children from Nigeria (Pela & Reynolds, 1982).

The internal consistency of the RCMAS factor scores has not been as extensively studied as that of the RCMAS total scale. The RCMAS manual (Reynolds & Richmond, 1985) reports alpha coefficients of .64 to .76 for each of the three anxiety factor scales across ages 6 to 19 for the standardization sample, with the Worry/Oversensitivity factor scale being the most consistent (alpha = .76). In addition, the standardization sample yielded alpha coefficients greater than .60 across gender and ethnicity for the Lie scale of the RCMAS (Reynolds & Paget, 1981; Reynolds & Richmond, 1985). These coefficients were slightly lower and somewhat more variable among children younger than 11 years of age.

In evaluating a scale's test–retest reliability, including that of the RCMAS, it is important to consider the influence of study design variables. These include the length of the retest interval, as well as the age of the participants. Consider, for example, the length of the retest interval. In a sample of 534 elementary school children in which a 9-month retest interval was used, reliability coefficients of .68 and .58 were found for the total scale and the Lie scale, respectively (Reynolds, 1981). In a sample of English-speaking Nigerian children in primary school in which a 3-week retest interval was used, reliability coefficients of .98 and .94 were found for the total scale and the Lie scale, respectively (Pela & Reynolds, 1982). In terms of age, higher reliability coefficients have been found with samples of older children than with younger children (e.g., Reynolds & Richmond, 1985).

The construct validity of the RCMAS has been examined by means of various research methods. One common method has been the use of factor analysis. The results of these factor-analytic studies have been generally consistent (e.g., Reynolds & Richmond, 1979; Reynolds & Paget, 1981; Reynolds & Scholwinski, 1985), as well as conforming to the factor structure reported earlier for the Children's Manifest Anxiety Scale (Finch, Kendall, & Montgomery, 1974). From principal-components factor analysis with varimax rotations, a three-factor solution (Worry/Oversensitivity, Physiological, Anxiety, and Social Concerns/Concentration) plus the Lie factor scale has emerged. This factor structure has been found in a variety of samples, including the standardization sample of over 4,900 children (Reynolds & Paget, 1981), school children diagnosed with learning disabilities (Paget & Reynolds, 1984), children viewed as "gifted" (Reynolds & Scholwinski, 1985), and children from an elementary school in Spain (with whom a Spanish version was used; Ferrando, 1994).

In terms of the convergent validity of the RCMAS, using a monomethod research strategy, Reynolds (1982) correlated the total RCMAS score with the scores obtained on another anxiety measure—namely, the STAIC (Spielberger, 1973; discussed below). A significant correlation was found ($r = .85$) between the RCMAS total score and the STAIC Trait scale score for 42 children aged 6 to 16, but not between the RCMAS total score and the State scale score. A similar pattern of correlations was found in additional studies conducted by Reynolds: one involving a sample of third- and fourth-graders (Reynolds, 1982), and one involving a sample of children and adolescents with "high IQs" (i.e., scores higher than 130) (Reynolds, 1985). Subsequent studies have since reported a positive association between total scores on the RCMAS and scores on other measures of trait anxiety, as well as scores reflecting related constructs such as fear (e.g., Hoehn-Saric, Maisami, & Wiegand, 1987; Lee, Piersel, Friedlander, & Collamer, 1988; Perrin & Last, 1992; Wisniewski, Mulick, Genshaft, & Coury, 1987).

Although results from the studies just cited are often taken as support for the validity of the RCMAS, it has been noted that these significant correlation coefficients may be spurious because the same source (i.e., the child) has completed the measures and/or because the same method (i.e., self-report) has been used (e.g., Finch et al., 1989). This has fueled investigations that have involved either multisource (e.g., child–parent, child–teacher; Moretti, Fine, Haley, & Marriage, 1985; Reynolds, 1982) or multimethod assessments (e.g., self-report and behavior observation; Hoehn-Saric et al., 1987). It has also fueled multitrait–multimethod investigations, along the lines described by Campbell and Fiske (1959).

A multitrait–multimethod assessment approach allows for the simultaneous evaluation of a scale's convergent and divergent validity. An example is a study conducted by Wolfe and colleagues (1987) with a sample of 102 inpatient children aged 6 to 16. Specifically, Wolfe et al. (1987) correlated the children's RCMAS total scores with their scores from other child self-rating scales of anxiety (the STAIC) and depression (the CDI; Kovacs, 1981) as well as with scores from a teacher rating scale (the Teacher's Report Form of the Child Behavior Checklist; Achenbach, 1991). Although the convergent validity of the RCMAS was supported by a significant and positive correlation between the RCMAS total scores and the STAIC Trait scale scores, the correlation between the RCMAS total scores and the teacher-rated anxiety scores was not significant. This finding supports the view that the demonstration of validity through significant correlations between child self-rating scales is problematic, because these correlations are likely to be spurious due to source variance. However, although a low correlation between ratings of different sources is often viewed as a demonstration of inadequate validity, it may also be a reflection of the different perspectives of sources. Generally speaking, confusion about "validity" lies with confusion about the "gold standard" or the final criterion of validity that will stand as the basis for all comparisons.

In addition to convergent validity, the findings of Wolfe et al. (1987) raise concerns about the divergent validity of the RCMAS (as well as the STAIC Trait scale and the CDI). Specifically, all of the children's total scores on the RCMAS, the STAIC Trait scale, and the CDI, respectively, were intercorrelated. Wolfe et al. (1987) discussed these findings in terms of the broad-band construct of negative affectivity, discussed earlier in this chapter. The authors further noted that the observed intercorrelations are not surprising, given the substantial overlap of many of the items contained on each measure.

Unlike the substantial amount of attention paid to the validity of the RCMAS total score, much less attention has been paid to the validity of the factor scale scores. One study examined the validity of the RCMAS Physiological Anxiety factor scale in a sample of 80 male students aged 10 to 17 (Lee, Piersel, & Unruh, 1989). Specifically, when behavioral ratings from parents and teachers were used as measures of comparison, neither convergent nor divergent validity was evidenced. This study was limited to male subjects, however, and lacked a more direct, objective index of physiological functioning. Additional research examining the validity of the RCMAS Physiological Anxiety factor scale and the other factor scales is needed.

Investigators have also examined whether the RCMAS total score is useful in discriminating among groups of children who would be expected to differ in their levels of anxiety, such as psychiatrically referred anxious children, psychiatrically referred nonanxious children, and nonreferred children. The ability of the RCMAS to do so has been used to support the measure's discriminant or descriptive validity; however, the findings in this area have been uneven (e.g., Bell-Dolan, Last, & Strauss, 1990; Hodges, 1990; Hoehn-Saric et al., 1987; Last, 1991; Last, Francis, & Strauss, 1989; Mattison & Bagnato, 1987; Mattison et al., 1988; Perrin & Last, 1992). For example, Mattison et al. (1988) reported that in a sample of 8- to 12-year-old outpatient boys, those diagnosed with DSM-III overanxious disorder scored significantly higher than boys with dysthymic disorder or attention deficit disorder on the Worry/Oversensitivity and Physiological Anxiety factor scales of the RCMAS. On the other hand, Hodges (1990), in her examination of several child self-rating scales (including the RCMAS) in anxious, depressed, and conduct-disordered psychiatric inpatients aged 6 to 13, reported that the RCMAS could not differentiate among these three groups. Perrin and Last (1992), using a sample of 213 outpatient boys aged 5 to 17, diagnosed with either DSM-III-R anxiety disorders, attention-deficit/hyperactivity disorder, or no psychiatric disorder, similarly found that the RCMAS could not differentiate between boys with anxiety disorders and boys with attention-deficit/hyperactivity disorder. However, the RCMAS could differentiate between boys with anxiety disorders and boys with no psychiatric disorder.

In both the Mattison et al. (1988) and the Hodges (1990) studies, the diagnostic utility of the RCMAS was further evaluated by calculating the scale's sensitivity and specificity (see earlier discussion). As noted earlier, both investigators found the RCMAS to be better at identifying "noncases" than "cases."

There are several reasons for the unevenness found in the discriminant validity and diagnostic utility of the RCMAS. As noted, one reason may be that the RCMAS primarily assesses the broad-band construct of negative affectivity. Another reason may be the high levels of comorbidity among clinic-referred participants (Costello & Angold, 1988). Yet another reason may be the presence of broad, nonanxious items in the scale (e.g., Finch et al., 1989).

In summary, when the validity of the RCMAS has been examined in ways that include both the simple monomethod approach and the multitrait–multimethod approach, the picture that has emerged is mixed. Studies that have compared different samples of children have similarly yielded mixed results with respect to the scale's discriminant validity. The diagnostic utility of the RCMAS, particularly in terms of identifying true cases, has been uneven as well. Finally, the validity of the RCMAS factor scales has been insufficiently studied by researchers.

State–Trait Anxiety Inventory for Children

The STAIC (Spielberger, 1973) is a downward extension of an anxiety inventory designed for adults, the State–Trait Anxiety Inventory (STAI; Spielberger, Gorsucth, & Lushene, 1970). (For a critique of the construct of trait anxiety, the reader is referred to Reiss, 1997.) The STAIC is made up of two 20-item scales, the Trait scale and the State scale. The Trait scale is designed to assess children's chronic, cross-situational anxiousness (e.g., "I worry about making mistakes"). Children are asked to rate on a 3-point scale ("hardly ever," "sometimes," "often") how often they experience these feelings. The State scale is designed to assess time-limited, transitory anxiousness (e.g., "I feel [very calm/calm/not calm] right now").

The internal consistency of the STAIC has been found to be satisfactory, with alpha coefficients in the .80 to .90 range for the State scale and approximately .80 for the Trait scale, based on a sample of 246 school children between the ages of 9 and 12 (Spielberger, 1973). Test–retest reliability estimates for the Trait scale have ranged between .45 (Finch, Montgomery, & Deardorff, 1974) and .71 (Spielberger, 1973), depending on the study design variables mentioned earlier (i.e., length of retest interval, age of subjects).

In terms of the validity of the STAIC, the picture that emerges is generally similar to that for the RCMAS. That is, monomethod research strategies in which STAIC scores are correlated with other anxiety self-rating scores yield significant and positive correlations (e.g., Hoehn-Saric et al., 1987; Perrin & Last, 1992; Spielberger, 1973). For example, Perrin and Last (1992) reported that scores on the STAIC State and Trait scales (which contained seven additional items that assessed somatic symptoms) correlated .62 and .36 with the RCMAS, respectively. Hoehn-Saric et al. (1987) also reported significant correlations between the STAIC and RCMAS in 63 inpatient children.

Another study evaluated the concurrent and factorial validity of the Trait scale of the STAIC among a nonclinical sample of 157 adolescents (Carey, Faulstich, & Carey, 1994). In a randomly selected subsample of 88 adolescents, statistically significant correlations were found between the total and factor scale scores of the STAIC and the RCMAS (r's ranged from .17 to .28; all p's < .006). The authors pointed out that these correlations, although significant, were lower than those found in earlier studies with younger children. In regard to the factorial validity of the Trait scale of the STAIC, principal-component analyses resulted in a factor structure similar to that found in previous factor-analytic studies with younger children (e.g., Finch, Kendall, & Montgomery, 1976). Specifically, a two-factor solution was found to be optimal; the first factor consisted of items assessing general unhappiness and indecisiveness (accounting for 29.5% of the variance), and the second factor consisted of items assessing physiological and cognitive aspects of anxiety (accounting for 8.1% of the variance). The investigators also examined the relations between the respective factor scores from the STAIC and the STAI and these relations were found to be low. For example, the correlation found between the children's total Trait scores accounted for only 21% of the variance. According to Carey et al. (1994), these findings raise questions about the comparability of the construct of trait anxiety when the STAIC and the STAI are used with adolescents, and they highlight the need for further research on the measurement of trait anxiety with this population.

For an evaluation of the STAIC's validity using a multitrait–multimethod approach, the reader is referred to the Wolfe et al. (1987) study described in connection with the RCMAS, as this study also included the STAIC. As noted, children's total scores on the RCMAS, the STAIC Trait scale, and the CDI, respectively, were intercorrelated. For example, the STAIC Trait and State subscale scores were highly correlated with scores on the CDI (r = .36 and .52, respectively).

The research findings are also uneven with respect to the STAIC's discriminant validity. For example, although Hodges (1990) found that the RCMAS could differentiate between the anxiety-disordered and non-anxiety-disordered children in an inpatient sample, the STAIC could not. Perrin and Last (1992), however, found that the STAIC, like the RCMAS, could not differentiate between boys with DSM-III-R anxiety disorders and boys with attention-deficit/hyperactivity disorder—only between boys with anxiety disorders and boys with no psychiatric disorders. Perhaps the different samples employed in these two studies (inpatient boys and girls aged 6 to 13 in Hodges, 1990; outpatient boys aged 5 to 17 in Perrin & Last, 1992) account for the different results.

Research examining the sensitivity and specificity of the STAIC has obtained findings similar to those for the RCMAS (e.g., the scale is better in identifying "noncases" than "cases"). For example, Hodges (1990) found the STAIC to have a sensitivity of 42% and a specificity of 79%.

In summary, the STAIC appears to be reliable, as evidenced by moderate to high coefficients of internal consistency and stability. As for the RCMAS, however, the findings are uneven with respect to validity, both in multitrait–multimethod research studies and in studies comparing groups of children who would be expected to differ in their levels of anxiety. Further research attention also needs to be paid to examining the scale's validity with adolescents. Research findings on the STAIC's sensitivity and specificity have found the scale to be better in identifying noncases than cases.

Specific Self-Rating Scales for Anxiety

For researchers and clinicians interested in assessing more specific facets of childhood anxiety, several self-rating scales exist. Some of the more commonly used scales include the Test Anxiety Scale for Children (Sarason, Davidson, Lighthall, Waite, & Ruebush, 1960), the Social Anxiety Scale for Children—Revised (La Greca & Stone, 1993), the Social Phobia and Anxiety Inventory for Children (Beidel, Turner, & Morris, 1995), and the Childhood Anxiety Sensitivity Index (Silverman, Fleisig, Rabian, & Peterson, 1991). With the exception of the Test Anxiety Scale for Children, all of these specific self-rating scales for anxiety have been developed relatively recently, and research on them is ongoing. The research findings that have been accumulating on these measures are positive, however, and provide supportive evidence for their utility in assessing specific facets of anxiety in children.

For example, the Childhood Anxiety Sensitivity Index, a downward extension of the Anxiety Sensitivity Index (Reiss, Peterson, Gursky, & McNally, 1986), was designed to assess children's fears of a variety of anxiety symptoms, in accordance with Reiss's (1991) expectancy theory of anxiety (see Silverman & Weems, 1999, for a review). The Childhood Anxiety Sensitivity Index has been found to possess satisfactory reliability and validity (Silverman et al., 1991), to predict variance beyond that explained by trait anxiety in both younger and older children (Weems, Hammond-Laurence, Silverman, & Ginsburg, 1998), to predict panic in adolescents (Lau, Calamari, & Waraczynski, 1996), to be capable of differentiating between children with and without panic disorder (Kearney, Albano, Eisen, Allan, & Barlow, 1997), to be significantly related to fear scores after an anxiety-evoking challenge procedure (Rabian, Embry, & MacIntyre, 1999), to have a hierarchical factorial structure similar to that of the adult version (Silverman, Ginsburg, & Goedhart, in press), and to be a sensitive index of clinical change in intervention outcome research (Eisen & Silverman, 1998; Ollendick, 1995).

Silverman also recently completed a study with colleagues Golda Ginsburg and Annette La Greca that provided support for the utility of the Social Anxiety Scale for Children—Revised (La Greca & Stone, 1993) in assessing social anxiety among a clinic sample of children aged 6 to 11 with anxiety disorders (n = 154) (Ginsburg, La Greca, & Silverman, 1998). Specifically, factor analysis supported the original three-factor solution, and internal consistencies were in the acceptable range. In addition, social anxiety was found to be associated with impairments in social and emotional functioning. Specifically, highly socially anxious children reported low levels of social acceptance and global self-esteem, as well as more negative peer interactions. Girls with high levels of social anxiety were also rated by parents as having poor social skills, particularly in the areas of assertive and responsible social behavior. These findings thus support the validity of the Social Anxiety Scale for Children—Revised as a measure of social anxiety for children with anxiety disorders.

Scales to Assess Related Constructs

Many researchers and clinicians interested in assessing childhood anxiety find it useful to assess related constructs. Of these, the construct of fear is perhaps most frequently assessed. Below we provide a brief description of the most widely used and extensively studied fear questionnaire, the Revised Fear Survey Schedule for Children (FSSC-R; Ollendick, 1983).

The FSSC-R, a revision of a scale developed originally by Scherer and Nakamura (1968), has been studied in American (Ollendick, 1983), Australian (Ollendick, King, & Frary, 1989), British (Ollendick, Yule, & Ollier, 1991), and Chinese (Dong, Yang, & Ollendick, 1994) children. The FSSC-R requires that children rate how much they fear 80 objects and events, using a 3-point scale ("none," "some," or "a lot"). Internal consistency coefficients for the FSSC-R range from .92 to .95; test–retest coefficients range from .55 (3 months) to .82 (1 week). In addition, significant correlations have been found between the FSSC-R and the anxiety self-rating scales, such as the Trait scale of the STAIC (r = close to .50; Ollendick, 1983).

In a study designed to investigate parameters of children's fear in terms of frequency of fearful thoughts and avoidance behavior (McCathie &

Spence, 1991), 376 non-clinic-referred children aged 7 to 12, were found to report high levels of fearful thoughts and avoidance behavior to those items that they rated highest on the FSSC-R, such as fears of injury, illness, death, and danger. However, many of these items were typically of low probability, leading the investigators to suggest that "everyday" sorts of fears may be overshadowed and underrated on the FSSC-R, and that children may rate items on the FSSC-R according to their affective response to the image or thought of the stimulus situations rather than their actual fear response. Further examination of this interesting hypothesis, using clinic-referred samples of children with anxiety disorders, would be worthwhile.

In a study of the FSSC-R with a clinical sample, Last, Francis, and Strauss (1989) found that although total fear scores on the FSSC-R did not differentiate children with different types of anxiety disorders (i.e., children with separation anxiety disorder vs. overanxious disorder vs. "phobia of school"), the specific types of fears endorsed by these children did differ. For example, children with separation anxiety disorder most commonly endorsed a fear of getting lost; children with overanxious disorder most commonly endorsed social and performance fears (e.g., "being teased").

In a recent study that extended the findings of Last et al. (1989), the discrimination of children's phobias was examined for children's and parents' ratings of the children's fear on the FSSC-R; a clinic sample of children who met DSM-III-R criteria for phobic disorders ($N = 120$) was used (Weems, Silverman, Saavedra, Pina, & Lumpkin, 1999). Specifically, discriminant function analyses and item analyses were conducted to determine whether children meeting diagnostic criteria for a primary disorder of social phobia, simple phobia of the dark/sleeping alone, simple phobia of animals, or a simple phobia of shots/doctors could be differentiated on the bases of FSSC-R subscale scores and items.

Results indicated that the child- and parent-completed FSSC-Rs were similarly useful in differentiating the specific types of phobias. Results of the item analyses further indicated that child-completed FSSC-R items could discriminate the different simple phobias but not social phobia, and that parent-completed FSSC-R items could discriminate not only the different simple phobias but social phobia as well. The results suggest that the FSSC-R shows promise in the assessment of clinically significant fears in children with phobic disorders, and that both child and parent ratings are likely to have relative utility in this assessment.

Self-Rating Scales for Depression

Children's Depression Inventory

The CDI (Kovacs, 1981) is the most widely used self-rating scale of depressed mood in children. A downward extension of the Beck Depression Inventory, the CDI consists of 27 items that reflect affective, cognitive, and behavioral symptoms of depression. Designed for use with children aged 7 to 17, each item on the CDI presents three sentences describing states that range from asymptomatic to clinically symptomatic. A sample item is as follows: "I am sad once in awhile," "I am sad many times," and "I am sad all the time."

The psychometric properties of the CDI have been studied extensively since its development, with early efforts focusing on the scale's internal consistency and test–retest reliability, and with more recent efforts focusing on the scale's validity. In terms of the CDI's internal consistency, the most recent revision of the CDI manual (Kovacs, 1992) reported an alpha coefficient of .86, based on the CDI's normative sample (1,266 students aged 7 to 16). Other researchers have reported similarly high coefficients in diverse samples (e.g., Finch, Saylor, & Edwards, 1985; Kovacs, 1983; Ollendick & Yule, 1990; Smucker, Craighead, Craighead, & Green, 1986; Weiss et al., 1991). For example, Ollendick and Yule (1990) reported alpha coefficients of .85 and .87 for samples of 336 American and 327 British school children (ages 8 to 10), respectively. Similarly, alpha coefficients greater than .80 were reported by Smucker et al. (1986) for three samples of Pennsylvania school children (aged 8 to 16). Internal consistency of the CDI has also been found in clinic samples of children. For example, in clinic samples of 515 children aged 8 to 12 and 768 adolescents aged 13 to 16, Weiss et al. (1991) found alpha coefficients (.86 and .88, respectively) similar to those found in nonclinic samples (e.g., Ollendick & Yule, 1990).

In terms of the CDI's test–retest reliability, once again the findings are influenced by study design variables, such as the length of the retest interval (e.g., Finch et al., 1987; Kovacs, 1981; Nelson & Politano, 1990). In Kovacs's (1992) review of this issue, the conclusion was that in studies in which the retest intervals were less than 1 month, the reliability coefficients were between .65 and .85; in studies in which the retest intervals were greater than 1 month, the reliability coefficients were between .40 to .55. Kovacs (1992) further pointed out that the CDI purportedly assesses a state, not a trait; thus the selection of an "appropriate" test–retest interval is questionable.

In addition to the length of the retest interval, another important study design contribution that influences the CDI's reliability is whether the sample used is clinic- or non-clinic-based. Test–retest reliability has been found to be higher in non-clinic-based samples than in clinic-based samples (e.g., Finch et al., 1987; Kazdin, French, Unis, & Esveldt-Dawson, 1983; Kovacs, 1983; Nelson & Politano, 1990; Smucker et al., 1986; Weiss & Weisz, 1988). Overall, additional research is needed on how these and other study design variables influence the reliability of CDI scores (Kazdin, 1990).

The construct validity of the CDI has been examined via factor-analytic procedures (e.g., Helsel & Matson, 1984; Hodges, Siegel, Mullins, & Griffin, 1983; Kovacs, 1985; Saylor et al., 1984; Weiss & Weisz, 1988). In general, inconsistencies have appeared across studies with respect to the most meaningful factor solution (solutions have ranged from three to eight factors). For example, Saylor et al. (1984), using a principal-component factor analysis with varimax rotation, reported a seven-factor solution for a sample of 269 psychiatric child inpatients and an eight-factor solution for a sample of 294 school children (ages 7 to 11). Carey, Faulstich, Gresham, Ruggiero, and Enyart (1987), using similar analytic procedures, reported a three-factor solution for a sample of 306 clinic and nonclinic children aged 9 to 17. In a maximum-likelihood factor analysis using oblique rotation, Kovacs (1992) reported a five-factor solution for the normative sample of 1,266 school children. These factors were Negative Mood, Interpersonal Problems, Ineffectiveness, Anhedonia, and Negative Self-Esteem.

As part of the validation of the CDI, attention has been paid to how the scale's internal structure may vary across groups, such as different age groups. Knowledge of the structure of the CDI for different age groups may provide information about whether it is appropriate to use a single total score to summarize the CDI responses of a child of a particular age, or whether scale scores should be derived and used to reflect various groups of symptoms (Weiss et al., 1991). Weiss et al. (1991) also pointed out that knowledge of the CDI's internal structure across different age groups can help in determining whether it is appropriate to compare or combine CDI scores from such groups. This is important to know, because the structure of a construct must be equivalent across groups if one is to compare or combine these groups' scores.

Thus Weiss et al. (1991) examined the CDI's factor structure in 515 children aged 8 to 12 and 768 adolescents aged 13 to 16, drawn from diverse clinical sites. Using a nonorthogonal rotation, the investigators performed separate exploratory factor analyses for the two groups. The degree of similarity in the factor patterns was evaluated via several techniques, including confirmatory factor analysis and goodness-of-fit indices. Like Kovacs (1992), Weiss et al. found five factors for both age groups. However, the composition of the factors varied. Specifically, the factors found for the children were (1) Negative Affect (sad, lonely) with Somatic Complaints; (2) Externalizing Problems and Negative Self-Image; (3) School Problems; (4) Unloved; and (5) Negative Affect (upset). The factors found for the adolescents were (1) Negative Affect (sad, upset) with Somatic Complaints; (2) Negative Self-Image; (3) Anhedonic, Socially Isolated; (4) Externalizing Problems; and (5) School Problems. In addition, both groups produced a second-order, general depression factor, but the items loading on the factor differed somewhat for the two groups. For children, several externalizing behavior items loaded on the general factor; for adolescents, several vegetative items loaded on this factor.

In addition to developmental differences in the factor structure of the CDI, research suggests that the CDI factor structure may be different for clinic and nonclinic children (e.g., Hodges et al., 1983; Kovacs, 1985), although not all studies have found differences (Carey et al., 1987). Additional research is needed to clarify this issue.

The validity of the CDI has also been examined with monomethod research strategies. For example, CDI scores have been correlated with other measures of depression, as well as with related constructs; the correlations obtained have been moderate to high (i.e., r's have ranged from .44 to .62) (e.g., Kazdin, Esveldt-Dawson, Sherick, & Colbus, 1985; Kazdin et al., 1983; Matson & Nieminen, 1987; Reynolds, Anderson, & Bartell, 1985; Weissman, Orvaschel, & Padian, 1980). For example, in a sample of 95 behavior-disordered school children aged 11 to 18, the CDI correlated significantly ($r = .62$) with the Reynolds Adolescent Depression Scale (Reynolds et al., 1985).

In studies that have employed multisource or multitrait–multimethod methodology, the validity picture has been uneven (e.g., Doerfler, Felner, Rowlinson, Raley, & Evans, 1988; Hodges, 1990; Kovacs, 1981; Matson & Nieminen, 1987; Saylor et al., 1984; Wierzbicki, 1987; Wolfe et al., 1987). For example, Kovacs (1981) found a correlation of .55 between CDI scores and clinician global ratings of depression for a mixed sample of 78 clinic and nonclinic children aged 8 to 13. Similarly, Wierzbicki (1987) found a correlation of .66 between CDI scores and parent ratings of child depression (on a parent version of the CDI) for 45 nonclinic children aged 8 to 14. Matson and Nieminen (1987), on the other hand, found a low but significant correlation ($r = .33$) between CDI scores and teacher ratings of depression. Wolfe et al. (1987) found a nonsignificant correlation ($r = .17$) between CDI scores and teacher ratings. Saylor et al. (1984) also found no relation between CDI scores and peer ratings of depression.

The research findings on the ability of the CDI to discriminate among different groups of children are also mixed. Although several investigators have found that the CDI can discriminate clinic children with depression from nonclinic children, as well as clinic children with other psychiatric diagnoses (e.g., Haley, Fine, Marriage, Moretti, & Freeman, 1985; Hodges, 1990; McCauley, Burke, Mitchell, & Moss, 1988; Moretti et al., 1985), several investigators have found that CDI cannot make the latter discrimination (i.e., clinic depressed children from clinic children with other diagnoses) (e.g., Asarnow & Carlson, 1985; Fristad, Weller, Weller, & Teare, 1991; Kazdin, 1987; Kazdin et al., 1983; Nelson, Politano, Finch, Wendal, & Mayhall, 1987; Saylor et al., 1984). For example, using the CDI to compare 79 depressed inpatient or outpatient children, 49 psychiatric controls, and 19 "normal" controls (6 to 12 years old), Fristad et al. (1991) found that CDI scores could differentiate the depressed and psychiatric control sample from the "normal" sample, but could not differentiate between the two psychiatric samples. Similarly, in a sample of 185 inpatient children with DSM-III diagnoses established via interviews, Kazdin (1987) found that the CDI scores of depressed children were not significantly higher than the scores of children diagnosed with other psychiatric disorders.

Furthermore, research findings on the sensitivity and specificity of the CDI suggest that like the anxiety scales, it is better in its ability to "rule out" rather than "rule in" particular diagnoses. For example, using a cutoff score of 15, Asarnow and Carlson (1985) found a sensitivity of 54% and a specificity of 91%. Using a higher cutoff score of 19, which has been recommended (Kovacs, 1992) as a marker of clinical significance, Hodges (1990) found roughly similar sensitivity and specificity rates.

In the earlier discussion on the anxiety measures, we offered several reasons to help explain why there may be unevenness in the research with respect to discriminant validity and diagnostic utility. These same reasons are relevant for the CDI as well. These include the extent to which the CDI is assessing the broad-band construct of negative affectivity; the influence of high levels of comorbidity among diagnosed participants; and the inclusion of broad, nondepressed items in the scale (e.g., Hodges & Craighead, 1990; Weiss et al., 1991).

Other Child Self-Rating Scales for Depression

At about the same time as the CDI was being developed, efforts were being made in diverse research sites across the United States to develop other child self-rating scales for depression. Like the CDI, these scales were designed to assess specific symptoms of depression in children, though some had other special features (e.g., a card-sorting format). The initial reports on these measures (e.g., psychometric properties) appeared promising. However, relative to the steady flurry of systematic research during the 1980s and into the 1990s on the CDI, the rate of systematic research on most of these other self-rating measures was lower. It currently appears as though either research on some of these measures has been curtailed altogether, or research may still be in progress, with the most recent findings not yet published. As a result, there is an inordinate imbalance in the literature, with research articles on the CDI predominant.

In previous reviews of children's depression self-rating scales (Costello & Angold, 1988; Kazdin, 1990a) detailed reviews of these other children's self-rating scales for depression were provided. Relatively few new empirical findings have appeared on these measures since those reviews. In Table 5.1, a brief summary of these other child self-rating scales is presented.

As the table indicates, most of the measures are relatively brief and can be quickly administered. The Children's Depression Scale, which contains 66 items, is an exception. Because of its length, this scale allows for the most detailed study of depressive symptomatology (e.g., affect, self-esteem), and it provides coverages in areas not sufficiently covered by the other scales (e.g., positive symptoms). In terms of age-appropriateness, three of these self-

TABLE 5.1. Other Children's Self-Rating Scales of Depression

Measure	Items/response format	Age range	Summary
Children's Depression Scale (Lang & Tisher, 1978)	66 items (48 depressive, 18 positive); symptoms over past week; available in card-sorting and paper-and-pencil formats; five depressive subscales	7 to 11	Fair coverage of DSM-II criteria; many items unique to this scale; high stability (.74 over 2 weeks) and internal consistency (>.90); high convergent validity with CDI (.70–.84); good discriminant validity for inpatients and outpatients
Center for Epidemiologic Studies Depression Scale (Weissman, Orvaschel, & Padian, 1980)	20 items assessing symptoms over past week, rated on 0–4 scale; child and parent forms; cutoff of 16	6 to 17	Only 8 items related to DSM-II; moderate stability (.51–.59); moderate convergent validity with CDI (.44, stronger for adolescents); unproven discriminant validity; low sensitivity
Depression Self-Rating Scale (Birleson, 1981; Birleson, Hudson, Buchanon, & Wolff, 1987)	18 items reflecting affective, cognitive symptoms over past week; scored on 3-point scale; child version only; recommended cutoff of 15	7 to 23	Empirically derived items; moderate to high reliability and internal consistency; high convergent validity with CDI (.81); cutoff of 13 to 15 yields sensitivity > 64%, specificity > 75%
Mood and Feelings Questionnaire (Angold, Costello, & Pickles, 1987)	32 items rated on a 3-point scale, covering symptoms over the past 2 weeks; child and parent versions; cutoff varies by version	8 to 17	Items based on DSM-III-R or clinical significance; no items unique to this scale; 1-week test–retest reliability of .72; Some evidence of discriminant validity for inpatients; screening efficiency of 32%
Reynolds Child Depression Scale (Reynolds, 1989)	30-item self-report format; 4-point Likert scale; child and parent versions	8 to 11	Assesses DSM-III-R criteria; large normative sample; adequate stability over 3–4 months (.85); high internal consistency (r = .88–92); moderate criterion validity (r = .68–.79); limited age range.

rating scales were designed for use with children in the middle age range (from ages 7 to 13), with the Reynolds Child Depression Scale having the most narrow age range (ages 8 to 11). Two of the rating scales—the Center for Epidemiologic Studies Depression Scale and the Mood and Feelings Questionnaire—are also appropriate for use with adolescents.

In terms of psychometric properties, the Children's Depression Scale has been (and continues to be) the most extensively studied. Studies have found that this scale possesses high stability and internal consistency (e.g., Clarizio, 1984; Kazdin, 1987), and that depressed samples score higher than nondepressed samples (e.g., Kazdin, 1987; Knight, Hensley, & Waters, 1988; for the most recent review, see Tisher, Lang-Takac, & Lang, 1992).

In sum, a handful of other child self-rating scales are available for assessing depression in children, but none of them have received as much systematic research attention as the CDI. More careful, systematic comparative studies of some of these measures are needed, to help clarify the specific functions or goals for which each may be most useful in the assessment of childhood depression.

Scales to Assess Related Constructs

Several measures exist for assessing constructs that relate to depression. The more commonly used measures include the Hopelessness Scale for Children (HSC; Kazdin, Rodgers, & Colbus, 1986), the Children's Attributional Style Questionnaire (Kaslow, Tanenbaum, & Seligman, 1981), and the Automatic Thoughts Questionnaire (Kazdin, 1990b).

Of these measures, the HSC has perhaps received the most research attention. Designed to measure "hopelessness," a construct that is central to cognitive theories of depression (Beck, 1967), this scale measures how much hope children have for themselves, the world, and the future. The 17-item true–false HSC has adequate internal consistency (>.69) for both clinic and nonclinic samples, and moderate stability (>.45) for periods of up to 10 weeks (Spirito, Williams, Stark, & Hart, 1988). The HSC has also been found to correlate significantly with children's ratings on the CDI ($r = .71$), and to differentiate suicide attempters from nonattempters (e.g., Kazdin, French, Unis, Esveldt-Dawson, & Sherick, 1983; Spirito et al., 1988). The evidence is mixed, however, as to whether the HSC can differentiate clinic children with depression from clinic children with other psychiatric disorders (Benfield, Palmer, Pfefferbaum, & Stowe, 1988; Kazdin et al., 1986).

FUTURE RESEARCH DIRECTIONS

Throughout this chapter, future avenues of research have been delineated. In our view, progress is most likely to be made if researchers adopt a pragmatic frame in their evaluation (and use) of assessment methods, including child self-rating scales for anxiety and mood disorders. That is, researchers should pay particular attention to discerning the particular contexts or settings wherein these scales can be used (i.e., clinical feasibility), and to discerning the specific goals (or problems) that child self-rating scales can achieve (or solve). A pragmatic frame should involve a careful examination of the actual and foreseeable alternatives (i.e., other possible methods of assessment) for achieving goals or solving problems. This will involve comparing child self-rating scales with other assessment procedures, including structured diagnostic interviews, parent/clinician symptom checklists, and behavioral observations, with an eye toward carefully specifying the types of problems that each of these assessment procedures can "best" solve.

The rating scales themselves also need to undergo systematic comparative analyses. We have noted earlier in the chapter, for example, that a scale that is useful for measuring symptoms will not necessarily perform well as a screen or criterion measure. Rating scales should be developed and evaluated differentially in terms of how well they fulfill specific goals and functions, and should be compared along these lines.

Moreover, it is evident that the results obtained from these types of studies will be influenced by various study design or contextual contributions, such as the population from which the sample has been drawn (e.g., inpatient vs. outpatient vs. nonclinic), the ages of the children, and so forth. Precise, systematic analysis is needed to determine how these design/contextual contributions differentially influence the various scales' scores. Once these issues are clarified, researchers can turn their attention to refining the child self-rating scales so that they can more successfully perform particular functions or meet certain goals. Watson and Kendall's (1988) suggestion regarding the improvement of the scales' distinctiveness in terms of the measurement of anxiety versus depression is one example of a refinement that may be worthwhile.

Research examining the application of computer-assisted rating scales is also warranted. There are several advantages of such application. For instance, printed reports that summarize the results of individual rating scales can be produced for clinicians immediately upon the completion of each scale, while data collected during the assessment process can be stored for later data analysis (Sawyer, Sarris, & Baghurst, 1991).

In addition, computer-assisted rating scales may, through graphics and printed reports, provide immediate feedback for children and families (Skinner & Pakula, 1986). Because of the advantages of computer-assisted methods, it is of interest whether computer-assisted rating scales yield the same information and scores as do rating scales administered in paper-and-pencil format. A study addressing this issue (Sawyer et al., 1991) found that the scores obtained with a computer-assisted parent rating scale (i.e., the Child Behavior Checklist) did not differ from the scores obtained with the standard written checklist. Whether such findings would be obtained for a child-completed rating scale would be well worth examining.

SUMMARY

In this chapter, we have described child self-rating scales for assessing anxiety and mood disorders. Within our pragmatic frame, we have discussed how child self-rating scales are better suited to meet certain goals or to perform certain functions than others. The ease with which self-rating scales can be administered to children and scored by researchers/clinicians makes these scales highly suitable for use in research and clinical settings. The use of these scales is apt to persist because they contain symptoms and behaviors that are of interest to most researchers and clinicians. We hope that researchers and clinicians alike will use the information provided in this chapter to guide their assessment efforts with anxious and depressed children. To the extent that these efforts also lead to the availability of children's self-rating scales that are more scientifically grounded and clinically relevant, then substantial strides can be made in the assessment realm.

ACKNOWLEDGMENT

Preparation of this chapter was supported by Grants No. 44781 and No. 49680 from the National Institute of Mental Health.

NOTES

1. The term "pragmatism" was originally coined by Charles Sanders Pierce, the American logician and philosopher of science, to describe his theory of meaning. Pierce's principle of pragmatism was subsequently translated by William James into a theory of truth and by John Dewey, often called the "dean of American philosophy," into a theory of value.

REFERENCES

Achenbach, T. M. (1991). *Manual for the Teacher's Report Form and 1991 Profile*. Burlington, VT: University of Vermont, Department of Psychiatry.

American Psychiatric Association. (1994). *Diagnostic and statistical manual of mental disorders* (4th ed.). Washington, DC: Author.

Angold, A., Costello, E. J., Pickels, A., & Winder, F. (1987). *The development of a questionnaire for use in epidemiological studies of depression in children and adolescents.* Unpublished manuscript, London University.

Asarnow, J. R., & Carlson, G. A. (1985). Depression Self-Rating Scale: Utility with child psychiatric inpatients. *Journal of Consulting and Clinical Psychology, 53,* 491–499.

Beck, A. T. (1967). *Depression: Clinical, experimental, and theoretical aspects.* New York: Harper & Row.

Beidel, D. C., & Turner, S. M. (1988). Comorbidity of test anxiety and other anxiety disorders in children. *Journal of Abnormal Child Psychology, 16,* 275–287.

Beidel, D. C., Turner, S. M., & Morris, T. L. (1995). A new inventory to assess childhood social anxiety and phobia: The Social Phobia and Anxiety Inventory for Children. *Psychological Assessment, 7,* 73–79.

Bell-Dolan, D. J., Last, C. G., & Strauss, C. C. (1990). Symptoms of anxiety disorders in normal children. *Journal of the American Academy of Child and Adolescent Psychiatry, 29,* 759–765.

Benfield, C. Y., Palmer, D. J., Pfefferbaum, B., & Stowe, M. L. (1988). A comparison of depressed and nondepressed disturbed children on measures of attributional style, hopelessness, life stress, and temperament. *Journal of Abnormal Child Psychology, 16,* 397–410.

Birleson, P. (1981). The validity of depressive disorder in childhood and the development of a self-rating scale. *Journal of Child Psychology and Psychiatry, 22,* 73–88.

Birleson, P., Hudson, I., Buchanon, D. G., & Wolff, S. (1987). Clinical evaluation of a self-rating scale for depressive disorder in childhood (Depression Self-Rating Scale). *Journal of Child Psychology and Psychiatry and Allied Disciplines, 28,* 43–60.

Birmaher, B., Khetarpal, S., Brent, D., Cully, M., Balach, L., Kaufman, J., & McKenzie Neer, S. (1997). The Screen for Child Anxiety Related Emotional Disorders (SCARED): Scale construction and psychometric characteristics. *Journal of the American Academy of Child and Adolescent Psychiatry, 36,* 545–552.

Campbell, D. T., & Fiske, D. W. (1959). Convergent and discriminant validation by the multitrait–multimethod matrix. *Psychological Bulletin, 56,* 81–105.

Carey, M. P., Faulstich, M. E., & Carey, T. C. (1994). Assessment of anxiety in adolescents: Concurrent and factorial validities of the trait anxiety scale of Spielberger's State–Trait Anxiety Inventory for Children. *Psychological Reports, 75,* 331–338.

Carey, M. P., Faulstich, M. E., Gresham, F. M., Ruggiero, L., & Enyart, P. (1987). Children's Depression Inventory: Construct and discriminant validity across clinical and nonreferred (control) populations. *Journal of Consulting and Clinical Psychology, 55,* 755–761.

Carson, T. P. (1986). Assessment of depression. In A. R. Ciminero, K. S. Calhoun, & H. E. Adams (Eds.), *Handbook of behavioral assessment* (pp. 404–445). New York: Wiley.

Castaneda, A., McCandless, B., & Palermo, D. (1956). The children's form of the Manifest Anxiety Scale. *Child Development, 27,* 317–326.

Clarizio, H. F. (1984). Childhood depression: Diagnostic considerations. *Psychology in the Schools, 21,* 181–197.

Costello, E. J., & Angold, A. (1988). Scales to assess child and adolescent depression: Checklists, screens, and nets. *Journal of the American Academy of Child and Adolescent Psychiatry, 27,* 726–737.

Cronbach, L. J. (1970). *Essentials of psychological testing* (3rd ed.). New York: Harper & Row.

Crowley, S. L., & Emerson, E. N. (1996). Discriminant validity of self-reported anxiety and depression in children: Negative affectivity or independent constructs? *Journal of Clinical Child Psychology, 25,* 139–146.

Doerfler, L. A., Felner, R. D., Rowlinson, R. T., Raley, P., & Evans, E. (1988). Depression in children and adolescents: A comparative analysis of the utility and construct validity of two assessment measures. *Journal of Consulting and Clinical Psychology, 56,* 769–772.

Dong, Q., Yang, B., & Ollendick, T. H. (1994). Fears in Chinese children and adolescents and their relations to anxiety and depression. *Journal of Child Psychology and Psychiatry, 35,* 351–363.

Eisen, A. R., & Silverman, W. K. (1998). Prescriptive treatment for generalized anxiety disorder in children. *Behavior Therapy, 29,* 105–121.

Feldman, L. A. (1993). Distinguishing depression and anxiety in self-report: Evidence from confirmatory factor analysis on nonclinical and clinical samples. *Journal of Consulting and Clinical Psychology, 4,* 631–638.

Ferrando, P. J. (1994). Factorial structure of the Revised Children Manifest Anxiety Scale in a Spanish sample: Relation with Eysenck personality dimensions. *Personality and Individual Differences, 16,* 693–699.

Finch, A. J., Kendall, P. C., & Montgomery, L. E. (1974). Multidimensionality of anxiety in children: Factor structure of the Children's Manifest Anxiety Scale. *Journal of Abnormal Child Psychology, 2,* 331–336.

Finch, A. J., Kendall, P. C., & Montgomery, L. E. (1976). Qualitative difference in the experience of state–trait anxiety in emotionally disturbed and normal children. *Journal of Personality Assessment, 40,* 522–530.

Finch, A. J., Lipovsky, J. A., & Casat, C. D. (1989). Anxiety and depression in children and adolescents: Negative affectivity or separate constructs? In P. C. Kendall & D. Watson (Eds.), *Anxiety and depression: Distinctive and overlapping features* (pp. 171–196). San Diego, CA: Academic Press.

Finch, A. J., Montgomery, L. E., & Deardorff, P. A. (1974). The Children's Manifest Anxiety Scale: Reliability with emotionally disturbed children. *Psychological Reports, 34,* 658.

Finch, A. J., Saylor, C. F., & Edwards, G. L. (1985). Children's Depression Inventory: Sex and grade norms for normal children. *Journal of Consulting and Clinical Psychology, 53,* 424–425.

Finch, A. J., Saylor, C. F., Edwards, G. L., & McIntosh, J. A. (1987). Children's Depression Inventory: Reliability over repeated administrations. *Journal of Clinical Child Psychology, 16,* 339–341.

Fristad, M. A., Weller, R. A., Weller, E. B., & Teare, M. (1991). Comparison of the parent and child versions of the Children's Depression Inventory (CDI). *Annals of Clinical Psychiatry, 3,* 341–346.

Ginsburg, G. S., La Greca, A. M., & Silverman, W. K. (1998). Social anxiety in children with anxiety disorders: Relation with social and emotional functioning. *Journal of Abnormal Child Psychology, 26,* 175–186.

Goldfried, M. R., & Kent, R. N. (1972). Traditional versus behavioral personality assessment: A comparison of methodological and theoretical assumptions. *Psychological Bulletin, 77,* 409–420.

Gotlib, I. H. (1984). Depression and general psychopathology in university students. *Journal of Abnormal Psychology, 93,* 19–30.

Gotlib, I. H., & Meyer, J. P. (1986). Factor analysis of the Multiple Affect Adjective Check List: A separation of positive and negative affect. *Journal of Personality and Social Psychology, 50,* 1161–1165.

Hagborg, W. J. (1991). The Revised Children's Manifest Anxiety Scale and social desirability. *Educational and Psychological Measurement, 51*, 1161–1165.

Haley, G., Fine, S., Marriage, K., Moretti, M., & Freeman, R. (1985). Cognitive bias and depression in psychiatrically disturbed children and adolescents. *Journal of Consulting and Clinical Psychology, 53*, 535–537.

Hanley, J. A., & McNeil, B. J. (1982). The meaning and use of the area under a receiver operating characteristic (ROC) curve. *Radiology, 143*, 29–36.

Hayes, S. C., Nelson, R. O., & Jarrett, R. B. (1987). The treatment utility of assessment: A functional approach to evaluating assessment quality. *American Psychologist, 42*, 963–974.

Helsel, W. J., & Matson, J. L. (1984). The assessment of depression in children: The internal structure of the Child Depression Inventory (CDI). *Behaviour Research and Therapy, 22*, 289–298.

Hodges, K. (1990). Depression and anxiety in children: A comparison of self-report questionnaires to clinical interview. *Psychological Assessment, 2*, 376–381.

Hodges, K., & Craighead, W. E. (1990). Relationship of Children's Depression Inventory factors to diagnosed depression. *Journal of Consulting and Clinical Psychology, 2*, 489–492.

Hodges, K., Siegel, L. J., Mullins, L., & Griffin, N. (1983). Factor analysis of the Children's Depression Inventory. *Psychological Reports, 53*, 759–763.

Hoehn-Saric, E., Maisami, M., & Wiegand, D. (1987). Measurement of anxiety in children and adolescents using semistructured interviews. *Journal of the American Academy of Child and Adolescent Psychiatry, 26*, 541–545.

Ialongo, N., Edelsohn, G., Werthamer-Larsson, L., Crockett, L., & Kellam, S. (1993). Are self-reported depressive symptoms in first-grade children developmentally transient phenomena?: A further look. *Development and Psychopathology, 5*, 433–452.

James, W. (1981). *Pragmatism*. Indianapolis, IN: Hackett. (Original work published 1907)

Jensen, B. J., & Haynes, S. N. (1986). Self-report questionnaires and inventories. In A. R. Ciminero, K. S. Calhoun, & H. E. Adams (Eds.), *Handbook of behavioral assessment* (pp. 150–175). New York: Wiley.

Kaslow, N., Tanenbaum, R., & Seligman, M. E. P. (1981). *The KASTAN* (rev. ed.). Unpublished manuscript.

Kazdin, A. E. (1987). Children's Depression Scale: Validation with child psychiatric inpatients. *Journal of Child Psychology and Psychiatry, 28*, 29–41.

Kazdin, A. E. (1990a). Assessment of childhood depression. In A. M. La Greca (Ed.), *Through the eyes of the child* (pp. 189–233). Needham Heights, MA: Allyn & Bacon.

Kazdin, A. E. (1990b). Evaluation of the Automatic Thoughts Questionnaire: Negative cognitive processes and depression among children. *Psychological Assessment: A Journal of Consulting and Clinical Psychology, 2*, 73–79.

Kazdin, A. E., Colbus, D., & Rodgers, A. (1988). Assessment of depression and diagnosis of depressive disorder among psychiatrically disturbed children. *Journal of Abnormal Child Psychology, 14*, 499–515.

Kazdin, A. E., Esveldt-Dawson, K., Sherick, R. B., & Colbus, D. (1985). Assessment of overt behavior and childhood depression among psychiatrically disturbed children. *Journal of Consulting and Clinical Psychology, 53*, 201–210.

Kazdin, A. E., French, N. H., Unis, A. S., & Esveldt-Dawson, K. (1983). Assessment of childhood depression: Correspondence of child and parent ratings. *Journal of the American Academy of Child Psychiatry, 22*, 157–164.

Kazdin, A. E., French, N. H., Unis, A. S., Esveldt-Dawson, K., & Sherick, R. B. (1983).

Hopelessness, depression, and suicidal intent among psychiatrically disturbed inpatient children. *Journal of Consulting and Clinical Psychology, 51*, 504–510.

Kazdin, A. E., Rodgers, A., & Colbus, D. (1986). The Hopelessness Scale for Children: Psychometric characteristics and concurrent validity. *Journal of Consulting and Clinical Psychology, 54*, 241–245.

Kearney, C. A., Albano, A. M., Eisen, A. R., Allan, W. D., & Barlow, D. H. (1997). The phenomenology of panic disorder in youngsters: An empirical study of a clinical sample. *Journal of Anxiety Disorders, 11*, 49–62.

Kearney, C. A., & Silverman, W. K. (1990). A preliminary analysis of a functional model of assessment and treatment for school refusal behavior. *Behavior Modification, 14*, 340–366.

Kearney, C. A., & Silverman, W. K. (1993). Measuring the function of school refusal behavior: The School Refusal Assessment Scale. *Journal of Clinical Child Psychology, 22*, 85–96.

Kearney, C. A., & Silverman, W. K. (1996). The evolution and reconciliation of taxonomic strategies for school refusal behavior. *Clinical Psychology: Science and Practice, 3*, 339–354.

Kearney, C. A., & Silverman, W. K. (in press). Functionally-based prescriptive and nonprescriptive for children and adolescents with school refusal behavior. *Behavior Therapy*.

Kendall, P. C., Cantwell, D. P., & Kazdin, A. E. (1989). Depression in children and adolescents: Assessment issues and recommendations. *Cognitive Therapy and Research, 13*, 109–146.

King, N. J., Ollendick, T. H., & Gullone, E. (1991). Negative affectivity in children and adolescents: Relations between anxiety and depression. *Clinical Psychology Review, 11*, 441–459.

Knight, D., Hensley, V. R., & Waters, B. (1988). Validation of the Children's Depression Scale and the Children's Depression Inventory in a prepubertal sample. *Journal of Child Psychology and Psychiatry, 29*, 853–863.

Kovacs, M. (1981). Rating scales to assess depression in school-aged children. *Acta Paedopsychiatrica, 46*, 305–315.

Kovacs, M. (1983). *The Children's Depression Inventory: A self-rated depression scale for school-aged youngsters*. Unpublished manuscript, University of Pittsburgh School of Medicine.

Kovacs, M. (1985). The Children's Depression Inventory (CDI). *Psychopharmacology Bulletin, 21*, 995–998.

Kovacs, M. (1992). *Children's Depression Inventory manual*. North Tonawanda, NY: Multi-Health Systems.

La Greca, A. M. (1990). Issues and perspectives on the child assessment process. In A. M. La Greca (Ed.), *Through the eyes of the child* (pp. 3–17). Needham Heights, MA: Allyn & Bacon.

La Greca, A. M., Dandes, S. K., Wick, P., Shaw, K., & Stone, W. L. (1988). Development of the Social Anxiety Scale for Children: Reliability and concurrent validity. *Journal of Clinical Child Psychology, 17*, 84–91.

La Greca, A. M., & Lopez, N. (1998). Social anxiety among adolescents: Linkages with peer relations and friendships. *Journal of Abnormal Child Psychology, 26*, 83–94.

La Greca, A. M., & Stone, W. L. (1993). Social Anxiety Scale for Children—Revised: Factor structure and concurrent validity. *Journal of Clinical Child Psychology, 22*, 17–27.

Lang, M., & Tisher, M. (1978). *Children's Depression Scale*. Victoria, Australia: Australian Council for Educational Research.

Lang, P. J. (1977). Imagery in therapy: An information processing analysis of fear. *Behavior Therapy, 8*, 862–886.

Last, C. G. (1991). Somatic complaints in anxiety disordered children. *Journal of Anxiety Disorders, 18*, 125–138.

Last, C. G., Francis, G., & Strauss, C. C. (1989). Assessing fears in anxiety-disordered children with the Revised Fear Survey Schedule for Children (FSSC-R). *Journal of Clinical Child Psychology, 18*, 137–141.

Lau, J. J., Calamari, J. E., & Waraczynski, M. (1996). Panic attack symptomatology and anxiety sensitivity in adolescents. *Journal of Anxiety Disorders, 10*, 355–364.

Lee, S. W., Piersel, W. C., Friedlander, R., & Collamer, W. (1988). Concurrent validity of the Revised Children's Manifest Anxiety Scale (RCMAS) for adolescents. *Educational and Psychological Measurement, 48*, 429–433.

Lee, S. W., Piersel, W. C., & Unruh, L. (1989). Concurrent validity of the physiological subscale of the Revised Children's Manifest Anxiety Scale: A multitrait–multimethod analysis. *Journal of Psychoeducational Assessment, 7*, 246–254.

Lehmann, H. E. (1959). Psychiatric concepts of depression: Nomenclature and classification. *Canadian Psychiatric Association Journal Supplement, 4*, 51–52.

Loeber, R., Green, S. M., & Lahey, B. B. (1990). Mental health professionals' perceptions of the utility of children, mothers, and teachers as informants on child psychopathology. *Journal of Clinical Child Psychology, 19*, 136–143.

Lonigan, C. J., Carey, M. P., & Finch, A. J. (1994). Anxiety and depression in children and adolescents: Negative affectivity and the utility of self-reports. *Journal of Consulting and Clinical Psychology, 62*, 1000–1008.

March, J. S., Parker, J. D. A., Sullivan, K., Stallings, P., & Conners, C. K. (1997). The Multidimensional Anxiety Scale for Children (MASC): Factor structure, reliability, and validity. *Journal of the American Academy of Child and Adolescent Psychiatry, 36*, 554–564.

Mash, E. J., & Terdal, L. G. (1997). *Assessment of childhood disorders* (2nd ed.). New York: Guilford Press.

Matson, J. L., & Nieminen, G. S. (1987). Validity of measures of conduct disorder, depression, and anxiety. *Journal of Clinical Child Psychology, 16*, 151–157.

Mattison, R. E., & Bagnato, S. J. (1987). Empirical measurement of overanxious disorder in boys 8 to 12 years old. *Journal of the American Academy of Child and Adolescent Psychiatry, 26*, 536–540.

Mattison, R. E., Bagnato, S. J., & Brubaker, B. M. (1988). Diagnostic utility of the Revised Children's Manifest Anxiety Scale in children with DSM-III anxiety disorders. *Journal of Anxiety Disorders, 2*, 147–155.

McCathie, H., & Spence, S. H. (1991). What is the Revised Fear Survey Schedule for Children measuring? *Behaviour Research and Therapy, 29*, 495–502.

McCauley, E., Burke, P., Mitchell, J., & Moss, S. (1988). Cognitive attributes of depression in children and adolescents. *Journal of Consulting and Clinical Psychology, 56*, 903–908.

Moretti, M. M., Fine, S., Haley, G., & Marriage, K. (1985). Child and adolescent depression: Child-report versus parent-report information. *Journal of the American Academy of Child Psychiatry, 24*, 298–302.

Nelson, W. M., & Politano, P. M. (1990). Children's Depression Inventory: Stability over repeated administrations in psychiatric inpatient children. *Journal of Clinical Child Psychology, 19*, 254–256.

Nelson, W. M., Politano, P. M., Finch, A. J., Wendal, N., & Mayhall, C. (1987). Children's

Depression Inventory: Normative data and utility with emotionally disturbed children. *Journal of the American Academy of Child and Adolescent Psychiatry, 26,* 43–48.

Norvell, N., Brophy, C., & Finch, A. J. (1985). The relationship of anxiety to childhood depression. *Journal of Personality Assessment, 49,* 150–153.

Ollendick, T. H. (1983). Reliability and validity of the Revised Fear Survey Schedule for Children (FSSC-R). *Behaviour Research and Therapy, 21,* 395–399.

Ollendick, T. H. (1995). Cognitive behavioral treatment of panic disorder with agoraphobia in adolescents: A multiple baseline design analysis. *Behavior Therapy, 26,* 517–531.

Ollendick, T. H., King, N. J., & Frary, R. B. (1989). Fears in children and adolescents: Reliability and generalizability across gender, age, and nationality. *Behaviour Research and Therapy, 27,* 19–26.

Ollendick, T. H., & Yule, W. (1990). Depression in British and American children and its relation to anxiety and fear. *Journal of Consulting and Clinical Psychology, 58,* 126–129.

Ollendick, T. H., Yule, W., & Ollier, K. (1991). Fears in British children and their relationship to manifest anxiety and depression. *Journal of Child Psychology and Psychiatry, 32,* 321–331.

Paget, K. D., & Reynolds, C. R. (1984). Dimensions, levels, and reliabilities on the Revised Children's Manifest Anxiety Scale with learning disabled children. *Journal of Learning Disabilities, 17,* 137–141.

Pela, O. A., & Reynolds, C. R. (1982). Cross-cultural application of the Revised Children's Manifest Anxiety Scale: Normative and reliability data for Nigerian primary school children. *Psychological Reports, 51,* 1135–1138.

Perrin, S., & Last, C. G. (1992). Do childhood anxiety measures measure anxiety? *Journal of Abnormal Child Psychology, 20,* 567–578.

Rabian, B., Embry, L., & MacIntyre, D. (1999). Behavioral validation of the Childhood Anxiety Sensitivity Index in children. *Journal of Clinical Child Psychology, 28,* 105–112.

Rachman, S. J., & Hodgson, R. I. (1974). Synchrony and desynchrony in fear and avoidance. *Behaviour Research and Therapy, 12,* 311–318.

Reiss, S. (1991). Expectancy model of fear, anxiety, and panic. *Clinical Psychology Review, 11,* 141–153.

Reiss, S. (1997). Trait anxiety: It's not what you think it is. *Journal of Anxiety Disorders, 11,* 201–214.

Reiss, S., Peterson, R. A., Gursky, D. M., & McNally, R. J. (1986). Anxiety sensitivity, anxiety frequency and the prediction of fearfulness. *Behaviour Research and Therapy, 24,* 1–8.

Rey, J. M., & Morris-Yates, A. (1991). Adolescent depression and the Child Behavior Checklist. *Journal of the American Academy of Child and Adolescent Psychiatry, 30,* 423–427.

Reynolds, C. R. (1981). Long-term stability of scores on the Revised Children's Manifest Anxiety Scale. *Perceptual and Motor Skills, 53,* 702.

Reynolds, C. R. (1982). Convergent and divergent validity of the Revised Children's Manifest Anxiety Scale. *Educational and Psychological Measurement, 42,* 1205–1212.

Reynolds, C. R. (1985). Multitrait validation of the Revised Children's Manifest Anxiety Scale for children of high intelligence. *Psychological Reports, 56,* 402.

Reynolds, C. R., Bradley, M., & Steele, C. (1980). Preliminary norms and technical data for use of the Revised Children's Manifest Anxiety Scale with kindergarten children. *Psychology in the Schools, 17,* 163–167.

Reynolds, C. R., & Paget, K. D. (1981). Factor analysis of the Revised Children's Manifest Anxiety Scale for blacks, whites, males, and females. *Journal of Consulting and Clinical Psychology, 49,* 352–359.

Reynolds, C. R., & Richmond, B. O. (1978). What I Think and Feel: A revised measure of children's manifest anxiety. *Journal of Abnormal Child Psychology, 6,* 271–280.

Reynolds, C. R., & Richmond, B. O. (1979). Factor structure and construct validity of "What I Think and Feel": The Revised Children's Manifest Anxiety Scale. *Journal of Personality Assessment, 43,* 281–283.

Reynolds, C. R., & Richmond, B. O. (1985). *Revised Children's Manifest Anxiety Scale: Manual.* Los Angeles: Western Psychological Services.

Reynolds, C. R., & Scholwinski, E. (1985). Dimensions of anxiety among high IQ children. *Gifted Child Quarterly, 29,* 125–130.

Reynolds, W. M. (1989). *Reynolds Child Depression Scale.* Odessa, FL: Psychological Assessment Resources.

Reynolds, W. M., Anderson, G., & Bartell, N. (1985). Measuring depression in children: A multimethod assessment investigation. *Journal of Abnormal Child Psychology, 13,* 513–526.

Roberts, R. E., Lewinsohn, P. M., & Seeley, J. R. (1991). Screening for adolescent depression: A comparison of depression scales. *Journal of the American Academy of Child and Adolescent Psychiatry, 30,* 58–66.

Rorty, R. (1979). *Philosophy and the mirror of nature.* Princeton, NJ: Princeton University Press.

Sarason, S. B., Davidson, K. S., Lighthall, F. F., Waite, R. R., & Ruebush, B. K. (1960). *Anxiety and elementary school children.* New York: Wiley.

Sawyer, M. G., Sarris, A., & Baghurst, P. (1991). The use of a computer-assisted interview to administer the Child Behavior Checklist in a child psychiatry service. *Journal of the American Academy of Child and Adolescent Psychiatry, 30,* 674–681.

Saylor, C. F., Finch, A. J., Spirito, A., & Bennett, B. (1984). The Children's Depression Inventory: A systematic evaluation of psychometric properties. *Journal of Consulting and Clinical Psychology, 52,* 955–967.

Scherer, M. W., & Nakamura, C. Y. (1968). A Fear Survey Schedule for Children: A factor-analytic comparison with manifest anxiety (CMAS). *Behaviour Research and Therapy, 6,* 173–182.

Seligman, L. D., & Ollendick, T. H. (1998). Comorbidity of anxiety and depression in children and adolescents: An integrative review. *Clinical Child and Family Psychology Review, 1,* 125–144.

Silverman, W. K. (1992). Taxonomy of anxiety disorders in children. In G. D. Burrows, R. Noyes, & S. M. Roth (Eds.), *Handbook of anxiety* (Vol. 5, pp. 281–308). Amsterdam: Elsevier Science.

Silverman, W. K., & Eisen, A. R. (1992). Age differences in the reliability of parent and child reports of child anxious symptomatology using a structured interview. *Journal of the American Academy of Child and Adolescent Psychiatry, 31,* 117–124.

Silverman, W. K., Fleisig, W., Rabian, B., & Peterson, R. A. (1991). Childhood Anxiety Sensitivity Index. *Journal of Clinical Child Psychology, 20,* 162–168.

Silverman, W. K., Ginsburg, G. S., & Goedhart, A. W. (in press). Factor structure of the Childhood Anxiety Sensitivity Index. *Behaviour Research and Therapy.*

Silverman, W. K., & Kurtines, W. M. (1996). *Anxiety and phobic disorders: A pragmatic approach.* New York: Plenum Press.

Silverman, W. K., & Kurtines, W. M. (1997). Theory in child psychosocial treatment research: Have it or had it? A pragmatic alternative. *Journal of Abnormal Child Psychology, 25,* 359–366.

Silverman, W. K., La Greca, A. M., & Wasserstein, S. B. (1995). What do children worry about? Worry and its relation to anxiety. *Child Development, 66*, 671–686.

Silverman, W. K., & Weems, C. F. (1999). Anxiety sensitivity in children. In S. Taylor (Ed.), *Anxiety sensitivity: Theory, research and the treatment of the fear of anxiety* (pp. 239–268). Mahwah, NJ: Erlbaum.

Skinner, H. A., & Pakula, A. (1986). The challenge of computers in psychological assessment. *Professional Psychological: Research and Practice, 17*, 44–50.

Smucker, M. R., Craighead, W. E., Craighead, L. W., & Green, B. J. (1986). Normative reliability data for the Children's Depression Inventory. *Journal of Abnormal Child Psychology, 14*, 25–39.

Spielberger, C. D. (1973). *Manual for the State–Trait Anxiety Inventory for Children*. Palo Alto, CA: Consulting Psychologists Press.

Spielberger, C. D., Gorsuch, R. L., & Lushene, R. E. (1970). *Manual for the State–Trait Anxiety Inventory (Self-Evaluation Questionnaire)*. Palo Alto, CA: Consulting Psychologists Press.

Spirito, A., Williams, C. A., Stark, L. S., & Hart, K. J. (1988). The Hopelessness Scale for Children: Psychometric properties with normal and emotionally disturbed adolescents. *Journal of Abnormal Child Psychology, 16*, 445–458.

Taylor, J. A. (1953). A personality scale of manifest anxiety. *Journal of Abnormal and Social Psychology, 48*, 285–290.

Tisher, M., Lang-Takac, E., & Lang, M. (1992). The Children's Depression Scale: Review of Australian and overseas experience. *Australian Journal of Psychology, 44*, 27–35.

Treiber, F. A., & Mabe, P. A. (1987). Child and parent perceptions of children's psychopathology in psychiatric outpatient children. *Journal of Abnormal Child Psychology, 13*, 115–124.

Vecchio, T. (1966). Predictive value of a single diagnostic test in unselected populations. *New England Journal of Medicine, 275*, 1171–1173.

Watson, D., & Kendall, P. C. (1989). Common and differentiating features of anxiety and depression: Current findings and future directions. In P. C. Kendall & D. Watson (Eds.), *Anxiety and depression: Distinctive and overlapping features* (pp. 493–508). San Diego, CA: Academic Press.

Weems, C. F., Hammond-Laurence, K., Silverman, W. K., & Ginsburg, G. S. (1998). Testing the utility of the anxiety sensitivity construct in children and adolescents referred for anxiety disorders. *Journal of Clinical Child Psychology, 27*, 69–77.

Weems, C. F., Silverman, W. K., Saavedra, L. M., Pina, A. A., & Lumpkin, P. W. (1999). The discrimination of children's phobias using the Revised Fear Survey Schedule for Children. *Journal of Child Psychology and Psychiatry, 40*.

Weiss, B., & Weisz, J. R. (1988). Factor structure of self-reported depression: Clinic-referred children versus adolescents. *Journal of Abnormal Psychology, 97*, 492–495.

Weiss, B., Weisz, J. R., Politano, M., Carey, M. P., Nelson, W. M., & Finch, A. J. (1991). Developmental differences in the factor structure of the Children's Depression Inventory. *Journal of Consulting and Clinical Psychology, 3*, 38–45.

Weissman, M. M., Orvaschel, H., & Padian, N. (1980). Children's symptom and social functioning self-report scales: Comparison of mothers' and children's reports. *Journal of Nervous and Mental Disease, 168*, 736–740.

Wierzbicki, M. (1987). A parent form of the Children's Depression Inventory: Reliability and validity in nonclinical populations. *Journal of Clinical Psychology, 43*, 390–397.

Wisniewski, J. J., Mulick, J. A., Genshaft, J. L., & Coury, D. L. (1987). Test–retest reliability of the Revised Children's Manifest Anxiety Scale. *Perceptual and Motor Skills, 65,* 67–70.

Wolfe, V. V., Blount, R. L., Finch, A. J., Saylor, C. F., Pallmeyer, T. P., & Carek, D. J. (1987). Negative affectivity in children: A multitrait–multimethod investigation. *Journal of Consulting and Clinical Psychology, 55,* 245–250.

6

Measures for Assessing Pervasive Developmental and Communication Disorders

✧

FRED R. VOLKMAR
WENDY D. MARANS

The pervasive developmental disorders (PDDs) and communication disorders share several features: They are of early onset, have strong developmental aspects, and are associated with a range of outcomes. In this chapter, we selectively review diagnostic and screening assessment instruments for these conditions. It is important to note that these instruments do not, of themselves, replace the need either for careful clinical evaluation or for the use of well-standardized, normative tests of intelligence and language in general (Sparrow, 1997). Such tests are essential for both diagnostic and educational purposes, and often establish eligibility for other services as well. Many of the instruments described subsequently require various levels of training, and, as with any instrument, there is the potential for inappropriate use or misuse. Individuals who undertake assessments with these instruments are obligated to be sufficiently aware of any special requirements for training and administration.

THE PERVASIVE DEVELOPMENTAL DISORDERS

The PDDs are a group of neuropsychiatric disorders characterized by patterns of both delay and deviance in the development of social, cognitive, communicative, and other skills (Volkmar, Klin, & Cohen, 1997a). Although these disorders are often associated with mental retardation, the patterns of delay and deviance observed do not simply reflect developmental level (Rutter, 1978). The validity of autistic disorder (also sometimes referred to as "Kanner's autism," "early infantile autism," or "childhood autism") is very well established, and there has been general agreement on features central to its definition. The validity and definition of the other PDDs have been controversial (Volkmar, Klin, & Cohen, 1997a).

Autism as a Diagnostic Concept

Present definitions of autism continue to be profoundly influenced by Leo Kanner's (1943) classic description, as subsequently modified by Rutter (1978). In his work, Kanner emphasized the centrality of two factors in the definition of autism: (1) "autism" per se, or an inborn disruption in the usual processes of socialization that characterize normal infant development; and (2) "insistence on sameness"—a term referring to a rather diverse group of behaviors that include not only literal insistence on sameness (e.g., taking the same route to school every day), but also other highly unusual behaviors (e.g., self-stimulation and stereotypy, unusual sensitivity to the inanimate environment, etc.). Early disagreements about the continuity of autism with childhood schizophrenia impeded initial research; the work of Kolvin (1971) and others was helpful in establishing the distinctiveness of the two conditions. In his 1978 synthesis of Kanner's definition and of subsequent research, Rutter emphasized that the social and communicative features are distinctive and not just secondary to any associated mental retardation. Rutter's 1978 definition and the large body of work that had accumulated on autism influenced the decision to include autism in the *Diagnostic and Statistical Manual of Mental Disorders*, third edition (DSM-III; American Psychiatric Association, 1980).

Given the general consensus on the validity of autism, its stability over time, and the reasonably good reliability with which the diagnosis can be made (Volkmar, Klin, et al., 1994), it is somewhat surprising that major changes were made in the definition in both DSM-III-R and DSM-IV (American Psychiatric Association, 1987, 1994). These reflect the issues associated with the broad range of expressions of the condition across both age and developmental level. These problems have been exemplified in the various changes in the definition of the condition from DSM-III to DSM-III-R and DSM-IV. For example, the DSM-III definition lacked a developmental orientation, whereas DSM-III-R appeared to overdiagnose autism in the very severely retarded. The DSM-IV definition was developed through a very large, international, multisite field trial. Consistent with previous definitions, it required disturbance in three broad areas of developmental dysfunction, all arising in the first 3 years of life (Volkmar et al., 1994). In addition to being based on a large body of empirical data, this system has the advantage of being conceptually identical with that employed in the *International Classification of Diseases*, 10th revision (ICD–10; World Health Organization, 1994).

"Nonautistic" PDDs

In addition to autism, various other disorders are now included within the PDD class in both DSM-IV and ICD–10. In childhood disintegrative disorder, children develop a condition that resembles autism, but do so after several years of normal development (Volkmar & Rutter, 1995). This fortunately rare condition differs from autism in its pattern of onset, its course, and its much worse outcome (see Volkmar, Klin, Marans, & Cohen, 1997b). The DSM-IV and ICD–10 criteria for the condition are largely compatible.

In Rett's disorder, so far observed only in females, a short period of normal development is followed by decelerated head growth, the loss of purposeful hand movements, and development of severe psychomotor retardation (van Acker, 1997). The condition is highly distinctive and various attempts have been made to provide guidelines for diagnosis (see van Acker, 1997). The major rationale for inclusion of the condition as a PDD was the potential for confusion with autism in the preschool years (see Rutter, 1994, and Gillberg, 1994, for opposing views on this issue).

Asperger's disorder was probably the most controversial of the "new" disorders included in DSM-IV (see Klin, 1997, for a discussion). ICD–10 explicitly notes that the validity of the category apart from high-functioning autism remains to be established firmly. Preliminary data suggest important points of difference. Consistent with Asperger's original report (1944), there appears to be a much stronger familial component than in high-functioning autism, and the condition is associated with some features that discriminate it from autism (e.g., neurocognitive profile and certain clinical features) (Klin, 1995).

The term PDD not otherwise specified (PDD NOS) encompasses the "subthreshold" PDD cases—that is, cases in which problems in social interaction, communication, or stereotyped behavior patterns or interest are present, but criteria for one of the explicitly defined PDDs are not met (see Towbin, 1997, for a review). Though this condition is probably much more common than autism, it is, paradoxically, more difficult to study; it is likely that multiple subtypes will eventually be recognized in this rather heterogeneous category.

Assessment Instruments Specific to Autism

Both categorical and dimensional approaches to the diagnosis of autism have been used (Lord, 1997; Volkmar et al., 1997a). As noted previously, categorical approaches have typically emphasized early onset of a disorder characterized by disturbances in the areas of social interaction and communication, as well as by various unusual behaviors. Usually the characteristic social and communicative deficits are noted to be deviant relative to the individual's overall developmental level, although explicit approaches to this problem are usually not specified (one exception is discussed subsequently). In contrast to categorical approaches, dimensional instruments have been designed for purposes of screening and monitoring change, as well as for diagnosis. In some instances categorical instruments have been explicitly "keyed" to categorical criteria, or standardized, dimensional assessments developed for other purposes have been used to generate categorical diagnoses or to screen children.

For both categorical and dimensional definitions and instruments, problems have been posed by several factors: (1) issues of continuity with other disorders (e.g., mental retardation); (2) the very broad range of syndrome expression; (3) changes in syndrome expression with age; (4) the lack of specificity of certain "autistic-like" features (e.g., stereotyped behaviors are very common among the severely mentally retarded, nonautistic population); (5) the relative infrequency of the disorder; and (6) the lack of good, developmentally based, metrics of social functioning (see Lord, 1997, and Volkmar, et al., 1997a, for detailed discussion).

Often, but not always, a child believed to have autism cannot be interviewed directly. Either of two approaches is usually employed: Either parents or teachers provide information via checklists, or an examiner interacts with or observes the individual. Both approaches have strengths and weaknesses. Although historical information is often critical for establishing a diagnosis, the use of parents as informants does raise issues of reliability. On the other hand, rating scales developed for teachers or others not experienced in work with autism may focus on highly unusual behaviors, so problems of standardization and reliability arise. The use of structured or unstructured observation is associated with still other problems (e.g., training the examiner to maintain reliability). With a few exceptions, the agreement of categorical with dimensional techniques and of parent reports with observation techniques has not been sufficiently addressed. For example, Stone and Lemanek (1990b) compared parent reports to the results of a structured interview based on DSM-III-R criteria and observed good agreement between the two methodologies for only 3 of the 16 DSM-III-R items: abnormal social play, stereotyped body movements, and restricted range of interests. The lack of good agreement reflects the facts that it can be difficult to disentangle highly deviant from delayed behaviors in younger children, and that the issue of context is critical in evaluating observed behaviors. Differentiation for adults between deficits specific to autism and those associated with any severe chronic psychiatric disorder that drastically limits social contact and everyday opportunities also becomes more difficult (see Howlin, 1998).

For higher-functioning individuals, the tensions between parent and child reports can be problematic. Higher-functioning children, adolescents, and adults can be asked to describe their own symptoms and concerns; such reports may be more accurate than parental ones. However, for some areas parent reports may be more valid and reliable (e.g., reports of friendships, historical information; Lord & Schopler, 1989). For lower-functioning or younger children, direct observational methods have important potential advantages (DiLavore, Lord, & Rutter, 1995). The use of multiple sources of information can help address some of these concerns. Other issues arise relative to the stringency of a diagnostic approach and the emphasis on screening (usually rather broad-gauged) or rigorous diagnostic ascertainment (usually narrow-gauged) (see Lord, 1997, for a review).

Several considerations can have an impact on the selection of the various assessment instruments. It is clear that the extremes of age and the range of symptom expression pose major problems for both categorical and dimensional assessment instruments—that is, among the very, very young and very old, and among the very mentally handicapped and the very high-functioning (see Lord, 1997). Classification is most robust in the verbal (even minimally verbal), mildly to moderately retarded school-age child. Unfortunately, the needs in terms of service are great both in lower-functioning preschool children and in adults; it is therefore important to consider the ages and developmental levels of the subjects used in developing a particular instrument. Similarly, although many instruments developed specifically for autism may have some utility for the "nonautistic" PDDs, it is important to realize that instruments developed specifically for the latter conditions are very uncommon, and that hasty generalizations or ad hoc uses of such instruments (e.g., to establish a diagnosis of Asperger's disorder or eligibility for services) should be avoided. Finally, as with all assessment instruments, the requirements of the instrument should be carefully adhered to—training of the examiner, methods of administration, and so forth.

Autism Behavior Checklist

The 57-item Autism Behavior Checklist (ABC) is one part of the Autism Screening Instrument for Educational Planning (Krug, Arick, & Almond, 1980). The dichotomous items are grouped into five areas (Sensory, Relating, Body and Object Use, Language and Social Interaction, and Self-Help). Items were derived from various sources, and the dichotomous items are assigned differential weights based on the strength of the item's association with a diagnosis of autism. On the basis of the ratings provided for a large (although not well characterized) sample of persons with autism, a total score of 67 or more is taken to suggest *probable* autism. Scores between 55 and 67 suggest *possible* autism. Information on various patient groups, including deaf, blind, and autistic children, is provided for various age ranges. The ABC was designed for use by teachers as one step in educational planning. No special training in scoring or administration is required. It has also been used with parents, who tend, on average, to produce higher scores than teachers (Volkmar, Cicchetti et al., 1988; Szatmari, Archer, Fisman, & Steiner, 1994).

Initial reports of reliability (Krug et al., 1980) were high but did not control for chance agreement. When the latter is controlled for, agreement is not as good, although still generally acceptable (Volkmar et al., 1988). Data on the ability of the instrument to discriminate autistic disorder from mental handicap are somewhat mixed. If the original guidelines for screening are used, the overlap between these two groups is relatively high, with both age and developmental level being related to diagnostic accuracy. On the other hand, authors who develop their own diagnostic thresholds or procedures report better results (Goodman & Minne, 1995; Wadden, Bryson, & Rodger, 1991; Yirmiya, Sigman, & Freeman, 1994). Issues in sample selection and study design, as well as the nature of the "gold standard" used for a diagnosis of autism, have probably influenced the results obtained; the ABC is in better agreement with a broad diagnosis of autism than with a narrow one.

Sturmey, Matson, and Sevin (1992) reported that the Relating and Body and Object Use scales of the ABC had the strongest internal consistency. Various reports have suggested that subsets of items may be as useful as the entire checklist in screening for autism (Oswald & Volkmar, 1991).

Convergence between the ABC and other instruments has not been good. It is possible that this reflects the ABC's rather broad-based symptom focus, as opposed to more recent diagnostic approaches, which have tended to center on abnormalities in socialization and communication as well as "insistence on samenesss." Sevin, Matson, Coe, Fee, and Sevin (1991) compared the ABC to the Real Life Rating Scale (RLRS) and the Childhood Autism Rating Scale (CARS) and found that the although the RLRS and CARS correlated moderately well, the ABC was not significantly correlated with either instrument. When the proposed scoring rules for the ABC were used, 50% of the sample was misclassified. Eaves and Milner (1993) reported a somewhat stronger association between the ABC and the CARS.

On the other hand, the ABC's focus on a number of behaviors associated with autism may make it useful as a dependent measure in research studies; it has not yet been utilized extensively for this purpose, however. The notion that the instrument might serve to document change in response to intervention does not, of course, suggest that it is ideal as a diagnostic instrument. Its ease of administration and rapid scoring are important advantages.

Autism Diagnostic Interview—Revised

The Autism Diagnostic Interview—Revised (ADI-R) is a semistructured, investigator-based interview for caregivers. The original version was developed for research purposes (Le Couteur, Rutter, Lord, & Rios, 1989), but the ADI-R addresses a broader age span and is linked explicitly to DSM-IV and ICD-10 criteria for autistic disorder (Lord, Rutter, & Le Couteur, 1994). Administration of the instrument entails participation in training workshops and the ability to establish reliability with other investigators. Although clinicians can use the instrument without extensive training, general experience in interviewing is needed, as well as experience in the area of autism and related disorders. Administration often takes several hours; although a "short" version of this research instrument is now available, even this version requires a considerable period of time (1½ hours).

The organization of the ADI-R around the conceptual model used in DSM-IV and ICD–10 is a significant advantage. Many items are arranged around the three behavioral areas relevant to diagnosis (problems in social reciprocity, communication problems, and restricted, repetitive behaviors); other items relate to the fourth diagnostic area (onset of the condition). The problem with developmental change is addressed, in that it is possible to score behaviors as current or as having "ever" occurred. Items are included that reflect the broad range of autism; in other words, the ADI-R encompasses various levels of severity.

Initial psychometric data for both the original interview and its revision, the ADI-R, have been very good although based on small samples. Interrater reliability has been good to excellent for individual items and overall scores (Yirmiya et al., 1994). Test–retest reliability and internal consistency have also been very good. In addition, these data have been supplemented by the generally very positive experience of researchers at various centers using the instrument (e.g., Smalley, Tanguay, Smith, & Gutierez, 1992).

Differentiation between autistic and mentally retarded children and adults is excellent, with the restriction that the instrument tends to be overinclusive for individuals with mental ages of less than 18 months (Lord, Storoschuk, Rutter, & Pickles, 1993). Yirmiya et al. (1994) reported that the original ADI tended to underdiagnose autism in higher-functioning children. On the other hand, for older children, the ADI-R shows excellent agreement with the CARS (Lord, 1997). Although its careful design, thorough coverage, and explicit relationships with DSM-IV and ICD–10 suggest the potential utility of the ADI-R for the diagnosis of "nonautistic" PDDs, scoring rules for such procedures have not yet been established. Convergence with a companion instrument, the Autism Diagnostic Observation Schedule (ADOS; see below), has been reported to be excellent.

Autism Diagnostic Observation Schedule (Original and Generic) and Pre-Linguistic Autism Diagnostic Observation Schedule

Two standardized observational protocols (Lord, Rutter, et al., 1989; DiLavore, Lord, et al., 1995) were originally developed for children with verbal communicative abilities (the ADOS) and for preschool children with little or no expressive speech (the Pre-Linguistic ADOS, or PL-ADOS). Developed as companions to the ADI, the two instruments have now been combined into a single instrument, the ADOS—Generic (ADOS-G; Lord, 1997), which is now composed of several "modules." Module 1, which includes most of the original PL-ADOS, is used for children with very little or no speech; Module 2 is used for children with some language but without spontaneous and fluent speech; Module 3, essentially including most of the previous ADOS, is used for individuals with fluent and spontaneous speech; and Module 4 is used for high-functioning adults and adolescents. The ADOS-G provides a series of structured and semistructured opportunities or "presses" for social interaction, communication, and play. These can be coded and scored directly, and a diagnostic algorithm for autism has been provided. For research purposes, both training and reliability establishment are essential; the ADOS-G usually takes 45 minutes to 1 hour to administer by an examiner who is familiar with working with autistic individuals.

Statistical information on the ADOS-G remains limited, although data on the ADOS and PL-ADOS are available. Interrater reliability for the earlier instruments was reported to be good as was internal consistency (Lord et al., 1989; DiLavore et al., 1995). Interrater reliability has been good for both instruments for items and excellent for totals. Internal consistency for both instruments within the domains of social communication and restricted, repetitive behaviors was good. Test–retest reliability for the ADOS was reported to be adequate, but this has not been tested for the PL-ADOS. The sensitivity and specificity of the ADOS-G have not yet been adequately evaluated. A major rationale for the expansion of the ADOS and PL-ADOS was concern about diagnostic coverage (i.e., concern that the PL-ADOS was underinclusive for children who had at least the capacity to speak in phrases, while the ADOS was somewhat overinclusive for lower-functioning children and underinclusive for higher-functioning children). Although the primary utility of the ADOS-G to date has been in research, it is likely that the instrument will be used clinically; expansion of the focus to include the various other PDDs will increase the value of the instrument.

Behavior Observation Scale and Real Life Rating Scale

The Behavior Observation Scale (BOS) provides for the ratings of various behaviors in a structured play setting (Freeman, Ritvo, Guthrio, Schroth, & Ball, 1978). This instrument was one of the first to provide real-time, quantitative ratings of behavior and to attempt to control for various situational factors. Several factors complicated the use of the instrument, however. For example, some behaviors were of great interest but occurred only rarely; frequencies of many behaviors were related to degree of mental handicap; and so on. This led to the development of the RLRS (Freeman, Ritvo, Yokota, & Ritvo, 1986). This scale is completed after a 30-minute period of observing a child in free play. Reliability of the instrument has been reported to range from adequate to marginal when chance-corrected statistics are used (Freeman et al., 1986; Sevin et al., 1991). Correlations with the CARS were, however, relatively high (Sturmey et al., 1992). As might be expected, many behaviors are not seen during the period of observation. The instrument is not designed to assign a diagnosis of autism, and it has most frequently been used as a measure to document change in response to treatment.

Behavior Rating Instrument for Autistic Adolescents and Children

The Behavior Rating Instrument for Autistic Adolescents and Children includes eight subscales that assess the severity of autistic behavior (on a continuum from normal to autistic (Ruttenberg, Dratman, et al., 1966; Ruttenberg, Kalish, et al., 1977). The scale is completed by a trained rater after considerable observation of a child. Several aspects of the scale were historically important—for example, the use of direct observation rather than parent report, reliance on standard descriptions, and attention to certain psychometric properties (Parks, 1983). Unfortunately, the scoring procedure is complex, and published data (Cohen, Caparulo, et al., 1978) have suggested some limitations of the instrument. Given its focus on current observation, it does, however, have the potential for use as a measure for evaluating therapeutic change. The lack of information on reliability is problematic (Lord, 1997).

Childhood Autism Rating Scale

The widely used CARS (Schopler, Reichler, DeVellis, & Daly, 1980), includes 15 items on which children and adults are rated on a 4-point scale. The problem of differences in developmental level is addressed through the use of specific anchor points for items. This scale has been extensively studied, although most of the research has been in the midrange of syndrome expression (i.e., among individuals with mild to moderate mental retardation). Some data suggesting discriminant validity of the instrument have been reported (Morgan, 1988; Teal & Wiebe, 1986). Internal consistency and interrater reliabilities have generally been reported to be good (Garfin, 1988; Sturmey et al., 1992; Sevin et al., 1991); however, interrater reliability has not been assessed with chance-corrected statistics such as kappa and is an area of concern.

Minimal training is required and can be obtained through videotapes or through workshops; some observation of the individual is required. Scores are summed over the items, and a cutoff of 30 has been used for a diagnosis of autism. There have been some suggestions that for the extremes of syndrome expression, some modification of the cutoff may be needed (Lord, 1995; Mesibov, Schopler, Schaffer, & Michal, 1989).

Relative to DSM-III-R, the CARS tends to be somewhat overinclusive (Mesibov et al., 1989); given that DSM-III-R was itself found to be overinclusive, this raises a concern about false-positive cases. Mentally retarded younger children who do not have autism may be particularly likely to be misdiagnosed (Lord, 1997), although convergence with other instruments, such as the ADI, is generally good (LeCouteur et al., 1989; Sevin et al., 1991; Venter, Lord, & Schopler, 1992). The tendency of the CARS to err on the side of being overinclusive makes it more appropriate for use as a screening instrument. It differs in its fundamental theoretical approach from current categorical definitions, which require deficits in specific areas.

Handicaps, Behavior, and Skills Schedule

The Handicaps, Behavior, and Skills Schedule was the first widely used semi-structured interview for parents or caregivers. Originally developed before the publication of DSM-III, it was used in Wing's epidemiological study of autism (Wing & Gould, 1979). The instrument is not a diagnostic instrument as such, but is used to obtain clinically relevant information, which can then be used in conjunction with psychological assessments for making a diagnosis. The instrument takes several hours to administer, and psychometric comparisons are based on a sample of nearly 200 children from an epidemiological sample receiving services in the London borough of Camberwell; many of the children had mental handicap without autism, and a small number had autism without mental handicap. Simple percentage of agreement was reported to be good; chance-corrected reliability has not been reported. A revised version of the instrument is presently being developed. The attention to agreement between the reports of parents and the observations of professionals is a unique aspect of the work on this scale; parents reported more unusual movements and responses to the inanimate environment, but also described the children as more socially responsive than the professionals did.

Rimland Forms E-1 and E-2

The Diagnostic Form for Behavior-Disturbed Children (generally referred to simply as Form E-1; Rimland, 1968) was the first instrument developed and widely used in the diagnosis of autism. A revised form, the E-2, was subsequently developed. The E-2 is designed to be completed by parents; the 80 multiple-choice questions are concerned with aspects of social interaction, speech, and symptom development. Items are scored +1 or −1 depending on whether the item is associated with the presence or absence of autism; a range of −42 to +45 has been reported, with a cutoff of +20 indicating autism (Rimland, 1971). Given its intended use, advantages of the E-2 include its selective focus on highly relevant behaviors and symptoms rather than more global constructs. The instrument tends to adopt a very strict approach to the diagnosis of autism, and agreement with other instruments is not high (Schopler, Reichler, DeVellis, & Daly, 1980; Cohen et al., 1978). Information on basic psychometric properties is lacking (Lord, 1997).

Other Approaches to Screening

Baron-Cohen and colleagues (Baron-Cohen, Allen, & Gillberg, 1992; Baron-Cohen, Cox, Baird, Swettenham, Nightingale, et al., 1996) developed a screening instrument called the Checklist for Autism in Toddlers. Designed to be completed as part of a broader screening, the instrument includes a short series of questions concerned with pretend play, protodeclarative pointing, joint attention, social interest, and social play. In their initial study, Baron-Cohen et al. (1992) evaluated 41 toddlers at high risk for autism and 50 randomly selected toddlers; 4 of the high-risk subjects failed in at least two of the areas assessed. At a 30-month follow-up, these 4 subjects were said to exhibit autism. Although the paper highlights the need to develop better approaches to screening for autism, several issues limit the apparent usefulness of this instrument. The exact procedures used are somewhat unclear as it appears that the original screen was supplemented by a phone interview (Baron-Cohen et al., 1996). In addition, it is not clear how representative the population was of children with autism, since children with mental handicap were apparently excluded from the sample.

Although the importance of standard, normative assessment instruments is well recognized, these have only rarely been used for purposes of diagnostic screening. For example, Volkmar, Sparrow, Goudveou, Cicchetti, Paul, et al. (1987) used measures of social development from the Vineland Adaptive Behavior Scales (Sparrow, Balla, & Cicchetti, 1984a, 1984b) to empirically evaluate Rutter's notion that social skills in autism are deviant relative to mental age. In this study, obtained levels of social ability were evaluated relative to either chronological or mental age by means of regression equations derived from a normative sample. In comparison to other children with developmental problems, greater-than-expected social deficits were observed (relative to predictions from either mental or chronological age) and could be used quite robustly for purposes of screening.

The development of screening instruments for PDDs other than autism is much less advanced. Mayes, Volkmar, et al. (1993) used a chart review to identify features that discriminated PDD NOS from autism and language disorders. Other attempts to differentiate autism and PDD NOS have been made (e.g., Serra, Minderaa van Geert, & Jackson, 1995; Van der Gaag, 1995). Efforts to develop screening approaches to Asperger's disorder are presently underway; the continued debate on the continuity–discontinuity of autism and Asperger's disorder presents a substantial problem for this effort.

COMMUNICATION DISORDERS

In preschool children, speech and language difficulties are the most commonly presenting developmental disorders, with reported prevalence rates ranging from 3% to 14% in children 3–5 years of age (Bax, Hart, & Jenkins,

1980; Silva, 1980; Stevenson & Richman, 1976). Epidemiological studies have documented the frequent co-occurrence of speech, language, and communication disorders and psychiatric disorders (Cantwell & Baker, 1987; Beitchman, Nair, Clegg, Ferguson, & Patel, 1986). Speech and language difficulties are significant risk factors for childhood psychopathology (Baltaxe & Simmons, 1988) and for subsequent learning disabilities (Aram & Nation, 1980; Aram, Ekelman, & Nation, 1984; Fundudis, Kolvin, & Garside, 1980; Tallal, 1988).

In 1975, the introduction of the Education for All Handicapped Children Act (P.L. 94-142) provided a federal mandate to identify communication disorders in children and to provide appropriate educational services for affected individuals. The 1986 amendment (P.L. 99-457) extended these provisions to include identification of children with special needs in the birth-to-3-years population. As a result, more effective, reliable, and valid ways of assessing this younger population were required—ways that took into account the rapidly changing nature of a child's developmental capacities during the first years of life, the variability in young children's early communicative styles, and the challenge involved in obtaining reliable data from this young population. Several newer assessment instruments have since been developed, ranging from linguistically based checklists with predictive value (Fenson et al., 1993; Rescorla, 1989; Reznick & Goldsmith, 1989) to assessments of a broad range of communicative and symbolic behaviors (Wetherby & Prizant, 1993; Lord et al., 1989). Many of these newer instruments reflect the increasing awareness of the interplay among social, communicative, and emotional development (Prizant & Wetherby, 1990a, 1992; Crais & Roberts, 1991); the need to consider the role of context, especially when testing younger children (Bates, 1976; Bloom & Lahey, 1978; Bruner, 1977, 1981); and/or the need to assess particular populations, such as children with autism and other PDDs (Wetherby & Prizant, 1993; Lord et al., 1993), where communication deficits are integral to the diagnosis (DSM-IV). These are welcome additions to the already existing tests available to researchers and clinicians.

Standard Assessment Instruments

As is the case in other developmental areas, standardized, normative assessments of speech, language, and communication are an essential part of a clinical evaluation. In some cases, test construction and standardization for speech and language instruments have not been as rigorous as for the more familiar psychological test batteries (Plante & Vance, 1994; McCauley & Swisher, 1984; Messick, 1989; Sattler, 1988), although this is less true of more recently developed or standardized instruments. In addition to psychometric properties, other factors to consider when selecting a test include multicultural issues and test bias. The validity and utility of the results obtained will depend on appropriate selection of tests for the given individual or population under study, with his/her or its specific cultural, ethnic and linguistic styles. For example, the ability to identify whether someone has a specific language impairment, as opposed to problems due to English as a second language, is essential in selecting a research population or, clinically, in planning for educational placement and programming (e.g., a communication class as opposed to a setting designed specifically for bilingual children). A number of rating scales are available to determine language dominance in bilingual children, so that testing can be conducted in the dominant language (see Paul, 1995, and Lund & Duchan, 1993, for reviews). Use of a translator is necessary in situations when a child's first language is not English and no instrument in the child's native language is available; this can be extremely useful, but it does not solve the problem of having very few assessment instruments developed specifically for individuals of different cultural/ethnic backgrounds. Tests standardized on American-English-speaking populations cannot always be directly or easily translated in ways that are valid. For instance, Spanish words frequently have more syllables than their English counterparts, so that word lists used to assess short-term auditory memory may not be equivalent when translated. Moreover, some vocabulary items may not have the same salience in a different culture; the choice of vocabulary items/depicted scenes may be biased toward the dominant culture and may be less relevant to some ethnic minorities. Similarly, when one is considering pragmatic skills, even nonverbal communication is culture-specific. For example, eye contact with a teacher or authority figure is considered respectful (and therefore appropriate) for many American children, but it may be the reverse in Asian American or some African American contexts (Paul, 1995).

Administration of assessments to children with particular disabilities, such as deafness or physical handicaps, presents other challenges. Unfortunately, although some tests may provide information regarding administration to such children, standardization sampling for both groups is rarely conducted.

The remainder of this chapter describes a number of assessment instruments (including checklists/rating scales, screening assessments, and more traditional tests) in terms of their purpose, design, standardization, and psychometric properties. This is not intended to be an exhaustive review. More detail is provided regarding recently developed tests, whereas those already well established are covered in less depth. In addition, we focus here on communication and language (receptive and expressive) rather than on speech (by which is meant the production and articulation of sounds) or reading and writing skills, although clearly these are frequently affected in children with language difficulties and will be relevant areas to consider for older children or high-functioning younger children on the autism spectrum, who may be able to utilize advanced reading decoding skills as a means of comprehension. Standard references (e.g., Paul, 1995) should be consulted for discussion of these issues.

Checklists and Rating Scales

Receptive Expressive Emergent Language Scale, Second Edition

The Receptive Expressive Emergent Language Scale, second edition (REEL; Bzoch & League, 1971) is a 132-item checklist used to identify major receptive and/or expressive language problems in children from birth to 36 months of age. This instrument is used (1) as a means of describing developmental status, (2) as an aid in development of intervention goals, (3) as a clinical research tool to help in differentiating between organic and environmental etiology, and (4) as a measure of change after intervention.

The authors' rationale assumes that there is a "universal and predictable pattern" (Bzoch & League, 1971, p. 18) for receptive and expressive language development during the first 36 months of life. Item selection for the REEL was based on a Piagetian language framework and on Lenneberg's linguistic milestones (Piaget, 1923; Lenneberg, 1967). Information is obtained directly from parent or caregiver report. Although interviewers are instructed to ask questions to elicit the desired information rather than reading items verbatim, the suggested questions are closed- rather than open-ended, which potentially biases or restricts the interviewees' responses.

Receptive and expressive lists are separate. In each, items are arranged three per age interval and age intervals increase from 1 month (Year 1) to 2 months (Year 2) to 3 months (Year 3). A ceiling is established as the highest age interval in which two of three items are passed. This age interval becomes the Receptive or Expressive Language Age, the mean of which yields the Combined Language Age. Language Quotients are derived via a ratio formula (Language Age ÷ Chronological Age × 100).

Psychometric data for the REEL are very limited. The standardization sample was limited to an unstated number of children from families "rich in linguistic stimulation patterns" (Bzoch & League, 1971, p. 19), with no sensory or organic disabilities. Studies of internal consistency and test–retest reliability yielded adequate correlation coefficients, but the groups used for validity studies were limited in both number and size. Predictive validity indicated that administration during the first and third years was more robust than during the second year. No explanation was given for this observation. An attempt to look at use of the scale with low-income families (Dickson, 1972) indicated a slight downward trend in the 12- to 24-month age group, as compared to the 0- to 12-month group. It was unclear whether this was an artifact of the test or the start of a downward trend in this group. Additional data based on a more representative demographic sample are needed. The nature of the scoring makes the REEL somewhat problematic for use as a screen for children whose language/communication skills may be disordered or atypical, as opposed to being delayed.

MacArthur Communicative Development Inventories

The MacArthur Communication Development Inventories (CDIs; Fenson et al., 1993) can be used for children from 8 to 30 months of age. Suggested clinical and research purposes include (1) screening, (2) delineation of strengths and weaknesses, (3) development of intervention strategies, (4) evaluation of treatment effects, and (5) screening for research purposes (in order to preselect children according to language age/levels or specific profiles).

The CDIs consist of two detailed checklists/forms: CDI Words and Gestures (CDI/WG; 8–16 months) and CDI Words and Sentences (CDI/WS; 16–30 months). Each is divided into several parts. The CDI/WG provides scores (percentile ranks) for Vocabulary Comprehension, Vocabulary Production, and Gestures. The CDI/WS yields scores for Vocabulary Production, Sentence Complexity, and Mean Length of (a child's longest) Utterance. Scores can be converted to percentile ranks.

Information is obtained from parental report. A recognition format was chosen (checklists), in order to circumvent the limitations inherent in a recall design (which is subject to inaccuracy). Though the CDIs are lengthy (the major section of the CDI/WG has 396 items, and that of the CDI/WS has 680), the authors report that completion of the forms averages 20 to 40 minutes. Scoring can be done by hand in 10 minutes, or through machine scanning in conjunction with computer support if large numbers of subjects are involved. In the latter case, approximately 10 minutes of form checking prior to scanning is required. Machine scanning is also recommended when individual item information is needed, as the risk of data entry errors is lower. Non-English versions are under development; preliminary data are already available for Spanish, Italian, and American Sign Language users.

Raw scores can be converted to percentile ranks for each part of the respective inventories, with separate tables for boys and girls, although few significant gender differences were found during standardization. Figures are also provided for comparison within each area over time and for information regarding standard errors of measurement. Additional tables provide mean, percentile, and distribution scores across ages for different linguistic behaviors under study.

Detailed documentation regarding standardization of the CDIs and other technical information is provided. Information regarding reliability and validity studies is extensive. Validity (convergent, concurrent, and predictive) and reliability correlations were generally modest to high, although the authors point out that it is typical of linguistic development at this age to have some variability across sections.

Several significant limitations regarding use of norms and potential weaknesses in the CDIs are addressed by the authors. First, although the sample sizes for the normative studies were large, the authors strongly caution users about applying the normative data to children who come from low-socioeconomic-status (low-SES) households or whose parents have a limited education. This is because the original sample included a skewed number of parents whose educational and occupational levels were above the national average. Second, the norms are inappropriate as a means of characterizing the language age level of an older child, although in these cases the inventories may help with profiling strengths and weaknesses and with of monitoring change after intervention. In some sections, prior to 18 months of age, small increments in raw scores lead to large percentile leaps (e.g., an additional point in the raw score for irregular nouns can shift the percentile rank from the 25th to the 50th percentile). The Sentence Complexity section is likely to differentiate children with advanced skills, but is less robust when it comes to establishing which subjects are "late bloomers" and which are at risk for continuing delay. Results on the Pretend Substitution section (obtained via parental recall as opposed to recognition) were found to be unreliable, and the authors suggest that this part be used with caution or dropped. Parents' responses to the Vocabulary Comprehension section were not commensurate with the literature regarding development of comprehension, and in terms of predictive validity, only those children exhibiting delays in both production and comprehension (as opposed to production alone) later continued to show delays. Modified versions of the test have been developed (Reznick & Goldsmith, 1989), in which several shorter lists have been utilized with some success, although the sample size ($n = 25$) was limited.

Language Development Survey

The Language Development Survey (LDS; Rescorla, 1989) is a vocabulary checklist developed as a screening tool to identify language delay in 2-year-old children and to determine whether early delays in productive vocabulary are predictive of more persistent language delays. In addition to serving as a screening tool, it is useful for epidemiological and longitudinal research studies.

The LDS consists of a single-page checklist of vocabulary items (309 words) grouped in semantic categories (14), to be completed by parents. Words that have been produced by a child are checked, and parents also provide information about two additional words and examples of the child's longest utterances (if the child is already combining words). Total time to complete the form is approximately 10 minutes. Item selection was based on studies of lexical development (Nelson, 1976; Rescorla, 1989). The initial pilot study consisted of 500 children recruited from pediatric settings covering a broad SES spectrum.

The utility of the LDS as an epidemiological tool across SES groups was assessed by using the instrument with children ($n = 351$) from five different pediatric catchment areas. A preliminary criterion for language delay of less than 30 words *or* no two-word combinations by 24 months was adopted; two other criteria (less than 30 words *and* no two-word combinations by 24 months, and less than 50 words *or* no combinations by 24 months) were also examined. Mean vocabulary size was calculated for the entire group and for each pediatric practice. Analysis of variance indicated a significant result, but only one pairwise comparison was significant (the two extreme groups on the SES spectrum). Across practices, the actual percentage of children with less than 50 words was not significantly different (range 13–16%). Gender and SES effects were noted. A second study was conducted to obtain prevalence data from an inner-city hospital setting ($n = 15$) and to assess use of a longer word list (353 words); 14% of the children had less than 50 words (as on the previous occasion) but twice as many (32%) had more than 200. Thus the longer list did not have an impact on the rate of reported delay, but it raised the ceiling for children with larger lexicons. The criterion of <30 words *or* no word combinations was met by 16% of the children, consistent with the first study, and most of these were boys. Application of the other two criteria yielded results similar to those obtained in the first study.

Concurrent validity was studied by comparing LDS scores for children ($n = 81$) with wide-ranging vocabulary sizes against their scores on two other expressive language measures—the Object and Picture Naming tasks from the Bayley Scales of Infant Development, and the Expressive portion of the Reynell Developmental Language Scales (Picture and Object Labeling). Children recruited for the study were divided into control (language development on target) and experimental (expressive vocabulary slow to emerge) groups, based on maternal report. Correlations were obtained between LDS vocabulary count and Bayley counts (.75), Reynell counts (.85), and combined Bayley–Reynell counts (.87; all p's < .001). The children were divided into "delayed" and "normal" groups according to the three LDS criteria described above. These groups were compared to the delayed versus normal groups as defined by the other tests used. Regardless of which criterion was used, the LDS "delayed" group labeled fewer objects and pictures on the Bayley and Reynell than did the LDS "normal" group (p < .001 by t test).

"Sensitivity" and "specificity" of the LDS were calculated using a "hit rate" analysis, in which the predictor was the LDS and the outcome was the Reynell score. A delay was defined as 6 months less than chronological age. Results ("sensitivity" refers to false negatives [misses], and "specificity" to false positives [false alarms] were as follows:

	Sensitivity	Specificity
1. <30 words *or* no combinations	76%	89%
2. <30 words *and* no combinations	53%	97%
3. <50 words *or* no combinations	86%	87%

Based on these findings, the third criterion was adopted as most valid. Internal consistency was very good (alpha = .99). Test–retest reliability correlations were high for the total LDS and for individual semantic word groups (.86 to .99). A final study of concurrent validity, using a brief screening as the additional language measure, was conducted with 58 mothers and their children (aged 18 to 33 months). The correlation between screening and mothers' LDS scores was .79. Other correlations were lower and were attributed to the smaller sample size.

Rescorla (1989) notes that these prevalence rates are somewhat higher than those reported in other prevalence studies, but suggests that a number of children evidencing delays at 24 months will be back on track at 36 months (the age for which prevalence rates from 3% to 5% have been reported; Silva, McGee, & Williams, 1983; Stevenson & Richman, 1978). Overall, the LDS differentiates children with delay from those developing normally across SES groups. It is also cost-effective and easy to complete, although adults with limited literacy skills may need support in completing the form.

Communication and Symbolic Behavior Scales

The Communication and Symbolic Behavior Scales (CSBSs; Wetherby & Prizant, 1993) constitute a systematic sampling procedure that examines communicative, social-affective, and symbolic functioning in children from 8 to 24 months of age, or in children from 9 months to 5 years who may be functioning developmentally within the targeted age range. The caregiver is an active participant in the process and is typically present throughout. The purposes of the CSBSs are to identify children at risk, to establish a profile that can be monitored over time, and to provide direction for intervention. The scales were developed from theories of communication and social-emotional development; they cover the communicative forms and functions served, reciprocity, and aspects of symbolic play known to parallel language closely.

The CSBSs include direct assessment (with a flexible yet standardized format) and a caregiver questionnaire that includes a perception rating (indicating the extent to which the child's performance during testing is representative of typical behavior). The direct assessment component (which is videotaped) takes approximately 60 minutes and moves from more to less structured contexts after the initial warmup. Components consist of elicitation of communicative acts (communicative temptations), sharing of books, symbolic play probes, language comprehension probes, and constructive play probes. Direct assessment is followed by completion of the Caregiver Perception Form, which consists of twenty-two 5-point scales providing both quantitative (developmentally organized) and qualitative behavioral data. Time taken by an experienced rater to score the scales is approximately 60 to 90 minutes. Based on cluster scores from the individual scales, the following parameters are considered: Communicative Functions, Gestural Communicative Means, Vocal Communicative Means, Verbal Communicative Means, Reciprocity, Social-Affective Signaling, and Symbolic Behavior.

All materials needed to conduct the assessment are provided, along with a detailed manual and training videotapes to ensure reliable and consistent administration and rating. Directions for administration of the communicative temptations are explicit. Raw scores are converted to scaled scores, cluster scores (percentile ranks or standard scores), and a communicative composite score. For scaled scores, there is a mean of 3 and a standard deviation of 1. Cluster scores have a mean of 10 and a standard deviation of 3. Finally, the composite can be presented as a cluster score or converted to a score with a mean of 100 and a standard deviation of 15. Either chronological age or language stage can be used to compute normed scores. For children aged 8 to 24 months, chronological age is used. Language stage is defined by whether a child uses single or multiple words during the communication sampling. If Comprehension is particularly low relative to other symbolic scales, an alternative symbolic cluster score can be obtained excluding Comprehension. Confidence intervals are provided to allow for more reliable interpretation of the results. When comparing standard scores, users should consider only cluster standard scores, should expect some variability, and should use confidence bands—not the standard scores alone.

Standardization sampling was limited to 282 subjects, and it included retest scores from a third of the group, who were retested 2 months after the initial administration. The age range sampled was from 8 to 24 months, but there was considerable variability in number of children per age group (from a low of 6 at 24 months to a high of 27 at 12 months). Scaling and norming analyses were therefore obtained via weighting, which was also used to balance for gender, race, and Spanish origin when demographics were considered. In developing the norms so that the various scales could be compared, a common metric was developed, so that a score metric was produced "based on equal contributions by children at each month of age within the sample" (Wetherby & Prizant, 1993, p. 66). Gender-based differences were insufficient to warrant construction of separate norms for boys and girls. Overall, the authors made excellent attempts to take into account the various issues in standardization, but the relatively small sample used may not sufficiently support the complex psychometrics applied.

Reliability across scales was variable, since not all scales were attempting to assess the same parameters. (The coefficient for the communicative composite score was .91, but the range was from .17 to .91.) As noted above, test–retest information was obtained on about 33% of the sample, with a mean age difference from Test 1 to Test 2 of 2.85 months ($SD = 2.05$).

Greater stability was found over short periods, and some scales proved more stable than others (Vocal and Verbal Communicative Means and Symbolic Behavior were more stable than Communicative Functions, Gestural Communicative Means, Reciprocity, and Social-Affective Signaling). Although the CSBSs can provide stable rankings of subjects, individual changes may be more variable.

Interrater reliability was high for most scales (.90, .88, and .83) but was dependent on rater training. Content and face validity concerns were addressed briefly, and little concurrent validity information was provided, as there are few similar assessment instruments available for this age group. Predictive validity was examined via a discriminant-function analysis to observe the test's ability to differentiate between children with PDDs and those with specific language impairment. Construct validity was demonstrated through gradual changes in scores with increasing age. Intercorrelations were more interpretable when the groups were divided by language stage (prelinguistic vs. linguistic) and suggested that the CSBSs constitute a more homogeneous measure for children who are talking. Factor analyses indicated that there was more than a single communication or symbolic trait being measured, as intended by the developers.

The CSBSs are a welcome addition to the available assessment tools, in that they provide a standardized means of evaluating important dimensions in the target population. The drawback for clinicians may be that the process is time-consuming and requires access to video equipment. In the long run, use of such methods will enhance the conceptual understanding of early communicative skills in practitioners and may foster development of more efficient educational programming.

Vocabulary Measures

A number of other types of instruments are available to measure receptive or expressive vocabulary. Methods range from picture identification and naming to providing definitions of words or demonstrating a range of semantic skills (providing antonyms, synonyms, defining, etc.). Caution should be taken in using scores from tests developed to tap a specific linguistic skill (in this case, vocabulary knowledge) as though they represent subjects' overall IQs (as in studies where groups are matched according to receptive vocabulary ability). Frequently, picture-cued vocabulary may not be reflective of spontaneous vocabulary usage/comprehension; most importantly, in some individuals the vocabulary measured through picture identification or naming may be comparatively much stronger than more broadly based language levels. For example, several studies of individuals with fragile X syndrome report that expressive vocabulary scores are as much as two standard deviations higher than formally assessed language or language level as based on spontaneous mean length of utterance.

Peabody Picture Vocabulary Scale—Revised

The Peabody Picture Vocabulary Scale—Revised (PPVT-R; Dunn & Dunn, 1981) was developed to measure receptive vocabulary for standard American English users (not as a test of general intelligence) from the ages of 2½ to adulthood. It consists of a picture identification task (four pictures to a page). Two alternative forms are available. Administration is individual and untimed, with basal and ceiling cutoffs that reduce administration time to approximately 15 minutes. No reading or writing is required. Raw scores are converted to standard scores, percentile ranks, or stanines, and age equivalents are provided. Age and grade reference groups are available. Standardization sampling consisted of 4,200 subjects, 200 per 6-month age interval from 2 years, 6 months to 18 years, 11 months (50% boys, 50% girls). Demographics matched the U.S. national demographics although data regarding ethnicity and community size were not available for 18- to 40-year-olds.

Internal consistency, split-half, and alternate-form reliabilities were established. Split-half reliabilities ranged from .61 to .88; immediate and delayed test–retest reliabilities (using alternative forms) ranged from .73 to .91 and .52 to .90, respectively. The manual reports that PPVT-R scores were found to change over time, the average being 4.5 points over a 6-year period. Disadvantaged subjects tended to have higher gains. Results were least stable for African American preschool girls.

Content validity was inherent in the research involved in item selection. As mentioned, construct validity is adequate as long as the test is not interpreted more broadly as a measure of general intelligence. Information regarding predictive and concurrent validity is not provided in the manual, but correlations with other vocabulary and intelligence tests are given and are higher for the former.

Peabody Picture Vocabulary Test, Third Edition

The third edition of the PPVT (PPPVT-III; Dunn & Dunn, 1997) has retained many features of the PPVT-R, but has added four items to each form to increase the number of easy and difficult items and has divided items into 17 sets of 12 pictures. Many of the illustrations have been modernized, and efforts have been made to improve the racial, ethnic, and gender balance represented in the pictures. A balance of verbs, nouns, and adjectives is used in multiple different categories, and updated items reflect new technologies. National norms were extended to cover ages from 2½ years to 90+ years, and the standardization sample of 2,752 people matched the 1995 Current Population Survey census data. Purposes of the test are (1) to measure receptive vocabulary and (2) to serve as a screening test of verbal ability. The authors caution against overgeneralizing on the basis of information from a screening instrument that looks at such a narrow area of linguistic ability. Its use as part of a test battery, however, is helpful, as long as an examinee has intact vision and hearing and is not limited in his/her proficiency with English.

Reliability studies were satisfactory and concluded that the PPVT-III is more reliable than its predecessor. Criterion (concurrent) validity studies were conducted during standardization. Correlations between the PPVT-III and the third edition of the Wechsler Intelligence Scale for Children (WISC-III; Wechsler, 1991) on standard scores ranged from .82 to .92, with WISC-III Verbal IQ scores correlating higher than Performance or Full Scale IQ scores. With the Kaufman Adolescent and Adult Intelligence Test (Kaufman & Kaufman,1993), corrected correlations ranged from .76 to .91, and higher correlations occurred with those subtests looking at verbal comprehension and general information (i.e., similar learned information skills). The authors conducted an equating study in order to allow for comparisons/conversions of scores on the PPVT-R and the PPVT-III, so that it is possible to use earlier data and gauge gain without having to resort to administering the previous version.

Expressive Vocabulary Test

The Expressive Vocabulary Test (EVT; Williams, 1997) is a welcome counterpoint to the PPVT-III. In fact, it was developed to be its expressive counterpart, and the same sampling population as that used in developing the PPVT-III was used. It is a norm-referenced assessment of expressive vocabulary and word retrieval for children and adults ranging from 2½ to 90+ years of age. Picture labeling is used for the earliest items, but then the task shifts to synonym naming in response to pictures plus verbal stimuli. The decision to use something other than simple object naming was based on research suggesting that naming of objects is based on information-processing skills that are typically established by the age of 7 years. The pictures provide sufficient contextual support for correct responses. Nouns, verbs, and adjectives are tapped. Word retrieval can be evaluated by examining standard score differences between the EVT and the PPVT-III.

Normative sampling for the EVT was extensive. As for the PPVT-III, 2,752 subjects were used and selected to meet the most recent U.S. census data on gender, race, ethnicity, region, and educational level. Results can be reported as standard scores, percentiles, normal curve equivalents, stanines, and test age equivalents. Users are cautioned against using normative scoring for people whose primary language is not English, although the test may be useful in establishing a baseline regarding word knowledge against which gains can be measured following intervention. The use of basal and ceiling rules ensures that only items that approximate the taker's ability level are administered, reducing the length of time needed.

Internal and test–retest reliability measures were high, and during validity studies control groups with specific clinical diagnoses took the test also (as well as the PPVT-III), although the sample sizes were small; the results are available in the EVT manual. The tests discriminated between controls and language-delayed/impaired students, students with mental retardation, and students with reading disability.

Test of Word Finding and Test of Adolescent/Adult Word Finding

The Test of Word Finding (TOWF; German, 1986) and the Test of Adolescent/Adult Word Finding (TOAWF; German, 1990) were developed as systematic procedures for the assessment of word-finding skills in children, adolescents, and adults. The TOWF is intended for students aged 6 through 12 years, and the TOAWF for students in 7th through 12th grades and for adults aged 20 through 80. Tasks include picture naming (nouns, verbs, categories), sentence completion naming, description naming, and a comprehension assessment (to rule out the possibility of failure on naming due to lack of familiarity with a word). Picture cues are utilized. Item selection was carefully researched, and consideration was given to demographic and age/grade bias. The standardization sample consisted of 1,200 children in first through sixth grades, whose composition matched demographic data from the 1980 U.S. census. Distribution across age and grade was equal (n's = 100 and 200, respectively). As recommended by Salvia and Ysseldyke (1981), 3% of the sample were identified as having linguistic deficits, and the manual provides data on this subgroup's performance. Results can be presented as standard scores or percentile ranks. Standard errors of measurement (SEMs) are given, and age equivalents can be obtained. Two indices of response time are provided. Reliability data include goodness-of-fit indices, SEMs, test–retest reliability, and correlations across the TOWF and the TOAWF.

Content and criterion validity were addressed. Correlations with other word-finding tests ranged from .75 (Expressive One-Word Picture Vocabulary Test—Revised) to .52 (Word Test—Antonyms) to –.54 (Producing Names on Confrontation, Clinical Evaluation of Language Fundamentals [CELF]). Specificity and sensitivity were also addressed, and only 1% of the normal subjects in the sample were misdiagnosed when a criterion of scores lower than a standard deviation below the sample mean was used. Final analyses allow for categorization of subjects into groups according to rate (slow vs. fast) and accuracy (accurate vs. inaccurate) of naming.

Expressive One Word Picture Vocabulary Test—Revised

Expressive One Word Picture Vocabulary Test—Revised (Gardner, 1987, 1990) is intended to provide a basal estimate of verbal IQ for subjects from 2 to 12 years of age (there is an upper extension for ages 12 years to 15 years,

11 months; Gardner, 1983) through a picture-naming task. The test has 110 items arranged developmentally and takes approximately 7 to 15 minutes to administer. The raw scores can be converted to age equivalents, standard and scaled scores, percentile ranks, and stanines. SEMs can be calculated.

The standardization sample consisted of 1,118 subjects ranging in age from 2 through 12 years (size per 6-month age groups, however, varied from 23 to 55, and no weighting of scores was utilized). Although gender was apparently balanced, some subjects' gender was unknown; all subjects were living in the San Francisco area, but other details regarding demographics are limited. The author evaluated the capacity of each item to differentiate age or ability levels, using a discrimination index and item–total correlations. Items were arranged according to when 40–60% of the children knew the word. (In spite of this, at face value it seems unlikely that "statues" would be known before some later items, such as "food," "tractor," or "drinks.")

Psychometric information is limited. Internal split-half consistency with a Kuder–Richardson formulation was .84 to .92. Some criterion-related correlations were reported, including correlations with the PPVT-R (.59) and the Wechsler Preschool and Primary Scale of Intelligence–Revised Vocabulary subtest (.48).

Other Vocabulary Tasks

Additional vocabulary tasks are often part of larger language batteries, such as the Test of Language Development—Primary—3 (Newcomer & Hammill, 1997) or the CELF-3 (Semel, Wiig, & Secord, 1995). Subtests of these larger tests evaluate vocabulary and semantic knowledge through more demanding tasks (e.g., requiring comparisons, retrieval, provision of definitions, etc.), and can shed useful light on the performance of students who may score more highly on simpler identification and naming tasks. Observation of vocabulary use and retrieval in conversational contexts (on preferred topics and those introduced by others) is also an essential source of information about day-to-day lexical capacities.

Measures of Broader Language Functions

Comprehension instruments utilize various tasks, including picture identification, toy identification, and object manipulation, and may require direct observation of the response or may allow credit based on parental report.

Test for Auditory Comprehension of Language—Revised

The Test for Auditory Comprehension of Language—Revised (TACL-R; Carrow-Woolfolk, 1985) assesses understanding of word meanings and relations (semantics); grammatical morphemes; and longer, more complex sentence forms through a picture identification task. Each test plate has three line drawings, one of which matches the stimulus that is read to the subject, the others being foils with semantic or grammatical contrasts. Normative data are available for subjects from 3 years to 9 years, 11 months of age, and can be presented as standard scores (z and T scores), percentile ranks, or age equivalents by age or grade level. Basal and ceiling rules are provided, and testing time is stated as 10 minutes. As with the PPVT-III (or any task relying on picture identification as a measure), supplementary information regarding a student's ability to demonstrate these comprehension skills in spontaneous interactions is needed for clinical purposes.

Subgrouping and item classification for the TACL-R were based on grammatical theory, research, and empirical observations of aphasic patients. Specific items were selected along developmental lines based on the child language literature (Brown, 1973). Attempts were made to reduce cultural, racial, gender, and age biases in the illustrations.

The TACL-R's standardization sample consisted of 1,003 children with normal language skills and was balanced according to 1981 U.S. Census Bureau data. Subdivisions according to parental occupation and SES were evaluated, in an attempt to observe the effect of presumed language level in the home.

Reliability information includes SEMs, internal consistency, and test–retest data. SEMs were low relative to the mean scores. Spearman–Brown split-half reliabilities ranged from .77 to .95, with lower correlations at older age levels (i.e., at the upper end of the test's utility). Test–retest reliability correlations ranged from .89 to .95.

Construct validity was indicated by the decreasing scores across sections (which increase in complexity), and by the intercorrelations between subsections and total scores (ranging from .80 to .96). Concurrent validity measures were conducted with small samples and with lengthy time lapses between testing. Generally, the TACL-R had higher correlations with tests tapping similar skills than with tests assessing expressive language tasks. In addition, information was obtained on language-disordered, hearing-impaired, mentally retarded, and aphasic subjects. Subjects ($n = 234$) with comprehension difficulties obtained lower scores than normal subjects or those with articulation problems. For subjects with severe developmental delays, non-normalized scores are available, although they are not for use in establishment of eligibility for services.

Token Test for Children

The Token Test was originally designed for testing receptive language in aphasic adults (DeRenzi & Vignolo, 1962). Various forms of the Token Test have been developed by researchers, including the Token Test for Children (DiSimoni, 1978). Studies comparing students' performance on the Token

Test for Children and other language measures have suggested it to be a sensitive indicator of receptive language function in children.

In this individually administered test, children from 3 years through 12 years, 5 months of age are asked to point to or move wooden shapes of different colors and sizes in relation to each other. Directions are divided into five parts, which become increasingly lengthy and complex (there are 61 items in all). Parts are presented in a specified sequence, with every item being administered. Responses are recorded as correct or incorrect, and an overall raw score is obtained that can be translated into standard scores (mean of 500, standard deviation of 5). The author suggests allowing some leeway in interpretation of standard scores and indicates the test to be a rapid screening of semantics. No quantification for the interpretative judgment is given.

Standardization for this version was based on a sample of 1,304 children from 3 years to 12 years, 6 months of age, who were not carefully matched to national demographic data and were not evenly distributed across the 6-month age group divisions. The author indicates that the numbers of subjects in the youngest and oldest age groups were too small for reliable data analysis, and that the standard scores for these groups should be interpreted with caution. Although test design, reliability, validity, and predictive value have been discussed in relation to other versions of the Token Test, the manual does not report on these psychometrics for this standardization sample.

Given the lack of basal and ceiling rules, younger children with language difficulties may tire of the task, and this is likely to interfere with reliability of the findings. In addition, the test is limited by the restricted nature of the task (picture identification/recognition), which fails to account for the range of variables influencing children's comprehension of language.

Tests of Auditory Comprehension and Expressive Language

Many tests either include auditory comprehension and expressive language scales or divide tasks according to theoretical models of language development. Some frequently used tests are presented here.

Illinois Test of Psycholinguistic Abilities

The Illinois Test of Psycholinguistic Abilities (ITPA; Kirk, McCarthy, & Kirk, 1968) was an early attempt to design an instrument based on a theoretical psycholinguistic model. Although it is not used extensively at present it is discussed here as an illustration of a tool whose development reflected an attempt to consider the processes potentially underpinning linguistic capacities.

The ITPA is based on an adaptation of Osgood's communication model and attempts to assess the psychological functions believed to be involved in communicative interactions. By defining specific aspects of these processes and developing tasks to tap these, the authors aimed at pinpointing specific psycholinguistic strengths and weaknesses. The following dimensions of cognitive abilities were considered central: channels of communication (auditory–vocal and visual–motor), psycholinguistic processes (comprehension, expression and central organizing processes), and levels of organization (representative and automatic). Based on these, 10 subtests and 2 supplementary subtests were developed—6 representational (Auditory and Visual Reception; Auditory–Vocal and Visual–Motor Association; Verbal and Manual Expression) and 6 automatic (Grammatic, Auditory, and Visual Closure; Sound Blending; Auditory and Visual Sequential Memory).

The test is for subjects from 2 years, 4 months to 10 years, 3 months of age, and subtest items are arranged in developmental sequence. Ceiling cutoff rules are provided, and the raw scores are converted to psycholinguistic language ages, standard score (mean of 36, standard deviation of 6), and composite psycholinguistic language age based on the 10 main subtests. A ratio method is used for computing a psycholinguistic language quotient. The test takes an hour to administer.

Standardization was conducted on 962 children from 2 years, 7 months through 10 years, 1 month of age, years with average IQ, school achievement, and SES, and without sensory or motor deficits. Subjects were from predominantly middle-class Midwestern communities, and fathers' occupations matched those of the population based on 1960 U.S. census data. Internal consistency reliabilities ranged from .67 to .95 for the 10 main subtests (Paraskevopoulos & Kirk, 1969). Test–retest reliabilities at 5- to 6-month intervals ranged from .28 to .90 for children aged 4 through 6 years.

Concurrent validity studies that used achievement tests as criteria had widely varying results (from nonsignificant to significant), while those using intelligence tests have frequently shown highly significant correlations. In studies looking for underlying factors, Verbal Comprehension, Vocal Motor Expression, and Meaningful Figural Comprehension have been identified.

Although some subtests from the ITPA yield useful information, there are some flaws both in item design and in standardization. In Auditory Reception, questions requiring yes–no responses are presented (e.g., "Do dogs eat?"), allowing for chance erroneous responses; some items in other subtests are likely to place students from less verbal backgrounds at a disadvantage (e.g., verbal analogies—"A daddy is big, a baby is _____"). Finally, the stimulus photographs are dated, and errors may reflect lack of familiarity with items rather than inability to do the task. The lack of a more representational population sample is also problematic.

Preschool Language Scale—3

The Preschool Language Scale—3 (PLS-3; Zimmerman, Steiner, & Pond, 1992) assesses receptive and expressive language skills in infants and young children aged 2 weeks to 6 years, 11 months. The third edition was developed specifically to comply with changes resulting from P.L. 99-457: It adds downward extensions and provides standardized, normative information in addition to age equivalents.

The PLS–3 has two subscales (Auditory Comprehension and Expressive Communication) and three supplemental measures (The Articulation Screener, Language Sample, and Family Information and Suggestions Form). The test takes less than 60 minutes to administer; it evaluates precursors to communication skills, such as attention, vocal development, and social communication; and it has tasks assessing semantics, structure, and integrative thinking skills (drawing on Bloom's theoretical model in regard to content, form, and use, although the last of these comes under less scrutiny). Tasks involve pictures and objects, and basal and ceiling rules are provided. In addition, certain items can be passed if skills are exhibited in observations of spontaneous behavior, in spite of failure to respond to the structured items. Parental report cannot be credited unless the behaviors under question are observed directly.

The standardization sample consisted of 1,200 children and was stratified by parent educational level, geographic region, and race, according to the 1986 update of the 1980 U.S. census. Data can be presented as standard scores, percentile ranks, and age equivalents for each subscale, and can be combined to yield a total language standard score or age equivalent. SEMs are provided for 68%, 80%, and 90% confidence bands.

Internal consistency was assessed with Cronbach's coefficient alpha, and the coefficients ranged from .47 to .88. Test–retest reliabilities for children aged 3, 4, and 5 were adequate (.82 to .94). No explanation was given as to why they were not established for younger subjects. Interrater reliabilities on items requiring subjective scoring were .89 to .98.

In order to assess validity, a discriminant-function analysis was conducted and a signal detection model applied. Accuracy of discrimination increased across ages 3 through 5 (66%, 80%, and 70%). The errors were usually due to the the the test's failure to identify children previously diagnosed with a communication disorder (i.e., false negatives—poor sensitivity). These results raise serious questions, given the need for accurate identification, particularly at earlier ages. Several concurrent validity studies are reported, although the numbers sampled are typically small.

Reynell Developmental Language Scales—U.S. Edition

The Reynell Developmental Language Scales were developed originally in England. The U.S. edition of this instrument (Reynell & Gruber, 1990) is an individually administered test of verbal comprehension and expressive language for children from 1 year to 6 years, 11 months of age. The 134-item battery is administered in under an hour, and the toy materials are particularly appealing and therefore motivating for younger children. Two separate normed versions are provided for the Comprehension scale—one for those able to provide oral responses, the other for children with physical impairments that may prevent oral responses or reduce manual dexterity. Information for administration and interpretation with hearing-impaired children is provided, although normative data on this population are not available.

Standard scores and percentile ranks are obtained, in addition to which a developmental age (actually a developmental language age; i.e., an age equivalent) can be established. An additional Ability/Difficulty scale is available to detect the presence of significant strengths or weaknesses. Confidence intervals for use with standard scores are recommended and are given at the 68% confidence level. This is particularly important for 5- and 6-year-olds, since reliability for these age groups was lower. Item interpretation is encouraged and explained in the manual. Standard scores do not go lower than 63; downward extensions would be helpful, in order to provide more specific information about those children falling into the lower ranges of language functioning.

Standardization sampling was conducted on 619 children from 1 year to 6 years, 11 months of age. Subjects were selected to match 1987 U.S. Census Bureau data on all demographic variables. Means and standard deviations were collected at 3-month intervals, and smoothing procedures (Tukey, 1977) were used to establish developmental trends. This process also provided evidence of construct validity. Normative tables were developed, and Spearman–Brown split-half reliability coefficients were calculated. Up to age 5 years, reliability was good (.80 to .93 range); from 5 years, 6 months through 6 years, 11 months, these coefficients declined to .70 (barely adequate). SEMs also increased as reliability decreased.

Issues of validity were addressed in a study (Silva, Bradshaw, & Spears, 1987) involving 225 children, which supported the concurrent validity and provided information regarding both divergent and convergent comparisons. Predictive validity in comparisons with the Stanford–Binet (.71) and the WISC (.69; $n = 185$) was high. A brief mention of discriminant validity was made.

Clinical Evaluation of Language Fundamentals—Revised

Developed as a clinical tool for the identification, diagnosis, and follow-up evaluation of language problems in children from kindergarten through 12th grade, the CELF-R (Semel, Wiig, & Secord, 1995) assesses semantics, morphology, syntax, and memory (recall and retrieval) in receptive and expressive language domains. The CELF-R consists of 11 subtests, but some are more discriminating at certain ages than others. For students aged 5 through 7 years, three subtests each yield receptive and expressive language ages and total language ages, although others can also be administered. Students aged 8 years and older take some of the same and some different subtests. Standard scores for receptive, expressive, and total language scores have means of 100 and standard deviations of 15; subtests have standard scores with means of 10 and standard deviations of 3. Age equivalent scores are available for the total language score only. SEMs are provided for 68%, 80%, and 90% confidence levels. Tables allow for comparison between subtest standard scores and also between each subtest. The mean score for all subtests thus gives information regarding significant strengths and weaknesses. Administration time depends on which subtests are given, but typically takes from 60 to 90 minutes. The standardization sample consisted of 2,426 subjects between the ages of 5 and 16 years. The demographic makeup of the group was representative of the 1980 U.S. census.

Test design and normative data are reported. Discriminant-function analyses of the items were conducted prior to standardization, to assess quality of items, ease of administration, and predictive power. Of 157 students assessed, 90.4% were diagnosed correctly (e.g., as either with or without communication disorders); of the 15 misclassified by the CELF-R, 3.2% were false positives and 6.4% were false negatives. Concurrent validity was measured against the original CELF and yielded a positive correlation of .49. Suggestions are given for extensive testing of areas falling below the average range.

Differences in performance between European American and African American subjects were assessed, and on the composite language score African Americans scored approximately one-third to one-half of a standard deviation lower than their European American matches. These discrepancies were less than those reported in most achievement tests, and significantly less than those observed between normally achieving and language-disabled students. Gender differences were minimal.

Generally, the CELF-R provides a range of tasks tapping different aspects of receptive and expressive skills, from which both quantitative data and qualitative information (i.e., clinical observations as to how a child approaches tasks and which are found easier or more difficult) can be obtained. The authors have also produced a preschool version for children from 3 to 5 years of age.

Clinical Evaluation of Language Fundamentals—3

The CELF-3 (Semel et al., 1995) was developed to identify language problems in students from 6 to 21 years of age. In this new edition, changes have been made in materials, content, and administration procedures, and normative scores have been updated. Test plates are in full color, contexts are updated, and gender and ethnic biases have been eliminated. An attempt is made to use basal and ceiling rules when possible, to reduce the frustration caused when students have to continue to the end of a series when they have already reached their top performance, or when students have to answer items well below their capacity. Dialectal variations and differences can be taken into account when they are part of an individual's language system. In addition, greater credit is allowed for partially correct responses in some subtests (e.g., Formulated Sentences and Recalling Sentences), while in others a 4-point scale has been reduced to a 3-point scale to reduce unreliable distinctions. The latter has led to increased reliability in scores (e.g., for 11-year-olds, from .70 on the CELF-R to .82 on the CELF-3).

The subtests attempt to assess the content and form aspects of language in listening (decoding) and speaking (encoding). Short-term auditory memory is also integral to several of the subtests, including following directions (Concepts and Directions), repeating sentences (Recalling Sentences), and listening comprehension (Listening to Paragraphs). Word retrieval is also tapped during a timed task.

Standardization sampling was conducted on 2,450 children, adolescents, and young adults. Participants were English-language-dominant and were not considered to have or have had any language difficulties; the sample matched the 1980 U.S. census demographics. As with the CELF-R, studies of reliability and validity were thorough.

The CELF preschool is a downward extension of the CELF-3, designed as a screening instrument for children from the ages of 3 years to 6 years, 11 months.

Test of Language Competence—Expanded Edition

The Test of Language Competence—Expanded Edition (Wiig & Secord, 1989) is a combination of the original test and a downward extension, such that it can now be used with children from 5 to 9 years of age (Level 1) and with children and adolescents aged from 9 years to 18 years, 11 months (Level 2). It was designed to identify children having difficulty with metalinguistic competence in semantics, syntax, or pragmatics, through tasks looking at nonliteral language, inference, attribution, and linguistic ambiguity. In addition, Level 2 has an optional supplementary task assessing memory strategy acquisition in a paired-word list formal. There are four subtests—two primarily receptive (interpretative) and two expressive—which yield individual standard scores (mean of 10, standard deviation of 3) and, in combination, yield receptive, expressive, and total language composite standard scores (mean of 100, standard deviation of 15). SEMs are available for confidence intervals, as are percentile ranks and age equivalents, although the authors stress the need for caution in interpretation of the latter. Tables are available for interpreting differences between subtest scores and establishing relative strengths and weaknesses. A shorter screening utilizing two subtests (one receptive and one expressive) can be used. The test takes a total of approximately 1 hour to administer, and discontinue rules are provided.

Tasks are presented differently in Levels 1 and 2, with greater use of pictorial stimuli in the former allowing for recognition responses as opposed to the greater demands of self-generated responses. In addition, several tasks incorporate interpretation and identification components, allowing for more insight into students' strategies and strengths (i.e., differences in performance when asked to generate ideas, as opposed to simply recognizing correct options). Suggestions for extension testing are given. The authors report on racial/ethnic minority differences (with black students scoring lower than their white matches) and advise users to be cautious when interpreting scores for minority students. Use of local norms is recommended.

Elementary Test of Problem Solving—Revised

The Elementary Test of Problem Solving —Revised (Zachman, Huisingh, Barrett, Orman, & LoGiudice, 1994) is a diagnostic test of problem solving and critical thinking for elementary school students from the ages of 6 years to 11 years, 11 months. It requires students to draw on their own experience, and questions require critical thinking skills such as clarifying, analyzing, generating solutions, evaluating, and affective thinking. A student responds orally to spoken questions that relate to photographic stimuli (scenes). There are no basal and ceiling rules, making this quite a long assessment for younger or less able students. The test consists of 14 photographs, for each of which there are six questions that typically begin at a concrete level (e.g., "What is happening in this picture?") and go on to test deduction, an appreciation of implications, or sensitivity to feelings. The test can therefore be an excellent opportunity to observe differences in response from the easiest (most concrete) to the more challenging (most abstract) questions, and also to see a student's capacity to draw on day-to-day knowledge to reach conclusions. Certain topics may be unfamiliar or less meaningful to younger students (e.g., a boy hitchhiking), and the photographs are quite dated. Guidelines are given regarding acceptable and unacceptable answers, and the test yields standard scores (mean of 100, standard deviation of 15), percentile ranks, and age equivalents.

This test is a useful tool in obtaining a sample of a student's expressive output during problem solving, and the pictures often provoke some interest.

Concluding Comments

Assessment tools tapping pragmatic and social skills have not been discussed in depth here, although there are various instruments available, many of which may be most helpful with students on the autistic spectrum. Some of these have been discussed earlier in this chapter (e.g., the ADOS, PL-ADOS, and ADI-R) and can be utilized by a speech pathologist trained to do so. They have the advantage of tapping many parameters, including nonverbal communication, prosodic features, and discourse skills; they also do so within the context of a semistructured play interview, which is a more naturalistic and often more accurate way of gauging skills than the more contrived tests designed to assess pragmatics. Direct observation is essential as a part of a broader communication evaluation and provides data that are unobtainable in an office evaluation, such as information about interactions with peers, participation and skill levels during group interactions, and differing capacities in structured versus unstructured activities.

As in any assessment, a battery of test instruments should be used in order to obtain comprehensive data regarding language/communication skills in a given subject. Spontaneous language sampling, though not discussed in detail here, should be utilized; various methods of computer-analyzing such data are available, some of which can be selected to identify given target structures/functions (e.g., verbs vs. nouns, responses vs. initiations in conversation, type–token ratios). Some of the more commonly used programs include the Systematic Analysis of Language Transcripts (Miller & Chapman, 1993) and the Child Language Analysis (Spektor & MacWhinney, 1991).

Members of a team working collaboratively—which may consist of a child psychiatrist, a psychologist, a speech language pathologist, an audiologist, a neurologist, an occupational therapist, a physical therapist, a special education teacher, and (always) the parents—can bring together their different areas of expertise in order to understand a given child's profile, to identify strengths and weaknesses, and to develop an effective educational plan. An understanding of the parameters to be considered in selecting tests is key, as is knowing what tests are available. However, equally important is to have a theoretical grasp of the aspects of functioning to be assessed, so that these things can also be observed in real-life situations. This is where the presence or absence of effective functioning is most critical, and where the team must concentrate its treatment efforts in order to provide a child with useful tools for living through communication and social skills development.

REFERENCES

Aram, D., Ekelman, B., & Nation, J. (1984). Preschoolers with language disorders: Ten years later. *Journal of Speech and Hearing Research, 27,* 232–244.

Aram, D., & Nation, J. (1980). Preschool language disorders: Subsequent language and academic difficulties. *Journal of Communication Disorders, 18,* 159–170.

American Psychiatric Association. (1980). *Diagnostic and statistical manual of mental disorders* (3rd ed.). Washington, DC: Author.

American Psychiatric Association. (1987). *Diagnostic and statistical manual of mental disorders* (3rd ed., rev.). Washington, DC: Author.

American Psychiatric Association. (1994). *Diagnostic and statistical manual of mental disorders* (4th ed.). Washington, DC: Author.

Asperger, H. (1944). Die "autistichen Psychopathen" im Kindersalter. *Archive fur psychiatrie und Nervenkrankheiten, 117,* 76–136.

Baltaxe, C., & Simmons, J. Q. (1988). Communication deficits in preschool children with psychiatric disorders. *Seminars in Speech and Language, 9,* 81.

Baron-Cohen, S., Allen, J., & Gillberg (1992). Can autism be detected at 18 months?: The needle, the haystack, and the CHAT. *British Journal of Psychiatry 161,* 839–843.

Baron-Cohen, S., Cox, A., Baird, G., Swettenham, J., Nightingale, N., Morgan, K., Drew, A., & Charman, T. (1996). Psychological markers in the detection of autism in infancy in a large population. *British Journal of Psychiatry, 168*(2), 158–163.

Bates, E. (1976). *Language in context: Studies in the acquisition of pragmatics.* New York: Academic Press.

Bax, M., Hart, H., & Jenkins, S. (1980). Assessment of speech and language development in the young child. *Pediatrics, 66*(3), 350–354.

Beichtman, J. H., Nair, R., Clegg, M., Ferguson, B., & Patel, P. G. (1986). Prevalence of psychiatric disorders in children with speech and language disorders. *Journal of the American Academy of Child Psychiatry, 25*(4), 528–535.

Bloom, L., & Lahey, M. (1978). *Language development and language disorders.* New York: Wiley.

Brown, R. (1973). *A first language: The early stages.* Cambridge, MA: Harvard University Press.

Bruner, J. (1977). *Early social interaction and language acquisition.* In M. Schaffer (Ed.), *Studies in mother–infant interaction* (pp. 155–178). New York: Academic Press.

Bruner, J. (1981). The social context of language acquisition. *Language and Communication, 1,* 155–178.

Bzoch, K., & League, R. (1971). *The Receptive Expressive Emergent Language Scale.* Gainesville, FL: Language Education Division, Computer Management Corporation.

Cantwell, D., & Baker, L. (1987). Clinical significance of child communication disorders: Perspectives from a longitudinal study. *Journal of Child Neurology, 2,* 257–264.

Carrow-Woolfolk, E. (1985). *Test for Auditory Comprehension of Language—Revised.* Allen, TX: DLM.

Cohen, D. J., Caparulo, B. K., Gold, J. R., Waldo, M. C., Shaywitz, B. A., Ruttenberg, B. A., & Rimland, B. (1978). Agreement in diagnosis: Clinical assessment and behavior rating scales for pervasively disturbed children. *Journal of the American Academy of Child Psychiatry, 17*(4), 589–603.

Crais, E., & Roberts, J. (1991). Decision making in assessment and early intervention planning. *Language, Speech, and Hearing Services in Schools, 22,* 19–30.

DeRenzi, E., & Vignolo, L. (1962). The Token Test: A Sensitive Test to detect receptive disturbances in aphasia. *Brain, 85,* 665–678.

Dickson, C. J. (1972). *Emergent language acquisition in children from low income families.* Unpublished masters thesis, University of Florida, Gainesville.

DiLavore, P. C., Lord, C., & Rutter, M. (1995). The Pre-Linguistic Autism Diagnostic Observation Schedule. *Journal of Autism and Developmental Disorders, 25*(4), 355–379.

DiSimoni, F. (1978). *Token Test for Children.* Austin, TX: Pro-Ed.

Dunn, L. M., & Dunn, L. (1981). *Peabody Picture Vocabulary Test—Revised.* Circle Pines, MN: American Guidance Service.

Dunn, L. M., & Dunn, L. (1997). *Peabody Picture Vocabulary Test* (3rd ed.). Circle Pines, MN: American Guidance Service.

Eaves, R. C., & Milner, B. (1993). The criterion-related validity of the Childhood Autism Rating Scale and the Autism Behavior Checklist. *Journal of Abnormal Child Psychology, 21*(5), 481–491.

Fenson, L., Dale, P., Reznick, S., Thal, D., Bates, E., Hartung, S., Pethick, S., & Reilly, J. (1993). *MacArthur Communicative Development Inventories.* San Diego, CA: Singular.

Freeman, B. J., Ritvo, E. R., Guthrie, D., Schroth, P., & Ball, J. (1978). The Behavior Observation Scale for Autism: Initial methodology, data analysis, and preliminary findings on 89 children. *Journal of the American Academy of Child Psychiatry, 17*(4), 576–588.

Freeman, B. J., Ritvo, E. R., Yokota, A., & Ritvo, A. (1986). A scale for rating symptoms of patients with the syndrome of autism in real life settings. *Journal of the American Academy of Child Psychiatry, 25*(1), 130–136.

Fundandis, T., Kolvin, L., & Garside, R. (1979). *Speech retarded and deaf children.* London: Academic Press.

Gardner, M. (1985). Receptive One Word Picture Vocabulary Test. Los Angeles: Western Psychological Services.

Gardner, M. (1990). *Expressive One Word Vocabulary Test—Revised.* Novato, CA: Academic Therapy.

Garfin, D. G., McCallon, D., & Cox, R. (1988). Validity and reliability of the Childhood Autism Rating Scale with autistic adolescents. *Journal of Autism and Developmental Disorders, 18,* 367–378.

German, D. (1986). *Test of Word Finding in Children.* Allen, TX: DLM.

German, D. (1990). *Test of Adolescent/Adult Word Finding.* Allen, TX: DLM.

Gillberg, C. (1994). Debate and argument: Having Rett syndrome in the ICD-10 PDD category does not make sense. *Journal of Child Psychology and Psychiatry and Allied Disciplines, 35*(2), 377–378.

Goodman, R., & Minne, C. (1995). Questionnaire screening for comorbid pervasive developmental disorders in congenitally blind children: A pilot study. *Journal of Autism and Developmental Disorders, 25*(2), 195–203.

Howlin, P. (1998). Outcome in autism and related conditions. In F. R. Volkmar (Ed.), *Autism and pervasive developmental disorders* (pp. 209–241). Cambridge, UK: Cambridge University Press.

Kanner, L. (1943). Autistic disturbances of affective contact. *Nervous Child, 2,* 217–250.

Kaufman, A., & Kaufman, N. L. (1983). *K-ABC: Kaufman Assessment Battery for Children.* Circle Pines, MN: American Guidance Service.

Kirk, S., McCarthy, J., & Kirk, W. (1968). *Illinois Test of Psycholinguistic Abilities* (rev. ed.). Urbana: University of Illinois Press.

Klin, A., Volkmar, F. R., Sparrow, S. S., Cicchetti, D. V., & Rourke, B. P. (1995). Validity and neuropsychological characterization of Asperger syndrome: Convergence with nonverbal learning disabilities syndrome. *Journal of Child Psychology and Psychiatry, 36*(7), 1127–1140.

Kolvin, I. (1971). Studies in childhood psychoses: I. Diagnostic criteria and classification. *British Journal of Psychiatry, 118,* 381–384.

Krug, D. A., Arick, J., & Almond, P. (1980). Behavior checklist for identifying severely handicapped individuals with high levels of autistic behavior. *Journal of Child Psychology and Psychiatry, 21*(3), 221–229.

Le Couteur, A., Rutter, M., Lord, C., & Rios, P. E. A. (1989). Autism Diagnostic Interview: A standardized investigator-based instrument. *Journal of Autism and Developmental Disorders, 19*(3), 363–387.

Lenneberg, E. H. (1967). *Biological foundations of language.* New York: Wiley.

Lord, C. (1995). Follow-up of two-year-olds referred for possible autism. *Journal of Child Psychology and Psychiatry, 36*(8), 1365–1382.

Lord, C. (1997). Diagnostic instruments in autism spectrum disorders. In D. J. Cohen & F. R. Volkmar (Eds.), *Handbook of autism and pervasive developmental disorders* (2nd ed., pp. 460–483). New York: Wiley.

Lord, C., Rutter, M., & Le Couteur, A. (1989). Autism Diagnostic Observation Schedule: A standardized observation of communicative and social behavior. *Journal of Autism and Developmental Disorders, 19*(2), 185–212.

Lord, C., Rutter, M., & Le Couteur, A. (1994). Autism Diagnostic Interview—Revised: A revised version of a diagnostic interview for caregivers of individuals with possible pervasive developmental disorders. *Journal of Autism and Developmental Disorders, 24*(5), 659–685.

Lord, C., & Schopler, E. (1989). The role of age at assessment, developmental level, and test in the stability of intelligence scores in young autistic children. *Journal of Autism and Developmental Disorders, 19*(4), 483–499.

Lord, C., Storoschuk, S., Rutter, M., & Pickles, A. (1993). Using the ADI-R to diagnose autism in preschool children. *Infant Mental Health Journal, 14*(3), 234–252.

Lund, N., & Duchan, J. (1993). *Assessing children's language in naturalistic contexts* (3rd ed.). Englewood Cliffs, NJ: Prentice-Hall.

Mayes, L., Volkmar, F., Hooks, M., & Cicchetti, D. (1993). Differentiating pervasive developmental disorder not otherwise specified from autism and language disorders. *Journal of Autism and Developmental Disorders, 23*(1), 79–90.

McCauley, R., & Swisher, L. (1984). Psychometric review of language and articulation tests for preschool children. *Journal of Speech and Hearing Disorders, 49,* 34–42.

Mesibov, G. B., Schopler, E., Schaffer, B., & Michal, N. (1989). Use of the Childhood Autism Rating Scale with autistic adolescents and adults. *Journal of the American Academy of Child and Adolescent Psychiatry, 28*(4), 538–541.

Miller, J., & Chapman, R. (1993). *MACSALT: Systematic Analysis of Language Transcripts for the Apple Macintosh Computer* [Computer software]. Madison: Language Analysis Laboratory, Waisman Center, University of Wisconsin.

Morgan, S. (1988). Diagnostic assessment of autism: A review of objective scales. *Journal of Psychoeducational Assessment, 6*(2), 139–151.

Nelson, K. (1976). Structure and strategy in learning to talk. *Monographs of the Society for Research in Child Development, 38*(Serial No. 149).

Newcomer, P. L., & Hammill, D. D. (1997). *Test of Language Development. Primary 3rd Ed.* Austin, TX: Pro-Ed.

Oswald, D. P., & Volkmar, F. R. (1991). Brief report: Signal detection analysis of items from the Autism Behavior Checklist. *Journal of Autism and Developmental Disorders, 21*(4), 543–549.

Paraskevopoulus, J. N., & Kirk, S. A. (1969). *The development and psychometric characteristics of the Revised Illinois Test of Psycholinguistic Abilities.* Urbana, IL: University of Illinois Press.

Parks, S. L. (1983). The assessment of autistic children: A selective review of available instruments. *Journal of Autism and Developmental Disorders, 13*(3), 255–267.

Paul, R. (1995). *Language disorders from infancy through adolescence: Assessment and intervention.* St. Louis, MO: Mosby.

Piaget, J. (1923) *The language and thought of the child.* London: Routledge & Kegan Paul.

Plante, E., & Vance, R. (1994). Selection of preschool language tests: A data based approach. *Language, Speech and Hearing Services in Schools, 25,* 15–24.

Prizant, B., & Wetherby, A. M. (1990). Toward an integrated view of early language, communication, and socio-emotional development. *Topics in Language Disorders, 10,* 1–16.

Rescorla, L. (1989). The Language Development Survey: A screening tool for delayed language in toddlers. *Journal of Speech and Hearing Disorders, 54,* 587–599.

Reynell, J., & Gruber, C. P. (1990). *Reynell Developmental Language Scales—U.S. Edition.* Los Angeles: Western Psychological Services.

Reznick, S., & Goldsmith, L. (1989). A multiple form word production checklist for assessing early language. *Journal of Child Language, 16,* 91–100.

Rimland, B. (1968). On the objective diagnosis of infantile autism. *Acta Paedopsychiatrica, 35*(4), 146–161.

Rimland, B. (1971). The differentiation of childhood psychoses: An analysis of checklists for 2,218 psychotic children. *Journal of Autism and Childhood Schizophrenia, 1*(2), 161–174.

Ruttenberg, B. A., Dratman, M. L., Frakner, T. A., & Wenar, C. (1966). An instrument for evaluating autistic children. *Journal of the American Academy of Child Psychiatry 5*(3), 453–478.

Ruttenberg, B. A., Kalish, B. I., Wenar, C., & Wolf, E. G. (1977). *Behavior rating instrument for autistic and other atypical children.* Philadelphia: Developmental Center for Autistic Children.

Rutter, M. (1978). Diagnosis and definition of childhood autism. *Journal of Autism and Childhood Schizophrenia, 8*(2), 139–161.

Rutter, M. (1994). Debate and argument: There are connections between brain and mind and it is important that Rett syndrome be classified somewhere [comment]. *Journal of Child Psychology and Psychiatry, 35*(2), 379–381.

Salvia, J., & Ysseldyke, J. (1981). *Assessment in special and remedial education.* Boston: Houghton Mifflin.

Sattler, J. M. (1988). *Assessment of children* (3rd ed.). San Diego, CA: Jerome M. Sattler.

Schopler, E., Reichler, R. J., DeVellis, R. F., & Daly, K. (1980). Toward objective classification of childhood autism: Childhood Autism Rating Scale (CARS). *Journal of Autism and Developmental Disorders, 10*(1), 91–103.

Semel, E., Wiig, E., & Secord, W. (1995). *The Clinical Evaluation of Language Fundamentals—3.* San Antonio, TX: Psychological Corporation.

Serra, M., Minderaa, R. B., van Geert, P. L., & Jackson, A. E. (1995). An exploration of person perception abilities in children with a pervasive developmental disorder not otherwise specified. *European Journal of Child and Adolescent Psychiatry, 4*(4), 259–269.

Sevin, J. A., Matson, J. L., Coe, D. A., Fee, V. E., & Sevin B. (1991). A comparison and evaluation of three commonly used autism scales. *Journal of Autism and Developmental Disorders, 21*(4), 417–432.

Silva, P. A. (1980). The prevalence stability and significance of developmental language delay in pre-school children. *Developmental Medicine and Child Neurology, 22*(6), 768–777.

Silva, P. A., McGee, R., & Williams, S. M. (1983). Developmental language delay from three to seven and its significance for low intelligence and reading difficulties at seven. *Developmental Medicine and Child Neurology, 18,* 431–441.

Silva, P. A., Bradshaw, J., & Spears, G. F. (1978). *A study of the concurrent and prediction validity of the Reynell Developmental Language Scales.* (A report from the Dunedin multidisciplinary child developmental study, University of Otago, New Zealand.) London: NFER-Nelson.

Smalley, S. L., Tanguay, P. E., Smith, M., & Gutierrez, G. (1992). Autism and tuberous sclerosis. *Journal of Autism and Developmental Disorders, 22*(3), 339–355.

Sparrow, S. S. (1997). Developmentally based assessments. In D. J. Cohen & F. R. Volkmar (Eds.), *Handbook of autism and pervasive developmental disorders* (pp. 411–447). New York: Wiley.

Sparrow, S. S., Balla, D., & Cicchetti, D. (1984a). *Vineland Adaptive Behavior Scales (Expanded Form)*. Circle Pines, MN: American Guidance Service.

Sparrow, S. S., Balla, D., & Cicchetti, D. (1984b). *Vineland Adaptive Behavior Scales (Survey Form)*. Circle Pines, MN: American Guidance Service.

Spiker, D., Lotspeich, L., Kraemer, H. C., Hallmayer, J., McMahon, W., Peterson, B., Nicholas, P., Pingree, C., Wiese-Slater, S., Chiotti, C., Lee Wong, D., Dimicelli, S., Ritvo, E., Cavalli-Sforza, L. L., & Ciaranello, R. (1994). Genetics of autism: Characteristics of affected and unaffected children from 37 multiplex families. *American Journal of Medical Genetics, 54*, 27–35.

Stevenson, J., & Richman, N. (1976). The prevalence of language delay in a population of three year old children and its association with general retardation. *Developmental Medicine and Child Neurology, 18*(4), 431–441.

Stevenson, J., & Richman, N. (1978). Behavior, language, and development in three year old children. *Journal of Autism and Childhood Schizophrenia, 8*, 299–313.

Stone, W. L., & Lemanek, K. L. (1990a). Play and imitation skills in the diagnosis of autism in young children. *Pediatrics, 86*(2), 267–272.

Stone, W. L., & Lemanek, K. L. (1990b). Parental report of social behaviors in autistic preschoolers. *Journal of Autism and Developmental Disorders, 20*(4), 513–522.

Sturmey, P., Matson, J. L., & Sevin, J. A. (1992). Brief report: Analysis of the internal consistency of three autism scales. *Journal of Autism and Developmental Disorders, 22*(2), 321–328.

Szatmari, P., Archer, L., Fisman, S., & Steiner, D. L. (1994). Parent and teacher agreement in the assessment of pervasive developmental disorders. *Journal of Autism and Developmental Disorders, 24*(6), 703–717.

Szatmari, P., Archer, L., Fisman, S., Steiner, D. L., & Wilson, F. (in press). Asperger's syndrome and autism: Differences in behavior, cognition, and adaptive functioning. *Journal of the American Academy of Child and Adolescent Psychiatry, 34*, 1662–1671.

Tallal, P. (1988). Developmental language disorders. In J. F. Kavanagh & T. J. Truss, Jr. (Eds.), *Learning disabilities: Proceedings of the National Conference* (pp. 181–272). Parkton, MD: York Press.

Teal, M. B., & Wiebe, M. J. (1986). A validity analysis of selected instruments used to assess autism. *Journal of Autism and Developmental Disorders, 16*(4), 485–494.

Towbin, K. E. (1997). Pervasive developmental disorder not otherwise specified. In D. J. Cohen & F. R. Volkmar (Eds.), *Handbook of autism and pervasive developmental disorders* (2nd ed., pp. 123–147). New York: Wiley.

Tukey, J. W. (1971). *Exploratory data analysis.* Reading, MA: Addison-Wesley.

van Acker, R. (1997). Rett's Syndrome, In D. J. Cohen & F. R. Volkmar (Eds.), *Handbook of autism and pervasive developmental disorders* (2nd ed., pp. 60–93). New York: Wiley.

Van der Gaag, R. J., Buitelaar, J., Van den Ban, E., Bezemer, M., Njio, L., & Van Engeland, H. (1995) A controlled multivariate chart review of multiple complex developmental disorder. *Journal of American Academy of Child and Adolescent Psychiatry, 34*(8) 1096–1106.

Venter, A., Lord, C., & Schopler, E. (1992). A follow-up study of high-functioning autistic children. *Journal of Child Psychology and Psychiatry and Allied Disciplines, 33*(3), 489–507.

Volkmar, F. R., Cicchetti, D. V., Dykens, E., Sparrow, S. S., Leckman, J. F., & Cohen, D. J. (1988). An evaluation of the Autism Behavior Checklist. *Journal of Autism and Developmental Disorders, 18*(1), 81–97.

Volkmar, F. R., Klin, A., et al. (1997a). Diagnosis and classification of autism and related conditions: Consensus and issues. In D. J. Cohen & F. R. Volkmar (Eds.), *Handbook of autism and pervasive developmental disorders* (2nd ed., pp. 5–40). New York: Wiley.

Volkmar, F. R., Klin, A., Marans, W., & Cohen, D. J. (1997b). Childhood disintegrative disorder. In D. J. Cohen & F. R. Volkmar (Eds.), *Handbook of autism and pervasive developmental disorders* (2nd ed., pp. 47–59). New York: Wiley.

Volkmar, F. R., Klin, A., Siegel, B., Szatmari, P., Lord, C., Campbell, M., Freeman, B. J., Cicchetti, D. V., Rutter, M., Kline, W., Buitelaar, J., Hattab, Y., et al. (1994). Field trial for autistic disorder in DSM-IV. *American Journal of Psychiatry, 151*(9), 1361–1367.

Volkmar, F. R., & Rutter, M. (1995). Childhood disintegrative disorder: Results of the DSM-IV autism field trial. *Journal of the American Academy of Child and Adolescent Psychiatry, 34*(8), 1092–1095.

Volkmar, F. R., Sparrow, S. S., Goudreau, D., Cicchetti, D. V., Paul, R., & Cohen, D. J. (1987). Social deficits in autism: An operational approach using the Vineland Adaptive Behavior Scales. *Journal of the American Academy of Child and Adolescent Psychiatry, 26*(2), 156–161.

Wadden, N. P., Bryson, S. E., & Rodgers, R. S. (1991). A closer look at the Autism Behavior Checklist: Discriminant validity and factor structure. *Journal of Autism and Developmental Disorders, 21*(4), 529–541.

Wechsler, D. (1991). *Wechsler Intelligence Scale for Children* (3rd ed.). San Antonio, TX: Psychological Corporation.

Wetherby, A., & Prizant, B. (1992). Profiling young children's communicative competence. In S. Warren & S. Reichler (Eds.), *Perspectives on communication and language intervention: Development, assessment, and intervention* (pp. 217–251). Baltimore: Brookes.

Wetherby, A., & Prizant, B. (1993). *Communication and Symbolic Behavior Scales—Normed Edition*. Chicago: Riverside.

Wiig, E. H., & Secord, W. (1989). *Test of Language Competence—Expanded Edition*. New York: Psychological Corporation.

Wing, L., & Gould, J. (1979). Severe impairments of social interaction and associated abnormalities in children: Epidemiology and classification. *Journal of Autism and Developmental Disorders, 9*(1), 11–29.

Williams, K. T. (1997) *The Expressive Vocabulary Test*. Circle Pines, MN: American Guidance Service.

World Health Organization. (1994). *International Classification of Diseases* (10th Ed.): *Diagnostic criteria for research*. Geneva: Author.

Yirmiya, N., Sigman, M., & Freeman, B. J. (1994). Comparison between diagnostic instruments for identifying high-functioning children with autism. *Journal of Autism and Developmental Disorders, 24*(3), 281–291.

Zachman, L., Huisingh, R., Barrett, B., Orman, J., & LoGiudice, C. (1994). *The Elementary Test of Problem Solving—Revised*. East Moline, IL: Linguisystems.

Zimmerman, I., Steiner, V., & Pond, R. (1992). *Preschool Language Scale—3*. San Antonio, TX: Psychological Corporation.

III

SPECIAL ASPECTS
OF ASSESSING
PSYCHIATRIC DISORDERS

✧

7

The Assessment
of Functional Impairment

✧

HECTOR R. BIRD

The assessment of functional impairment has become increasingly important in the ascertainment of psychopathology in clinical practice, as well as in epidemiological research. Functional impairment has implications for treatment decisions at the individual level, as well as for service planning based on epidemiological data. Clinicians need to identify those individuals whose mental health is a cause for concern and who are considered to be in need of mental health services. Epidemiological studies must provide estimates of the prevalence of psychiatric disorders that indicate the proportion of truly ill or handicapped individuals, in terms that are broadly used by and acceptable to other researchers as well as clinicians.

It is no longer adequate for case ascertainment merely to detect those individuals who meet symptomatic criteria for one or more psychiatric disorders; it is equally important to assess the degree to which those individuals are dysfunctional or impaired. The determination of "caseness" requires a method for assessing impairment attributable to psychiatric morbidity as a fundamental element of case detection. This is true for clinical, research, and administrative purposes.

"CASENESS" AND THE ASSESSMENT
OF FUNCTIONAL IMPAIRMENT

Three fundamental notions enter into, but also complicate, the determination of caseness. One is the presence of specifically stipulated operational criteria that are requirements for classifying an individual as having a particular disorder; another is the presence of impairment or disability associated with, but assessed independently from, the symptomatology; the third is the presence of distress associated with the condition. The first complication to this scheme is that it aims to operationalize disorders as categorical phenomena that are either present or absent, whereas the clinical reality is that most disorders occur along dimensions of symptomatology. The symptom thresholds established by the existing nosology to distinguish between presence and absence of a disorder are generally arbitrary and not based on empirical data, although the two most recent modifications of the *Diagnostic and Statistical Manual of Mental Disorders* (DSM; American Psychiatric Association, 1987, 1994) have attempted to enhance its empirical basis. Another complication is that level of functional impairment depends to a great extent on other issues, such as personal role definitions and the individual's as well as society's goals and expectations. "Functional impairment" is therefore a relative concept that is difficult to operationalize for either clinical or research purposes with any degree of precision. Finally, the experience of distress and the extent to which it occurs are highly subjective epiphenomena that also depend on other factors in the individual, such as psychological defenses, intelligence, competence, and vulnerabilities. This fact also makes distress difficult to operationalize and to ascertain reliably.

For nearly two decades, the DSM taxonomy has been consistent in requiring that the concept of mental disorder be applied to those who both meet the symptomatic criteria for a psychiatric diagnosis, *and* have associated distress and disability or functional impairment (American Psychiatric Association, 1980, p. 6; American Psychiatric Association, 1987, p. xxii; American Psychiatric Association, 1994, p. xxi). The notion that diagnostic considerations need to include a measure of severity or of level of impairment, or both, follows DSM stipulations and is consonant with the clinician's tendency to evaluate and to make treatment decisions along dimensional rather than along categorical lines (Robins, 1985).

Despite numerous attempts to derive an assessment of functional impairment empirically, the determination of "caseness" is ultimately an issue of clinical judgment. A clinician may base a conclusion that an individual is a case or in need of clinical attention on the severity of the person's symptomatology, or on the degree of impairment or distress associated with the symptomatology, rather than on whether criteria for a particular diagnosis are or are not fully met. This kind of clinical latitude in the procedures to ascertain caseness poses a significant problem in research, where diagnostic assessments typically attempt to adapt the clinical method. Notwithstanding the fact that assessing the presence or absence of symptomatic criteria has reached a moderate level of precision and sophistication through the use of standardized measures, it has been difficult to develop a systematic way of operationalizing and measuring functional impairment for research purposes. Determining level of functional impairment continues to be particularly problematic in any research that relies on standardized assessments of large samples done by laypersons, who are generally not qualified to assess these domains from a clinical perspective. Furthermore, while the notion of "clinical significance" is explicit in the DSM definition of mental disorder, the diagnostic criteria stipulated for specific disorders rarely if ever specify what makes a symptom "clinically significant." As a result, this aspect of diagnosis is seldom operationalized in diagnostic instruments and also remains, in essence, a clinical judgment.

It is useful to define and to classify disorder by combining categorical criteria with a measure of impairment (Bird et al., 1988, 1990); nevertheless, the level of impairment necessary to define a "case" may vary with the purpose at hand. For example, an estimate of the prevalence of general distress may be higher than an estimate of the number of children who require mental health services, and certainly higher than the proportion of those who actually receive them. Estimates are more meaningful, however, when they relate disorder either to severity and impaired functioning, to need for services, or to personal distress.

THE DOMAINS OF FUNCTIONAL IMPAIRMENT

"Adaptive functioning" has been defined as the interplay between the social environment and the individual (Weissman & Paykel, 1974) and can be conceptualized in terms of role performance and role satisfaction. Its assessment is more complex than the determination of levels of symptomatology; it is even more complex in children, for whom developmental factors also need to be considered to judge whether their functioning is at an age-appropriate level. Adaptation can be broadly seen as a composite of three major dimensions. One is interpersonal relations, including both the qualitative and the quantitative aspects of how a child relates to peers, to family members, and to other adults outside the family. Another is performance in school (or, in an older adolescent, at work)—more specifically, the ability to perform comfortably and without undue anxiety, at a level commensurate with the individual child's potential. Last is the capacity to enjoy life and to use leisure time for self-fulfillment through a broad range of recreational activities, interests, or hobbies. Specific areas that relate to these major dimensions of functioning and that need to be assessed in children and adolescents include cognitive level, verbal abilities, academic achievement, social interactions, and an age-appropriate capacity for self-care.

Severity is another element that typically enters into the evaluation of caseness. Although they are closely related concepts, "impairment in adaptive functioning" and "severity" are not interchangeable concepts. "Severity" is a characteristic of a disorder that indicates the extent to which the disorder is manifested or the level of seriousness of the disorder itself. The symptomatology of some disorders (e.g., autistic disorder) makes the disorders severe by their very nature. Other disorders are inherently less severe. When the symptomatology of a specific disorder is not pervasive or frequent in occurrence, one may find a mild or milder case of a severe disorder; there may also be severe cases of relatively mild disorders (e.g., oppositional defiant disorder). A simple way for determining the severity of a given disorder is to sum up its symptomatic criteria, setting thresholds of severity at various points along the spectrum in which the symptomatology is manifested. However, even this oversimplified approach has limitations. For example, in a disorder such as conduct disorder, which is defined by the presence of 3 out of 15 criteria, it is conceivable that one could find an individual adolescent who manifests only 3 of the criteria, but each of these can be quite serious (e.g., stealing with confrontation, destroying other people's property, setting fires). By contrast, another adolescent may exceed the number of symptoms required for the diagnosis and have a larger number of less serious behaviors, each occurring at a lesser level of severity. It is not possible to make a statement of the severity of the disorder on the basis of the number of criteria alone, and it is not possible to make a statement of the level of functional impairment based purely on the assessment of severity. By contrast to severity, impairment in adaptive functioning is a characteristic of the subject under investigation, rather than of the disorder itself. In that sense, impairment in adaptive functioning is much more of a global notion and is perhaps best measured globally.

THE ASSESSMENT OF "CASENESS" AND FUNCTIONAL IMPAIRMENT IN RECENT EPIDEMIOLOGICAL RESEARCH

Diagnostically driven child psychiatry epidemiological surveys reported over the past decade and a half (Verhulst, Berden, & Sanders-Woudstra, 1985; Anderson, Williams, McGee, & Silva, 1987; Cohen, Velez, Kohn, Schwab-Stone, & Johnson, 1987; Cohen, Cohen, Kasen, et al., 1993; Cohen, Cohen, & Brook, 1993; Offord et al., 1987; Kashani et al., 1987; Costello et al., 1988; Bird et al., 1988; Fergusson, Horwood, Shannon, & Lawton, 1989; Fergusson, Horwood, & Lynskey, 1993; Esser, Schmidt, & Woerner, 1990; Fombonne, 1994; Jensen et al., 1995; Costello et al., 1996; Costello, Farmer, Angold, Burns, & Erkanli, 1997; Verhulst, van der Ende, Ferdinand, & Kasius, 1997) have generally revealed that rates of disorders in children and adolescents are higher than would have been expected from previous reports about rates of disorders in the younger age groups (see Gould, Wunsch-Hitzig, & Dohrenwend, 1981, for a review of studies prior to 1980). Prevalence estimates prior to DSM-III and ICD-9 were based on a broad variety of definitions of "maladjustment" primarily derived from symptom scales.

Recent investigations cited above have provided rates of disorder based on the diagnostic nosology embodied in DSM-III (American Psychiatric Association, 1980) or DSM-III-R (American Psychiatric Association, 1987) and ICD-9 (World Health Organization, 1977). From one-third to one-half of children and adolescents in these population studies have been found to meet criteria for one or more diagnostic categories. It is unclear whether the high rates of diagnoses obtained are a function of an overinclusive nosology or actually reflect the rates of disturbed children.

We are presently at the threshold of a new wave of studies that will use the diagnostic modifications made for DSM-IV (American Psychiatric Association, 1994). The inclusion of a threshold of impairment or dysfunctionality in the operational definition of "caseness" is particularly important for studies in the community, where disorders tend to appear at or slightly above the diagnostic threshold (Bird et al., 1990), and where most individuals meeting diagnostic criteria are not receiving or even seeking help and many are functioning relatively well.

Most recent surveys have devised ways to incorporate severity or level of impairment into the operational definition of "caseness." When this is done, the rates of disordered children and adolescents considered to be "cases" are reduced two- or threefold below the rates of those meeting diagnostic criteria for disorders. Different investigations have employed different methods to achieve this objective. Anderson et al. (1987) used the level of concordance on diagnosis among three separate groups of informants (parents, youth, and teachers) as a gauge of the pervasiveness, and therefore the seriousness, of a disorder. They identified four levels of certainty of "caseness." The most certain level was present when each of two or more informants independently fulfilled diagnostic criteria; the least certain level indicated that diagnostic criteria were not met by any single informant and were only arrived at by aggregating multi-informant data. Cohen et al. (1987) combined categorical DSM diagnostic criteria with statistical criteria to set a threshold of disorder. In their study, a "case" was defined as a child who was at or above the threshold of DSM-III or DSM-III-R criteria and whose total symptom count for that disorder was two standard deviations above the sample mean. The Ontario Child Health Study (Offord et al., 1987; Boyle et al., 1987) determined caseness through a combination of clinical judgment and statistical procedures that balanced false positives and false negatives to set cutoff scores on diagnostic symptom scales at levels that concurred with clinicians' assessments of certain DSM-III disorders; these cutoff scores were subsequently applied to determine the number of cases in the sample.

Other groups of investigators (Bird et al., 1988; Costello et al., 1988; Fombonne, 1994; Jensen et al., 1995; Verhulst et al., 1997) have combined diagnostic assessments with global measures of impairment such as the Children's Global Assessment Scale (CGAS; Shaffer et al., 1983; Bird, Canino, Rubio-Stipec, & Ribera, 1987), to define a case; others (Esser et al., 1990;

Verhulst et al., 1985) have used diagnosis and global ratings of severity to distinguish cases from noncases, from among those meeting symptomatic criteria for the disorder. In a Dutch study (Verhulst et al., 1985), clinical raters doing second-stage assessments administered the Child Assessment Schedule (Hodges, McKnew, Cytryn, Stern, & Kline, 1982) and at the end of the interview provided clinical global ratings of severity of psychopathology ranging from "no disorder" through "ambiguous or trivial," "mild" and "moderate" to "severe disorder." Only the moderate and severe ratings were considered to be "cases" of psychiatric disorder for reporting prevalence. Some investigators have used clinical outcome as an indicator of severity or impairment. For example, Kashani et al. (1987) developed a scale to score an adolescent's need for treatment based on a clinician's assessment, and defined "caseness" by the presence of a psychiatric diagnosis coupled with moderate or severe impairment that was judged to be present based on the need for treatment.

The methods to assess severity and/or impairment are as varied as the surveys that have employed them. The field of child psychiatric epidemiology lacks a systematic way of assessing impairment or dysfunctionality that can be used in large community surveys. The absence of a uniform methodology limits the studies' ability to compare findings in different settings. It is not possible to determine whether any of the methods employed can be recommended over the others. Furthermore, it is still not possible to ascertain the "clinical significance" of most childhood disorders in large-scale epidemiological surveys of the population with any of the methods available, particularly when structured diagnostic interviews are administered by laypersons. Although lay interviewers can be trained in the administration of diagnostic instruments and scales, they generally lack the level of expertise necessary to make such clinical judgments.

MEASURES TO ASSESS FUNCTIONAL IMPAIRMENT

Measures of Symptom-Specific Impairment

Several global measures of impairment have been employed in recent child psychiatry research (Bird & Gould, 1995). Some recent methodological attempts have also been made to develop measures of symptom- or diagnosis-specific impairment, embedded in the diagnostic schedules of structured or semistructured instruments (Shaffer et al., 1996; Angold & Costello, 1995). These measures are intended to determine the degree to which functional impairment is associated with a particular diagnosis or symptomatology; they directly ask the subjects or their parents whether the symptoms reported have led to difficulties in interpersonal relations or in school.

One instrument, the Child and Adolescent Psychiatric Assessment

(CAPA; Angold et al., 1995; Angold & Costello, 1995), determines the clinical level of severity by training interviewers to rate symptoms as present only when they are clinically significant. Purportedly, through this method only those symptoms of consequence are rated as present, and thus the subjects who meet criteria for disorders are by definition functionally impaired from a clinical standpoint. Notwithstanding its appeal, this promising methodology still lacks a rigorous test of its validity and replicability.

A further development, which also seems to hold promise, is the attempt to arrive at an informant-based rating of impairment attributable to specific syndromes of symptomatology. Such an attempt was made in the Diagnostic Interview Schedule for Children (DISC) and was initially tested in the DISC-2.3 (Shaffer et al., 1996; Schwab-Stone et al., 1996). These informant-based ratings have been improved for the most recent revision of the instrument, the DISC-IV (Fisher et al., 1997). The method does not require the interviewer to make a clinical judgment, but it does require the subjects to make an attribution of impairment to specific constructs of symptomatology that they have endorsed as present. The experience in the Methods for Epidemiology in Children and Adolescents (MECA) study, where the use of this device in the DISC-2.3 was tested, suggested that subjects or their parents may find it difficult to make accurate attributions of impairment to specific constructs of symptomatology (Bird, Cohen, Narrow, Dulcan, & Hoven, 1994). For example, in subjects with comorbidity, when impairment was attributed to one diagnosis, there was a strong likelihood that it was also attributed to the comorbid disorders; in other words, when impairment was reported for one specific set of endorsed symptoms, it was likely that the same impairment would be reported for any other set of symptoms endorsed. Although this approach is promising, it still requires further methodological refinements, and the validity of respondent attributions of impairment to specific symptomatic clusters needs to be further assessed before this method becomes widely used. The discussion in the remainder of this chapter has been restricted to global measures of impairment, and it focuses on the four instruments that have been most widely used.

Children's Global Assessment Scale

The CGAS (Figure 7.1) was devised by Shaffer et al. (1983) as an adaptation of the Global Assessment Scale (GAS) for adults (Endicott, Spitzer, Fleiss, & Cohen, 1976). Both the adult GAS and the CGAS have received a rigorous psychometric assessment. Both scales reflect a subject's lowest level of functioning during a specified time period and are used as measures of impaired functioning.

Scores on the CGAS can range from 1 (for the most impaired child or adolescent) to 100 (for a child or adolescent at the healthiest level of adaptive functioning). For each decile, the CGAS contains descriptions of behaviors

CHILDREN'S GLOBAL ASSESSMENT SCALE

For children 4–16 years of age

David Shaffer, MD, Madelyn S. Gould, PhD,
Hector Bird, MD, Prudence Fisher, MA

Adaptation of the Adult Global Assessment Scale
(Robert L. Spitzer, MD, Miriam Gibbon, MSW, Jean Endicott, PhD)

Rate the subject's most impaired level of general functioning for the specified time period by selecting the *lowest* level which describes his/her functioning on a hypothetical continuum of health–illness. Use intermediary levels (e.g., 35, 58, 62).

Rate actual functioning regardless of treatment or prognosis. The examples of behavior provided are only illustrative and are not required for a particular rating.

Specified time period: 1 month

100–91 Superior functioning in all areas (at home, at school, and with peers), involved in a range of activities and has many interests (e.g., has hobbies or participates in extracurricular activities or belongs to an organized group such as Scouts, etc.). Likeable, confident, "everyday" worries never get out of hand. Doing well in school. No symptoms.

90–81 Good functioning in all areas. Secure in family, school, and with peers. There may be transient difficulties and "everyday" worries that occasionally get out of hand (e.g., mild anxiety associated with an important exam, occasional "blow-ups" with siblings, parents, or peers).

80–71 No more than slight impairment in functioning at home, at school, or with peers. Some disturbance of behavior or emotional distress may be present in response to life stresses (e.g., parental separations, deaths, birth of a sibling) but these are brief and interference with functioning is transient. Such children are only minimally disturbing to others and are not considered deviant by those who know them.

70–61 Some difficulty in a single area, but generally functioning pretty well (e.g., sporadic or isolated antisocial acts, such as occasionally playing hooky or petty theft; consistent minor difficulties with schoolwork, mood changes of brief duration; fears and anxieties which do not lead to gross avoidance behavior; self-doubts). Has some meaningful interpersonal relationships. Most people who do not know the child well would not consider him/her deviant but those who do know him/her well might express concern.

60–51 Variable functioning with sporadic difficulties or symptoms in several but not all social areas. Disturbance would be apparent to those who encounter the child in a dysfunctional setting or time but not to those who see the child in other settings.

50–41 Moderate degree of interference in functioning in most social areas or severe impairment of functioning in one area, such as might result from, for example, suicidal preoccupations and ruminations, school refusal and other forms of anxiety, obsessive rituals, major conversion symptoms, frequent anxiety attacks, frequent episodes of aggressive or other antisocial behavior with some preservation of meaningful social relationships.

40–31 Major impairment in functioning in several areas and unable to function in one of these areas, that is, disturbed at home, at school, with peers, or in the society at large (e.g., persistent aggression without clear instigation; markedly withdrawn and isolated behavior due to either mood or thought disturbance, suicidal attempt with clear lethal intent). Such children are likely to require special schooling and/or hospitalization or withdrawal from school (but this is not a sufficient criterion for inclusion in this category).

30–21 Unable to function in almost all areas, for example, stays at home, in ward or in bed all day without taking part in social activities OR severe impairment in reality testing OR serious impairment in communication (e.g., sometimes incoherent or inappropriate).

20–11 Needs considerable supervision to prevent hurting others or self, for example, frequently violent, repeated suicide attempts OR to maintain personal hygiene OR gross impairment in all forms of communication, for example, severe abnormalities in verbal and gestural communication, marked social aloofness, stupor, etc.

10–1 Needs constant supervision (24-hour care) due to severely aggressive or self-destructive behavior or gross impairment in reality testing, communication, cognition, affect, or personal hygiene.

FIGURE 7.1. Children's Global Assessment Scale (CGAS).

and life situations applying to subjects who would be scored in that decile. Using these descriptors, a rater is expected to synthesize his/her knowledge about a subject's psychological and social functioning, and to assign a single numerical global score of psychological impairment that can lie at any point within the spectrum. There are no specific items of information directly asked of the subject in order to score the CGAS, and for that reason it can be scored in a few seconds. However, the score is assigned in the context of a broader evaluation in which the rater needs to have gathered clinical information about the child's past history, symptomatology, behavior at school and at home, and social relations. With such an information base, the rater then assigns the global score of functioning to the child either for the present or for a specified recent time period, such as the last 3 or 6 months. The score, based on the descriptors or examples provided by the scale, is given in the context of what the rater knows about the child and obviously requires a synthetic process and a clinical judgment by the rater. Nevertheless, if a measure of impairment that is independent of other data is required, the advantage that the CGAS provides because of its brevity is offset by the fact that other contextual information must be obtained in order to provide a score.

The initial report on the psychometric properties of the CGAS (Shaffer et al., 1983) showed high interrater reliability and adequate discriminant and concurrent validity. A repeated analysis of variance showed no significant differences by rater or across time, or any interaction between rater and time. A subsequent report (Bird et al., 1987), based on the data collected during the pilot phase of the Child Psychiatry Epidemiologic Study in Puerto Rico, also demonstrated high interrater reliability and both concurrent and discriminant validity. A discriminant function was generated that highly correlated with other predictors of impairment, such as service utilization, measures of overall severity, and scores obtained on the Child Behavior Checklist (CBCL; Achenbach & Edelbrock, 1983, 1986).

Shaffer et al. (1983) had recommended a cutoff score of 70 to distinguish a "case" from a "noncase." Their recommendation was based on the descriptors provided. A subsequent study using the data from the Puerto Rico field study (Bird et al., 1990) looked for the optimal threshold for "caseness" on the CGAS score that had been independently assigned to the child by a child psychiatrist. The exploration of a threshold was done by means of a discriminant-function analysis that looked for the optimal threshold to discriminate within other external validators, such as service utilization, parental perceived need for mental health services, and behavior problem scores on the CBCL. The threshold on the CGAS that best distinguished between what was considered a case and a noncase occurred at scores in the decile between 60 and 70. On the basis of these analyses, it was recommended that any child in the community with a CGAS score below 61 be considered a "definite" case; that any child with a score from 61 to 70 be considered a "probable" or "possible" case of disorder; and that any child with a score of

71 or above be considered a "noncase," regardless of whether or not the child met criteria for a DSM-III diagnosis.

A global measure of impairment, such as the CGAS, adds a dimension to the definition of disorder that goes beyond categorical diagnostic ratings or syndrome-specific scales. The instrument's greatest strength may be its multidimensional or global nature. In general, global ratings such as the CGAS have demonstrated more sensitivity to change over time than have other ratings of severity or specific psychopathological categorizations.

The CGAS has proven to be useful in epidemiological investigations employing clinicians. The recent multisite study funded by the National Institute of Mental Health to develop an optimal protocol for epidemiological research of children and adolescents (the MECA study; Lahey et al., 1996) explored the possibility of modifying the descriptors on the CGAS so that a nonclinical person with some knowledge of a child could be asked to provide a Nonclinician CGAS score (see Figure 7.2). The descriptors were simplified to enhance a rater's understanding of the anchor points, and the level of dif-

---

NONCLINICIAN CHILDREN'S GLOBAL ASSESSMENT SCALE
For children 9–17 years of age
Stephen Setterberg, MD, Hector Bird, MD,
Madelyn Gould, PhD, David Shaffer, MD,
Prudence Fisher, MA

Adaptation of the Clinician Children's Global Assessment Scale
(David Shaffer, MD, Madelyn S. Gould, PhD,
Hector Bird, MD, Prudence Fisher, MA)

Specified time period: 6 months

100–91	DOING VERY WELL in all areas; no problems at home, at school, or with friends; likeable, confident, involved in activities and interests. Functioning is superior or above average.
90–81	DOING WELL in all areas; secure at home, at school, and with friends. There may be occasional minor upsets or everyday worries, but in general her/his functioning is good.
80–71	DOING ALL RIGHT at home, at school, and with friends; some trouble or upset may occur after a stressful situation, but those who know the child well would find the child's reaction completely understandable. Any problem with functioning is temporary and mild.
70–61	SOME PROBLEMS; most people who do not know the child very well would not notice the problems, but people who know her/him well could be concerned.
60–51	SOME NOTICEABLE PROBLEMS; in some situations the problems are noticeable to anyone, but in other situations the child could seem fine.
50–41	OBVIOUS PROBLEMS; several problems that cause trouble in most situations, at home, at school, or with [her/his] friends; or one very disruptive problem.
40–31	SERIOUS PROBLEMS; very seriously disturbed at home, at school, with peers, and/or with society at large. Major functional impairments and in some situations is unable to function.
30–21	SEVERE PROBLEMS; unable to function in almost all situations.
20–11	VERY SEVERELY IMPAIRED; so impaired that considerable supervision is required for safety.
10–1	EXTREMELY IMPAIRED; so impaired that constant supervision is required for safety.

FIGURE 7.2. Nonclinician Children's Global Assessment Scale (CGAS).

ficulty in comprehension was reduced to obtain responses that would agree with a clinician's independent clinical assessment of the child's CGAS score. This instrument was tested during the MECA study field trials, and the results showed good psychometric properties (Bird & Gould, 1995; Bird et al., 1996). The CGAS provided by the rater who interviewed the child's parent also provided evidence of validity (discriminating between clinical and nonclinical subjects), and particularly of concurrent validity (correlating moderately with a child psychiatrist's CGAS score; intraclass correlation coefficient [ICC] = .65, p < .001).

Columbia Impairment Scale

The Columbia Impairment Scale (CIS; Figure 7.3) is a 13-item scale whose scoring is respondent-based. It was devised to tap four major areas of functioning: interpersonal relations (items 2, 3, 7, 9, and 10); certain broad areas of psychopathology (items 1, 4, 8, 13); functioning at school or work (items 5, 12); and use of leisure time (items 6 and 11). Items are scored on a Likert scale ranging from 0 ("no problem") through 2 ("some problem") to 4 ("a very bad problem"); thus the total score can range from a minimum of 0 to a maximum of 52. The instrument was developed in two almost identical versions—one that can be administered directly to a child or adolescent respondent, and another that can be administered to a parent or other informant who knows the child or adolescent well. The respondent is either provided with a card, so that he/she can point to the score given to each item, or asked actually to give a score to each item from 0 to 4; therefore, the CIS provides a respondent-based rating that is independent from the clinical judgment of the person administering the instrument. It takes approximately 3 minutes to administer.

The results of the pilot study at the Columbia University site of the MECA study (Bird et al., 1993) indicated that the CIS has excellent psychometric properties when applied to a population of children ranging in age from 9 through 17 years. These results were replicated in the subsequent field survey at all four sites of the MECA study (Bird et al., 1996) with a much larger sample. In both the pilot study and the field survey, the internal consistency of the scale was high, with the parent scale showing greater internal consistency (alphas = .89 and .82, respectively) than the child scale (alpha = .78 in both the pilot study and the field survey). A factor analysis of the scale did not replicate the four conceptual domains that guided its design, and only a single and well-differentiated factor was extracted (eigenvalue = 4.9). The test–retest reliability of the scale was high, with the reliability of the parent scale (ICC = 0.89, p < .001) again somewhat better than that of the child scale (ICC = .63, p < .001). The mean scores on both the parent CIS and the child CIS were found to be significantly higher (indicating more problems in functioning) in clinical subjects than in community respondents, providing

THE COLUMBIA IMPAIRMENT SCALE (CIS)
(Parent Version)

In general how much of a problem do you think (she/he) has with:

1) getting into trouble?	0	1	2	3	4			9
2) getting along with (you/[her/his] mother/mother figure)?	0	1	2	3	4	8		9
3) getting along with (you/[her/his] father/father figure)?	0	1	2	3	4	8		9
4) feeling unhappy or sad?	0	1	2	3	4			9

How much of a problem would you say [she/he] has:

5) with [her/his] behavior at school (or at [her/his] job)?	0	1	2	3	4	8		9
6) with having fun?	0	1	2	3	4			9
7) getting along with adults other than (you and/or [her/his] mother/father)?	0	1	2	3	4			9

How much of a problem does [she/he] have:

8) with feeling nervous, or afraid?	0	1	2	3	4			9
9) getting along with [her/his] [sister(s)/brother(s)]?	0	1	2	3	4	8		9
10) getting along with other kids [her/his] age?	0	1	2	3	4			9

How much of a problem would you say [she/he] has:

11) getting involved in activities like sports or hobbies?	0	1	2	3	4			9
12) with [her/his] school work (doing [her/his] job)?	0	1	2	3	4	8		9
13) with [her/his] behavior at home?	0	1	2	3	4			9

RESPONSE OPTIONS PROVIDED
0   No problem
1
2   Some problem
3
4   A very bad problem
8   (not applicable)
9   Don't know

CARD

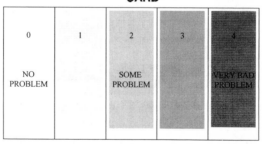

FIGURE 7.3. Columbia Impairment Scale (CIS), parent version.

evidence of the instrument's discriminant validity. This difference was greater in the parent CIS than in the child CIS. The correlation of the CIS score with the clinician's CGAS score was considerably better for the parent instrument (Pearson's $r = .68$) than for the child instrument (Pearson's $r = .58$). In general, it was noted that the parent CIS had better psychometric properties than the child CIS. It is therefore likely that the parent instrument is also useful for school-age children under the age of 9 years. The parent CIS also showed moderate to high correlations with other specific indicators of psychological dysfunction, such as referral for mental health services, academic performance and school difficulties, and low scores in measures of competence. The values obtained for the child CIS were uniformly lower. The correlations obtained for the parent CIS (Bird et al., 1996) were comparable to those reported for the CGAS (Bird et al., 1987) when similar indicators of psychological dysfunction were used.

To address the issue of a threshold on the parent CIS, a discriminant-function analysis using all 10 variables indicative of impairment simultaneously was carried out. The results of these analyses indicated that any child with a parent CIS score of 15 or greater can be considered impaired. The instrument appears to be useful as a brief measure of impairment that can be used in large-scale community studies. It has the advantage of being respondent-based, and therefore neither clinical judgment nor a broad information base is required to obtain a score. Its potential as a screening device or as a means of monitoring change over time has not been determined.

Social Adjustment Inventory
for Children and Adolescents

The Social Adjustment Inventory for Children and Adolescents (SAICA; John, Gammon, Prusoff, & Warner, 1987) is an extensive, semistructured instrument to assess adaptive functioning in children and adolescents. It has been used for children aged 6 to 18 years. Trained mental health professionals can administer the interview, which obtains data on current and/or past functioning and summarizes social functioning.

The items in the SAICA cover a broad spectrum of behaviors in four major role areas: school, peer relations, home life, and spare time activities. It consists of 77 items designed to assess observable social transactions (or outcomes of transactions) and social self-evaluations applicable to children and adolescents aged 6 through 18. There are 35 competence items and 42 problem behavior items. The scores from responses to items in each of the major role areas have been broken down into 11 subscales, including School Academic, School Social, Social Problems, Spare Time Activities, Peer Relationships, Peer Problems, Peer Heterosexual Adjustment, Sibling Relationships, and Home Problems. The item scores are respondent-based and do not require interviewer judgment. They range from 1 ("best adjustment") to 4 ("worst adjustment"). The time frame is adjustable to the period covered by the study at hand. The instrument is completed by a child or adolescent as a self-report, or by a parent about the child or adolescent.

The authors of the SAICA have reported on the psychometric properties of the instrument, and have noted that it shows acceptable levels of inter-rater reliability, internal consistency, and concurrent validity (John et al.,

1987). This single report on the use of the SAICA suggests that the subscales were based on content/face validity rather than on factor-analytic methods. The qualifications that a rater must have are somewhat vague. John et al. (1987) stated that its administration and coding requires interviewers "who are knowledgeable about child development and who have clinical or testing experience with children and adolescents" (p. 899). The SAICA performed adequately when used by interviewers with these characteristics, but there is a need for further testing of the instrument if it is to be administered by lay interviewers and useful for epidemiological field surveys. Nevertheless, the instrument has some potential for epidemiological use, with straightforward instructions and easy adaptability for individual administration to children and their parents. One of its main drawbacks is that although it is rich in content, it is lengthy. When used directly with a child or adolescent, administration time ranges between 30 and 75 minutes, depending on the age of the subject. It also mixes issues of social competence (e.g., school achievement, sociability, and enjoyment of leisure time) with ratings of specific deviant behaviors and symptoms (e.g., bullying, excessive anxiety, inattention, and negativism). In this sense, it is redundant with some elements of diagnosis and does not strictly provide a measure of functional impairment that would complement more precise diagnostic assessments.

Child and Adolescent Functional Assessment Scale

The CAFAS was originally described by its author (Hodges, 1990) as a clinician-rated instrument used to record the extent to which a youth's mental health/substance use disorder is disruptive of functioning in each of five psychosocial areas. More recently the qualifications of the rater have been expanded to include other "trained raters" as well. The instrument is an adaptation for children and adolescents of the North Carolina Functional Assessment Scale (North Carolina Department of Human Resources, 1989, 1994) for adults. It provides five main scales reflecting a child's or adolescent's functioning and psychopathology in areas that include Role Performance (subdivided into subscales for Home, School, and Community), Behavior Towards Others, Moods/Self-Harm (subdivided into Emotions and Self-Harmful Behavior), Substance Use, and Thinking. The instrument has two additional scales, which are optional and which apply to the caregiver rather than to the youth. The latter two scales score the caregiver's resources in terms of his/her ability to meet the youth's basic needs and to provide a home setting free of known risk factors. A total CAFAS score is obtained by adding the five main scores.

Examples of different levels of functional impairment or psychopathology are provided for each of the areas rated. The rater is expected to give a score for the subject based on these examples. Therefore, like the CGAS, the CAFAS requires the rater to make clinical judgments. Each scale is scored in the direction of deviance, with a score of 0 being indicative of the norm and implying minimal or no impairment. The most severe or worst score on each scale is a score of 30, with a score of 20 indicating moderate impairment, and a score of 10 mild impairment. A total score is estimated by a simple summation of all the scales.

Of the different scales in the CAFAS, those that come closest to providing some measurement of impaired functioning are the two Role Performance subscales. For the other scales, the descriptors in the CAFAS are linked to symptomatology rather than to the dysfunctional outcomes of symptomatology. The Thinking scale scores symptomatology characteristic of psychoses (hallucinations, delusions, loose associations, magical thinking, etc.); the Behavior Towards Others scale and the Self-Harmful Behavior subscale of the Moods/Self-Harm scale inquire about patterns of social interaction and interpersonal problems, but also go into symptomatology (e.g., self-mutilation, social withdrawal, avoidance, dangerous behavior toward self); the Emotions subscale of the Moods/Self-Harm scale focuses on symptoms of anxiety and depression (e.g., sleep, eating, energy level, concentration); and the Substance Use scale rates the use of drugs on the basis of frequency, ranging from none through sporadic use, habituation, and addiction. The different behaviors are classified on each of the scales under the headings of "severe," "moderate," "mild," or "minimal/no impairment." Therefore, by definition the presence of a behavior or emotion determines the level of impairment, and thus the score assigned on the scale.

A fairly extensive information base is required in order to score the CAFAS. The instrument was originally designed to be employed in conjunction with the CAPA (Angold et al., 1995; Angold & Costello, 1995). Although scoring can be done in approximately 5–10 minutes, administering the full CAPA to elicit the information required to score the CAFAS takes considerably longer. To overcome this limitation, the author has developed a concise interview that can be administered in person or by telephone to elicit the information necessary to score the instrument. The time needed for administration of this interview has been estimated to be approximately 30 minutes. Scoring of many of the items in the interview requires a clinical judgment as to the age-appropriateness or age-inappropriateness of the behavior or social interaction. In this respect, it is doubtful that a rater without some background in child development and psychopathology can score the instrument reliably. A score of 0 is considered the average or the norm. Therefore, any score on the instrument is in the direction of deviance, and the instrument does not allow for a rating of superior functioning.

The reliability of the CAFAS was tested with 20 written case vignettes, to which 45 graduate and undergraduate psychology students and 9 clinical staff working in child service agencies provided ratings (Hodges & Wong, 1996). ICCs were used to estimate agreement between raters at each level of clinical expertise and were found to be good (generally > .75) at all levels of expertise, including that of the undergraduate students, who for practical purposes would be considered lay interviewers. Thus far, there are no published reports describing a formal reliability study of the instrument with live subjects and actual test–retest of subjects in either clinical or community settings. Tests of the instrument's validity were reported in the same publication (Hodges & Wong, 1996) with a larger sample of actual subjects enrolled in a demonstration project conducted at three U.S. Army bases. Validity was assessed by correlating the CAFAS total score with scores that the subjects obtained on the parent, teacher, and youth versions of the CBCL (Achenbach & Edelbrock, 1983, 1986; Achenbach, 1991); with their scores on a Burden of Care Questionnaire developed by the investigators, which assesses the impact on a family of having a child with serious emotional or behavioral problems; and with their results on using the Child Assessment Schedule (Hodges et al., 1982). The total score on the CAFAS correlated well with all of these instruments, with zero-order correlations ranging from .36 to .59.

There are some caveats about interpreting these results as evidence of the reliability and validity of the CAFAS as a measure of functional impairment. As noted above, with the exception of the two Role Performance subscales (which together provide one of the six scaled scores that enter into the total score), the items in the remaining scales of the CAFAS ascertain psychiatric symptomatology, and the score of the level of impairment is dictated by which behavior or emotion is ascertained. It is therefore expectable that if subjects are consistent in their reports of deviant behavior and emotional symptoms, the score on the CAFAS will be strongly correlated with scores on scales and instruments that also consist of items designed to measure deviant behaviors and symptomatology. The results so far could be interpreted as providing evidence that the CAFAS has concurrent validity as a measure of the presence and severity of psychopathology, but further assessment of its test–retest reliability and of its validity as a measure of functional impairment will be necessary.

The CAFAS potentially provides a useful instrument for assessing severity in clinical practice or in studies that require extensive or in-depth evaluations of relatively small samples, with ratings done by clinically trained interviewers. The time required for its administration and its complexity do not seem to recommend its use in broader and more extensive community studies in which many other measures are to be administered, particularly when these are to be administered by lay interviewers.

CONCLUSION

The assumption that all of the syndromes applicable to children are truly "mental disorders" has been questioned (Garmezy, 1978). Many child psychiatric conditions, some with elevated prevalence rates in the community (e.g., separation anxiety disorder, oppositional defiant disorder, specific phobias) may be phase-specific, transitory phenomena, which resolve by themselves through the natural course of child development and without clinical intervention. It is questionable whether such conditions, in their milder forms and without perceptible impairment, should be considered pathological or enter into the counts of the prevalence rates of childhood disorders in the community.

Many of the children who meet diagnostic criteria are not severely impaired, and when evaluated clinically are not deemed to be in need of services. Their disorders may be transient and may not persist, and their functioning may not be affected in any major way. It can be argued that at least some if not all of such children, who would not be considered "cases" on clinical grounds, should also not be considered as "cases" for epidemiological purposes. If all these children were considered as "cases," we would be impelled toward the implausible conclusion that nearly half of the children in the community are psychiatrically disturbed. When we take into account the limitations inherent in our present categorical diagnostic systems, the results of recent community studies lend weight to the idea that estimation of the prevalence of childhood psychiatric disorders in the community is enhanced and made more meaningful by incorporating a measure of impairment into the operational definition of "caseness." Moreover, functional impairment has gained increasing relevance in determining the eligibility for managed care mental health services, and rates of persons with impairment are required components of applications for federal block grants and other entitlements.

Rates of maladjusted children in the community are more plausible when the criterion for morbidity or "caseness" is diagnosis combined with impairment. The notion that diagnosis needs to include a measure of severity, or of level of impairment, is consonant with the clinician's tendency to evaluate and to make treatment decisions along dimensional rather than categorical lines (Robins, 1985).

Several measures of impairment have proven useful for both research and clinical purposes. In research, the decision as to which instrument to use cannot be based merely on psychometric considerations, but on the research questions to be addressed and the methodology to be employed in the study. The choice of instrument largely depends on design constraints, such as how old the children or adolescents to be studied are, whether lay interviewers or clinicians will administer or rate the instruments, or whether lifetime assessments are needed. The most widely used measure of impairment has been the CGAS. An adaptation of the CGAS designed to be rated by nonclinicians, and a new instrument, the CIS, were developed for the MECA study (Bird et al., 1996; Lahey et al., 1996; Shaffer et al., 1996; Schwab-Stone et al., 1996). Both seem to be acceptable as global measures of impairment suitable for epidemiological and other research purposes. Two other measures, the SAICA and the CAFAS, provide adequate measures of severity of psychopathology rather than of functional impairment; their usefulness in large-scale epidemiological studies, especially when rated by laypersons, is questionable. Although severity of disorder has often been used as a proxy for impairment, severity and functional impairment are not identical concepts, although they may strongly overlap with each other. Severity is a characteristic of the disorder itself, whereas functional impairment addresses the individual's functioning in different social contexts and psychological domains.

Although the CGAS provides a global score, its rating involves a clinical decision and is dependent on a rater's having access to other information that enters into that decision, such as a child's adaptive capabilities and observational as well as symptomatic data. More objective measures of impairment—ones that take into account not only recalled behavior and symptomatology but also children's functioning in other areas (e.g., school performance, relationships to others, interests, use of leisure time), and that do not require a clinician's judgment—are necessary. The CIS shows some promise in this respect. Even more intriguing, is the possibility of linking impairment to the syndrome of psychopathology that is causing it. Particularly in epidemiology, it is of importance to count as cases of a disorder those to whom the disorder is causing a certain level of difficulty in adaptive functioning. However, further methodological work is necessary before such measures of specific impairment can be employed.

The relative importance of functional impairment cannot be addressed fully with the cross-sectional data that are currently available. Longitudinal research with larger community samples is necessary to evaluate the stability of psychiatric conditions, as well as of the instruments that measure them over time—and, indeed, to learn whether stability of diagnosis is in some way related to the level of functional impairment.

REFERENCES

Achenbach, T. M. (1991). *Manual for the Child Behavior Checklist/4–18 and 1991 Profile.* Burlington: University of Vermont, Department of Psychiatry.

Achenbach, T. M., & Edelbrock, C. S. (1983). *Manual for the Child Behavior Checklist and Revised Child Behavior Profile.* Burlington: University of Vermont, Department of Psychiatry.

Achenbach, T. M., & Edelbrock C. S. (1986). *Manual for the Teacher's Report Form and Teacher Version of the Child Behavior Profile.* Burlington: University of Vermont, Department of Psychiatry.

American Psychiatric Association (1980). *Diagnostic and statistical manual of mental disorders* (3rd ed.). Washington, DC: Author.

American Psychiatric Association (1987). *Diagnostic and statistical manual of mental disorders* (3rd ed., rev.). Washington, DC: Author.

American Psychiatric Association (1994). *Diagnostic and statistical manual of mental disorders* (4th ed.). Washington, DC: Author.

Anderson, J. C., Williams, S., McGee, R., & Silva, P. A. (1987). DSM-III disorders in preadolescent children. *Archives of General Psychiatry, 44,* 69–76.

Angold, A., & Costello, E. J. (1995). A test–retest reliability study of child-reported psychiatric symptoms and diagnoses using the Child and Adolescent Psychiatric Assessment (CAPA-C). *Psychological Medicine, 25,* 755–762.

Angold, A., Prendergast, M., Cox, A., Harrington, R., Simonoff, E., & Rutter, M. (1995). The Child and Adolescent Psychiatric Assessment (CAPA). *Psychological Medicine, 25,* 739–753.

Bird, H. R., Andrews, H., Schwab-Stone, M., Goodman, S., Dulcan, M., Richters, J., Rubio-Stipec, M., Moore, R., Chiang, P., Hoven, C., Canino, G., Fisher, P., & Gould, M. S. (1996). Global measures of impairment for epidemiologic and clinical use with children and adolescents. *International Journal of Methods in Psychiatric Research, 6,* 1–13.

Bird, H. R., Canino, G., Rubio-Stipec, M., Gould, M. S., Ribera, J., Sesman, M., Woodbury, M., Huertas, S., Pagan, A., Sanchez-Lacay, A., & Moscoso, M. (1988). Estimates of the prevalence of childhood maladjustment in a community survey in Puerto Rico. *Archives of General Psychiatry, 45,* 1120–1126.

Bird, H. R., Canino, G., Rubio-Stipec, M., & Ribera, J. (1987). Further measures of the psychometric properties of the Children's Global Assessment Scale (CGAS). *Archives of General Psychiatry, 44,* 821–824.

Bird, H. R., Cohen, P., Narrow, W., Dulcan, M., & Hoven, C. (1994). Global impairment and impairment attributed to specific disorders: A comparison of available measures. In N. Alessi & S. Porter (Eds.), *Scientific proceedings: 41st Annual Meeting of the American Academy of Child and Adolescent Psychiatry, New York, NY* (p. 12). Washington, DC: American Academy of Child and Adolescent Psychiatry.

Bird, H. R., & Gould, M. (1995). The use of diagnostic instruments and global measures of functioning in child psychiatry epidemiological studies. In F. C. Verhulst & H. M. Koot (Eds.), *The epidemiology of child and adolescent psychopathology* (pp. 86–103). New York: Oxford University Press.

Bird, H. R., Shaffer, D., Fisher, P., Gould, M. S., Staghezza, B., Chen, J. Y., & Hoven, C. (1993). The Columbia Impairment Scale (CIS): Pilot findings on a measure of global impairment for children and adolescents. *International Journal of Methods in Psychiatric Research, 3,* 167–176.

Bird, H. R., Yager, T., Staghezza, B., Gould, M., Canino, G., & Rubio-Stipec, M. (1990). Impairment in the epidemiological measurement of childhood psychopathology in the community. *Journal of the American Academy of Child and Adolescent Psychiatry, 29*(5), 796–803.

Boyle, M. H., Offord, D. R., Hoffman, H. G., Catlin, G. P., Byles, G. A., Cadman, D. T., Crawford, J. W., Links, P. L., Rae-Grant, N. I., & Szatmari, P. (1987). Ontario Child Health Study: I. Methodology. *Archives of General Psychiatry, 44,* 826–831.

Cohen, P., Cohen, J., & Brook, J. (1993). An epidemiological study of disorders in late childhood and adolescence: II. Persistence of disorders. *Journal of Child Psychology and Psychiatry, 34*(6), 869–877.

Cohen, P., Cohen, J., Kasen, S., Velez, C. N., Hartmark, C., Johnson, J., Rojas, M., Brook, J., & Struening, E. L. (1993). An epidemiological study of disorders in late childhood and adolescence: I. Age- and gender-specific prevalence. *Journal of Child Psychology and Psychiatry, 34*(6), 851–867.

Cohen, P., Velez, N., Kohn, M., Schwab-Stone, M., & Johnson, J. (1987). Child psychiatric diagnosis by computer algorithm: Theoretical issues and empirical tests. *Journal of the American Academy of Child and Adolescent Psychiatry, 26*(5), 631–638.

Costello, E. J., Angold, A., Burns, B. J., Stangl, D. K., Tweed, D. L., Erkanli, A., & Worthman, C. M. (1996). The Great Smoky Mountains Study of Youth: Goals, design, methods, and the prevalence of DSM-III-R disorders. *Archives of General Psychiatry, 53*(12), 1129–1136.

Costello, E. J., Costello, A. J., Edelbrock, C., Burns, B., Dulcan, M., Brent, D., & Janiszewski, S. (1988). Psychiatric disorders in pediatric primary care: Prevalence and risk factors. *Archives of General Psychiatry, 45,* 1107–1116.

Costello, E. J., Farmer, M. Z., Angold, A., Burns, B. J., & Erkanli, A. (1997). Psychiatric disorders among American Indian and white youth in Appalachia: The Great Smoky Mountains study. *American Journal of Public Health, 87*(5), 827–832.

Endicott, J., Spitzer, R., Fleiss, J., & Cohen, J. (1976). The Global Assessment Scale: A procedure for measuring overall severity of psychiatric disturbance. *Archives of General Psychiatry, 33,* 766–771.

Esser, G., Schmidt, M. H., & Woerner, W. (1990). Epidemiology and course of psychiatric disorders in school-age children: Results of a longitudinal study. *Journal of Child Psychology and Psychiatry, 31*(2), 243–263.

Fergusson, D. M., Horwood, L. J., & Lynskey, M. T. (1993). Prevalence and comorbidity of DSM-III-R diagnoses in a birth cohort of 15 year olds. *Journal of the American Academy of Child and Adolescent Psychiatry, 32,* 1127–1134.

Fergusson, D. M., Horwood, L. J., Shannon, F. T., & Lawton, J. M. (1989). The Christchurch Child Development Study: A review of epidemiological findings. *Paediatric and Perinatal Epidemiology, 3,* 302–325.

Fisher, P., Lucas, C., Shaffer, D., Schwab-Stone, M., Dulcan, M., Graae, F., Lichtman, J., Willoughby, S., & Gerald, J. (1997). The Diagnostic Interview Schedule for Children, Version IV (DISC-IV): Test–retest reliability in a clinical sample. In M. Schwab-Stone (Ed.), *Scientific proceedings: 44th Annual Meeting of the American Academy of Child and Adolescent Psychiatry, Toronto, Ontario, Canada* (p. 141). Washington, DC: American Academy of Child and Adolescent Psychiatry.

Fombonne, E. (1994). The Chartres Study: I. Prevalence of psychiatric disorders among French school-aged children. *British Journal of Psychiatry, 164,* 69–79.

Garmezy, N. (1978). Never mind the psychologists: Is it good for the children? *Clinical Psychologist, 31,* 3.

Gould, M. S., Wunsch-Hitzig, R., & Dohrenwend, B. (1981). Estimating the prevalence of childhood psychopathology: A critical review. *Journal of the American Academy of Child Psychiatry, 20,* 462–476.

Hodges, K. (1990). *The Child and Adolescent Functional Assessment Scale: Self-training manual.* Unpublished manuscript, Eastern Michigan University.

Hodges, K., McKnew, D., Cytryn, L., Stern, L., & Kline, J. (1982). The Child Assessment Schedule (CAS) diagnostic interview: A report on reliability and validity. *Journal of the American Academy of Child Psychiatry, 21*(5), 468–473.

Hodges, K., & Wong, M. M. (1996). Psychometric characteristics of a multidimensional measure to assess impairment: The Child and Adolescent Functional Assessment Scale. *Journal of Child and Family Studies, 4,* 445–467.

Jensen, P. S., Watanabe, H. K., Richters, J. E., Cortes, R., Roper, M., & Liu, S. (1995). Prevalence of mental disorder in military children and adolescents: Findings from a two-stage community survey. *Journal of the American Academy of Child and Adolescent Psychiatry, 34,* 1514–1524.

John, K., Gammon, G. D., Prusoff, B. A., & Warner, V. (1987). The Social Adjustment Inventory for Children and Adolescents (SAICA): Testing of a new semistructured interview. *Journal of the American Academy of Child and Adolescent Psychiatry, 26,* 898–911.

Kashani, J. H., Beck, N. C., Hoeper, E. W., Fallahi, C., Corcoran, M. A., McAllister, J. A., Rosenberg, T. K., & Reid, J. C. (1987). Psychiatric disorders in a community sample of adolescents. *American Journal of Psychiatry, 144,* 584–589.

Lahey, B., Flagg, E., Bird, H., Schwab-Stone, M., Canino, G., Dulcan, M. K., Leaf, P. L., Davies, M., Brogan, D., Bourdon, K., Horwitz, S. M., Rubio-Stipec, M., Freeman, D. H., Lichtman, J., Shaffer, D., Goodman, S. H., Narrow, W. E., Weissman, M. M., Kandel, D., Jensen, P. S., Richters, J. E., & Regier, D. A. (1996). NIMH Methods for Epidemiology in Children and Adolescents (MECA) study: Background and methodology. *Journal of the American Academy of Child and Adolescent Psychiatry, 35*(7), 855–864.

North Carolina Department of Human Resources. (1989a). North Carolina Functional Assessment Scale (NCFAS). In *Funding system operating manual: Vol. 3. Level of eligibility* (pp. 10–25). Raleigh: Author.

North Carolina Department of Human Resources. (1989b). North Carolina Functional Assessment Scale (NCFAS). In *Funding system operating manual: Vol. 3. Level of eligibility* (3rd ed., p. 10–12). Raleigh: Author.

Offord, D. R., Boyle, M. H., Szatmari, P., Rae-Grant, N., Links, P., Cadman, D. T., Byles, J. A., Crawford, J. W., Munroe Blum, H., Byrne, C., Thomas, H., & Woodward, C. A. (1987). Ontario Child Health Study: II. Six month prevalence of disorder and rates of service utilization. *Archives of General Psychiatry, 44,* 832–836.

Robins, L. N. (1985). Epidemiology: Reflections on testing the validity of psychiatric interviews. *Archives of General Psychiatry, 42,* 918–924.

Schwab-Stone, M., Shaffer, D., Dulcan, M. K., Jensen, P., Fisher, P., Bird, H. R., Goodman, S. H., Lahey, B. B., Lichtman, J. H., Canino, G., Rubio-Stipec, M., & Rae, D. S. (1996). Criterion validity of the NIMH Diagnostic Interview Schedule for Children Version 2.3 (DISC 2.3). *Journal of the American Academy of Child and Adolescent Psychiatry, 35*(7), 878–888.

Shaffer, D., Fisher, P., Dulcan, M. K., Davies, M., Piacentini, J., Schwab-Stone, M., Lahey, B. B., Bourdon, K., Jensen, P., Bird, H. R., Canino, G., & Regier, D. (1996). The NIMH Diagnostic Interview Schedule for Children Version 2.3 (DISC–2.3): I. Description, acceptability, prevalence rates, and performance in the MECA study. *Journal of the American Academy of Child and Adolescent Psychiatry, 35*(7), 865–877.

Shaffer, D., Gould, M. S., Brasic, J., Ambrosini, P., Fisher, P., Bird, H., & Aluwahlia, S. (1983). A Children's Global Assessment Scale (CGAS). *Archives of General Psychiatry, 40,* 1228–1231.

Verhulst, F. C., Berden, G. F. M., & Sanders-Woudstra, J. (1985). Mental health in Dutch children: II. The prevalence of psychiatric disorder and relationship between measures. *Acta Psychiatrica Scandinavica, 72*(Suppl. 324), 1–45.

Verhulst, F. C., van der Ende, J., Ferdinand, R. F., & Kasius, M. C. (1997). The prevalence of DSM-III-R diagnoses in a national sample of Dutch adolescents. *Archives of General Psychiatry, 54,* 329–336.

Weissman, M. M., & Paykel, E. S. (1974). *The depressed woman: A study of social relationships.* Chicago: University of Chicago Press.

World Health Organization. (1977). *International classification of diseases* (9th rev.). Geneva: Author.

8

Assessment of Family History of Psychiatric Disorder

✧

RICHARD RENDE
MYRNA M. WEISSMAN

It is not an overstatement to suggest that most forms of psychopathology run in families. Indeed, it would be a challenge to document psychiatric disorders that are not in part familial. A recent review has suggested significant familial aggregation for essentially every childhood psychiatric disorder (Rutter, Silberg, O'Connor, & Simonoff, 1999b). Given the accumulating evidence for familial aggregation of most if not all psychiatric disorders, including those that arise in childhood or adolescence, the uninitiated reader might wonder why there is a need for further family studies. For example, an often-noted limitation of family studies is that they cannot disentangle genetic and environmental influences; more specialized methodologies, such as twin and adoption designs are necessary for that purpose. Furthermore, molecular genetic techniques are recognized as a critical component of psychiatric research (Rutter, Silberg, O'Connor, & Simonoff, 1999a). Such tides of interest might seem to diminish the need for future family studies of psychiatric disorders, including child and adolescent psychopathology.

We believe, however, that family studies may continue to have an important role in psychiatry. First, although many studies have provided evidence of familial aggregation of childhood and adolescent psychopathology, they have not adhered to the contemporary standards of methodological rigor (see Rutter et al., 1990, 1999b). Hence, firm conclusions cannot readily be drawn from these studies, and there is a need for more carefully designed studies (e.g., ones that use appropriate control groups, take comorbidity into account, and ensure so-called "blindness" on the part of raters) to provide data on the precise risk and specificity involved in the familial transmission of disorders.

Second, family studies may provide information that will prove invaluable in defining diagnostic boundaries between disorders. To take a classic example, family studies have demonstrated that although affective illness and schizophrenia sometimes co-occur within individuals, these disorders do not cluster within families and hence appear to have different etiological bases (e.g., Guze, Cloninger, Martin, & Clayton, 1983; Kendler, Gruenberg, & Tsuang, 1985; Weissman et al., 1984). In addition, family studies may extend traditional diagnostic boundaries to include a broader range of problems. A notable example is that social and cognitive abnormalities are found in the relatives of autistic individuals, suggesting that genetic influence on autism may affect these areas of functioning (Folstein & Rutter, 1988). Hence family studies of psychopathology in childhood and adolescence not only may indicate the precise risk involved for specific disorders, but also may provide important data on the diagnostic specificity involved within and between different disorders.

Third, the heightened interest in molecular genetic approaches to adult psychiatric disorders has been tempered by the lack of replicated findings of linkage. Because molecular genetic approaches to adult disorders will involve more complexity than originally thought, clearly applications to childhood and adolescent disorders will not take place immediately. The identification of highly familial phenotypes may aid in the search for specific genes by highlighting potential subtypes of disorders that may have genetic causes (see Rutter et al., 1999a). Family studies will also provide valuable data on persons at increased risk, which will be useful for targeting secondary prevention. Furthermore, most psychiatric disorders involve the expression of environmental as well as genetic factors. Because of this, family studies should be viewed as a resource for studying environmental risk factors.

The primary purpose of this chapter is to describe the designs and methods used to conduct family studies, especially those designed to examine the familiarity of childhood and adolescent psychopathology. We discuss research designs, assessment of family members, issues of data analysis, and the role of family studies in disentangling genetic and environmental influences on psychopathology.

RESEARCH DESIGNS

Top-Down, Bottom-Up, and High-Risk Designs

A prototypical family study is the "family retrospective cohort design," in which subjects are asked to recall their lifetime course of psychiatric disorders. As a first step, an "affected proband" (i.e., case with the disorder under investigation) is identified and matched to a "control proband," who is an individual not affected with the disorder but matched to the affected proband on other salient characteristics (e.g., age, sex, socioeconomic status) that may influence the rates of disorders in relatives. As a second step, all living and willing first-degree relatives (i.e., biological parents, siblings, and offspring) are assessed to determine their lifetime course of disorders, and family history information is obtained for deceased relatives or for relatives who cannot be interviewed directly. All assessments of relatives are conducted by evaluators who are unaware of ("blind" to) the probands' status (i.e., affected vs. control). The prevalence of the disorder under study in first-degree relatives of affected probands is then compared with its prevalence among relatives of control probands. If the prevalence is statistically greater in the relatives of affected probands, then the disorder under investigation is considered to aggregate within families. Second-degree (grandparents, aunts, uncles) and third-degree (cousins) relatives can also be studied, but the number of subjects in such a study will become very large, and cooperation will usually decrease. (However, see below.)

There are a few variants of this approach, which are especially relevant to the study of psychopathology in childhood and adolescence. An important distinction is made between "top-down" and "bottom-up" designs when children and adolescents are included in family studies (Puig-Antich, 1984; Strober, 1984; Strober & Carlson, 1982). Family studies that begin with adult probands and study psychopathology among their offspring as well as other relatives are known as "top-down" studies, which is the design just described. In contrast, "bottom-up" studies identify children or adolescents as the probands, and their relatives are then examined for lifetime rates of psychiatric disorders.

Top-down and bottom-up designs are different because the rates of disorders are calculated for relatives of different ages, and these designs thus require different types of controls. In a bottom-up design, the parents are the ones who bring affected child probands for treatment and who grant permission for the children to be included in the study. This creates a potential bias in the family design, because parents who have psychiatric disorders themselves may be more likely than unaffected parents whose children have a disorder to bring their children to treatment and to consent to the children's inclusion in a study. This sampling bias can artificially produce high rates of disorders in the child's adult relatives. One method used to control for this referral bias is to include a control proband group of children with another psychiatric disorder where the same bias of selection for psychopathology may exist. That is, the rates of psychiatric disorders will also tend to be higher in the adult relatives of this comparison group. Hence differences in either the types or rates of disorders between the adult relatives of the cases and the relatives of the psychiatric control group may provide useful information on the familial nature of the disorder under study.

The "high-risk" design is a variant of the family study; specifically, it is a modification of the top-down design. In the high-risk design, the focus is usually limited to the young offspring of affected probands, and strong efforts are made to interview both biological parents and offspring (and, as discussed in detail later, other adults in the children's lives, such as nonbiological rearing parents). Ideally, the offspring are identified before the age of onset of the disorder in question and studied longitudinally, so that the early signs and first episodes of the disorder may be examined. In addition, a focus on offspring at high risk for a disorder also permits potential investigation of salient risk and protective factors, which may be more obvious in younger individuals through childhood and adolescence. In general, high-risk studies have been developed after the familial nature of a disorder has been established by means of the family case–control and top-down designs.

One additional design should be mentioned. A few family studies of psychiatric disorders have widened their focus from first-degree relatives (i.e., parents, siblings, offspring) to include second- and third-degree relatives (i.e., aunts, uncles, grandparents, grandchildren). In general, the assessment of extended pedigrees is used in order to develop statistical genetic models of the way in which a disorder is transmitted across generations. For example, inclusion of second- and third-degree relatives may be useful for developing genetic models of psychiatric disorders, because their resemblance would not be due to common family experiences shared by first-degree relatives. Although this method has not been used very frequently in the study of child and adolescent psychopathology, there is increasing interest in this approach (Todd, Neuman, Geller, Fox, & Hickok, 1993).

Family History versus Family Study

A traditional method for collecting family data in clinical psychiatry has been to ask a patient about psychiatric illness in the family. This approach has been standardized, so that the questions and relatives included are precise, and it is referred to as the "family history method" (Andreasen, Endicott, Spitzer, & Winokur, 1977). Here the goal is to gather systematic information on the psychiatric history of family members (the specific methods used are discussed in the next section of this chapter), whether the design is top-down, bottom-up, or high-risk. One difficulty with the family history method is that it underreports rates of disorders in family members. One way to correct this problem is to obtain family history from multiple informants and piece together a picture on each noninterviewed relative. Using more than two informants can produce results approaching those obtained through a direct interview (Thompson, Kidd, & Weissman, 1979).

Although the family history method represents an important approach to assessing family history of psychiatric disorders, a more powerful and preferable approach is to interview the family members directly. This approach, referred to as the "family study method," attempts to use direct interviews with all available family members under study, in order to gather sufficient diagnostic information from each individual. This approach is preferred because direct interviews have been found to provide more complete diagnostic information on individuals within a family (see Weissman et al., 1986). Again, the family study method can be used within top-down, bottom-up, or high-risk paradigms. The one difficulty with this approach, however, is the pragmatic problem of being able to conduct direct interviews with all family members, for reasons including refusal to participate in the study, unavailability due to geographic distance, or death. It is for these reasons that the family history method has a place along with the family study method in the assessment of family history of psychiatric disorders.

GENERAL PROCEDURES

Selection of Affected Probands

Family studies begin with the identification of affected probands, or index cases with the disorder under investigation. The criteria for including or excluding these probands should be well defined, as they form the sampling frame for a study; such criteria include demographic variables (e.g., including/excluding probands of certain ages or one gender) or diagnostic considerations (e.g., including/excluding probands with comorbid conditions). Probands should be selected without knowledge of family history, and probands without family members should be omitted from a study.

With rare exceptions, affected probands in family studies of psychiatric disorders are patients receiving psychiatric treatment. This situation represents a potential bias in family studies, as a majority of individuals with psychiatric disorders never receive treatment (e.g., Shapiro et al., 1984). Hence questions may be raised about the generalizability of findings to the population as a whole. For example, such a bias may influence results in regard to severity, as treated individuals are generally among the more severely affected. If severity is related to familial aggregation, then the findings based on treated samples of affected probands may not extend readily to the full range of the disorder in the population. Moreover, patients with ill family members may be more likely to come to treatment—a bias that could result in increased rates of illness in relatives. However, it should be noted that in one family study of panic disorder and major depression, patterns of familial aggregation were not affected by whether affected probands came from treatment clinics or a community sample (Weissman et al., 1993).

Selection of Control Groups

The reason for inclusion of control groups is to permit comparison of the rates of the disorder among relatives, in order to obtain data on relative risk. Although earlier studies have compared rates of disorders in relatives of affected probands to population rates (see Weissman et al., 1986), the use of a control group allows a more stringent testing of the hypothesis of no familial aggregation: Data on relatives of affected and control probands are collected in an identical manner, reducing possible sources of bias introduced by using different diagnostic instruments. In addition, affected and control probands may be matched on likely confounding factors, which may affect the rates of disorders in relatives. Such basic confounding factors include age, sex, socioeconomic status, race, and ethnicity.

The types of control groups used in family studies of psychopathology vary according to the purpose of the study. Many family studies have used a "normal" control group, consisting of individuals who have never had a psychiatric disorder. Such a control group can be randomly sampled from the community (e.g., Weissman et al., 1984). Another approach is the "acquaintanceship" procedure, in which relatives of probands are asked to name acquaintances who of are the same gender and of about the same age and socioeconomic status as themselves; then their relatives are interviewed. In this method, it is important to screen for mental illness in the acquaintances, in order to create a control group without lifetime histories of psychiatric disorders (Mannuzza et al., 1992).

There have been suggestions that the use of a normal control group may lead to inflated rates of familial aggregation, and that a population control group would be more informative (Kendler, 1990). Such a bias could theoretically occur if affected probands in a family study have a secondary disorder that is also associated with the primary disorder in relatives (see Weissman et al., 1993). However, relying on population control groups could also result in overestimating the degree of familial aggregation; thus multiple control groups offer the best alternative. Normal controls may be used to study the aggregation of the primary disorder in the absence of a secondary disorder, and comorbid groups may serve as appropriate controls for studying the effects of a secondary disorder on the aggregation of the primary disorder in affected probands and relatives (Weissman et al., 1993).

Other control groups may serve more specialized purposes in family studies. A control group of individuals who have a disorder other than that of interest, and who have sought treatment for this disorder, provides a test of the hypothesis that the rate of the primary disorder in relatives of affected probands "breeds true" (i.e., is specific to that particular type of disorder). In addition, an inclusion of a medically, but not psychiatrically, ill control group allows a test of the hypothesis that high rates of psychopathology reflect dysfunction due to major psychosocial stressors resulting from having any form of illness. One example of a study involving children using multiple control groups was conducted by Hammen, Burge, Burney, and Adrian (1990); the controls included psychiatric, medical, and normal controls.

Identification of Relatives

Relatives can be first-, second-, or third-degree, depending on the study design. The ascertainment of relatives should be systematic, and methods for eliciting and recording the pertinent information on relatives (or "pedigree") have been developed to ensure complete and unambiguous data, which can be transferred directly to a computer file (Thompson et al., 1979; see Weissman et al., 1986). Such a process is essential to the proper conduct of family studies: The database for such studies may be quite large, and it is crucial to identify all family members, living or deceased, by sex, current age (or age at death), and precise biological relationship (e.g., "grandfather" rather than "second-degree relative"). As will be discussed below, the various types of family structures observed in contemporary society also require that systematic methods be used for identifying all members of non-nuclear families, and especially for defining the precise relationship of each family member to each proband. Several data management systems that monitor the collection of pedigree data, check for errors, and track persons as they progress through data collection are now available (Adams, 1994).

DIRECT INTERVIEW OF FAMILY MEMBERS

As discussed previously, the preferred method for collecting information on the lifetime psychiatric status of relatives is the family study method, in which all relatives of interest are assessed through direct interview. A few specific guidelines should be followed in choosing the most appropriate diagnostic assessment procedure for a family study. One essential feature is to use a structured or semistructured interview that assesses the lifetime history of a variety of diagnoses, such as the instruments discussed below. An important feature is that widely used methods should be chosen in order to facilitate comparability with other studies. No matter what instrument is used, it is essential that all interviewers of family members be unaware of probands' clinical status, so that bias does not influence the interviews.

Assessment of Adults

It is important to note that as yet no methodological studies have compared the utility of different instruments for diagnosing disorders in adults within family studies. Rather, the emphasis in family studies has been on choosing a method that meets the fundamental requirements indicated above—primarily the capacity to indicate *lifetime history* of psychiatric disorders. Many studies utilize criteria that fit either with a given diagnostic system (e.g., the *Diagnostic and Statistical Manual of Mental Disorders* [DSM] or the *International Classification of Diseases* [ICD]) or with the well-established Research Diagnostic Criteria (RDC). In general, studies also usually rely on structured diagnostic interviews that systematically elicit signs and symptoms of disorders, such as the Schedule for Affective Disorders and Schizophrenia—Lifetime (SADS-L; Mannuzza, Fyer, Klein, & Endicott, 1986) and the Structured Clinical Interview for DSM-III-R (SCID; Spitzer, Williams, Gibbon, & First, 1992). Other measures include the Diagnostic Interview Schedule (DIS; Robins, Helzer, Croughan, & Ratcliff, 1981), which was designed as a diagnostic interview to be used by lay interviewers.

A fairly recent methodological development has been the introduction of the Diagnostic Interview for Genetic Studies (DIGS), which was designed specifically for psychiatric genetic studies (Nurnberger et al., 1994). The DIGS, which focuses on the assessment of major mood and psychotic disorders, was developed (1) to ensure a broad sampling of possible diagnoses, with maximum comparability across data sets; (2) to provide detailed information on the phenomenology of mood and psychotic disorders (not typically assessed with other instruments); (3) to allow for quantitative assessments of the relevant phenotypes, in addition to diagnoses; and (4) to incorporate an algorithmic scoring capability. An initial study using the DIGS reports satisfactory reliabilities for most disorders of interest, and in fact reports that the algorithmic approach produced test–retest coefficients superior to those obtained with more traditional measures such as the SCID and SADS (Nurnberger et al., 1994).

Assessment of Children and Adolescents

Family studies assessing psychopathology in children and adolescents have also used structured and semi-structured diagnostic instruments. These instruments have been designed for assessing children's and adolescents' presentation of psychopathological symptoms in a systematic fashion. Three instruments that may be put to such use in family studies are the Diagnostic Interview Schedule for Children (DISC-2.3; Schwab-Stone et al., 1996), the Child and Adolescent Psychiatric Assessment (CAPA: Angold et al., 1995), and the Schedule for Affective Disorders and Schizophrenia for School-Age Children (K-SADS-PL; Kaufman et al., 1997). These instruments are of interest because they all have a standard set of questions as well as specific criteria for each question, include a wide range of syndromes and disorders, and include both child and parent versions. The CAPA and K-SADS-PL are designed to be administered by clinicians, whereas the DISC was developed for use by lay interviewers. Hence, in choosing an interview for a family study involving children and adolescents, researchers must keep in mind the time demands of the various interviews available. Again, it is essential to note that there are no studies which compare the utility of different instruments in the assessment of children and adolescents in family studies.

Choice of Informants

One issue that arises when assessing children and adolescents is the choice of informants. To date, most family studies have collected diagnostic information on a child directly from the child and from at least one parent, given the considerable discrepancy found between parent and child reports (e.g., Andrews, Garrison, Jackson, Addy, & McKeown, 1993; Ivens & Rehm, 1988; Orvaschel, Puig-Antich, Chambers, Tabrizi, & Johnson, 1986; Weissman et al., 1987). Children have been found to be better informants about their own internal feelings, whereas parents underreport affective disorders in their children (Weissman et al., 1987). Parents are essential as informants, however, for very young children. Parental reports are necessary for externalizing disorders such as attention-deficit/hyperactivity disorder, and teacher reports are also useful in making diagnoses (Biederman, Faraone, Milberger, & Doyle, 1993). Hence a general principle is to acquire information from as many relevant sources as possible (e.g., Rutter, 1988). Various strategies for combining the information from different informants are available (e.g., Bird, Gould, & Staghezza, 1992).

Telephone Interviews

Another method that aids in the collection of direct interview data from relatives is to conduct interviews by telephone. Since family members often live at great distances from one another, it is not feasible to conduct in-person interviews with everyone. Even when probands are able and ready to be interviewed in person, their family members may be less invested in or less available for research. Telephone interviewing is a practical solution to these problems and may reduce the costs of a study, and information is becoming available on how information derived from telephone interviewing compares to that acquired through face-to-face interviews. One study compared the diagnostic results obtained from relatives of probands who were interviewed in a family genetics study either via telephone or face to face (Sobin et al., 1993). No significant differences in the rates of disorders or in the patterns of familial aggregation were found between the two interview methods, suggesting that telephone interviewing may represent a valid way of conducting direct interviews with relatives in family studies.

Brief Assessments

A direct and extensive interview with each relative is the ideal method for assessing lifetime psychiatric status in a family study. However, in large-scale investigations (such as epidemiological studies), the time constraints and costs of conducting direct interviews may prohibit the use of a family study component. Hence there is a need for instruments that can serve as screens for psychopathology in large studies. One such instrument that has potential is the Family History Screen for Epidemiologic Studies (FHE), which was developed as a brief, structured, computer-scorable instrument to screen for 15 DSM-III diagnoses. In one study, the FHE was administered to one informant in each of 77 families in which pedigrees had been collected by clinically trained interviewers, and in which 316 relatives had been interviewed with the SADS and diagnosed "blindly" and independently by doctoral-level clinicians (Lish, Weissman, Adams, Hoven, & Bird, 1995). For adults reporting on themselves, the FHE showed excellent specificity and fair to excellent sensitivity. Hence the FHE is a potentially useful method as a screen for psychiatric disorders in a subject's adult relatives. For studies of children and adolescents, it has potential utility for obtaining family psychiatric history of parents and/or relatives if each relative is directly screened.

Locating Relatives

A difficulty often encountered in using the family study method is locating family members, especially when populations with unstable living patterns are under investigation. There are now several strategies that may be used to help locate family members. A first strategy is to mail recruitment letters both to the subjects' last known addresses and to contacts identified in a thorough review of case records (if any such contacts are available). A powerful method is to gain low-cost access to electronic nationwide databases that provide address information on the basis of last known address, Social Security number, surname, and/or phone number. Such databases also provide the names of the current residents of a given address and neighbors in close proximity to an address. Other potential strategies include developing contacts with departments of motor vehicles, as well as state agencies such as departments of criminal justice and departments of income maintenance, all of which have guidelines concerning record searches for address information (Denny, n.d.).

Training Interviewers

Whichever instrument is used in a family study, certain standard procedures should be followed to ensure the integrity of the data collected. All interviewers should undergo a period of training sufficient for the instrument of choice. Formal training manuals are available that explain methods for contacting subjects, scheduling appointments, conducting interviews, and checking errors; such manuals also provide instructions for completing diagnostic assessment, obtaining family history and pedigree, assessing social functioning, and writing narratives. Training can include lectures, small-group workshops, viewing of videotaped interviews, role-playing practice, assigned homework, and supervised interviews (see Weissman et al., 1993). Formal interrater reliability studies should also be conducted, as different interviewers will be assessing different families. Interviewers should also be monitored periodically for reliability (e.g., by having two interviewers assess the same individual) to avoid rater drift, which can skew the results of a family study.

FAMILY HISTORY METHOD

As discussed earlier, although the family study method is the preferred methodology for determining familial aggregation, pragmatic issues often require the use of the family history method. The basic procedures that have been used to date are described in Weissman et al. (1986) and are summarized here. The best-known procedure is the Family History Research Diagnostic Criteria (FH-RDC) method, in which structured family history interview methods are used systematically to obtain the data necessary to make RDC diagnoses in family members (Andreasen et al., 1977). The FH-RDC approach has been updated in a new format—the Family Informant Schedule and Criteria (FISC; Mannuzza, Fyer, Endicott, & Klein, 1985). The basic procedure is as follows. First, basic information on first- and second-degree relatives is listed on a pedigree collection form, as described previously. Second, the proband completes a direct diagnostic interview about himself/herself. Third, the proband then serves as an informant about his/her first-degree relatives (and possibly second-degree relatives as well, depending on the design of the study), as the interviewer asks the informant whether each relative (one by one and by name) has had any of the problems that were just mentioned in the interview about himself/herself. This approach ensures that the informant is well acquainted with the symptoms that he/she is asked to identify in his or her family members. When the informant indicates that a relative has had a problem, the interviewer is instructed to probe for the information necessary to generate diagnoses by using the diagnostic interview as a guide and by completing symptom checklists for relevant disorders. It should be noted that this overall procedure may also be carried out with relatives who have completed direct diagnostic interviews, so that multiple sources of information are collected about relatives unavailable for direct interview.

Studies have converged on the finding that the family history method leads to underestimation of the frequencies of disorders in both adult and child relatives (Andreasen et al., 1977; Weissman et al., 1986). A few suggestions have been made for increasing the sensitivity of the family history method, such as using multiple informants, which increases the sensitivity of the method (Orvaschel, Thompson, Belanger, Prusoff, & Kidd, 1982). A new twist in this area, however, is the suggestion that the family history method may add unique information not discerned through personal interviews (Kendler & Roy, 1995). For example, these authors report that family history diagnoses of major depression, though agreeing poorly with personal interview diagnoses, nonetheless are predictive of risk for subsequent episodes of major depression (even after personal interview diagnoses are statistically controlled for). Hence Kendler and Roy (1995) suggest that a multimethod approach—one that incorporates both family history methods and direct interview—may yield a more accurate measure of psychopathology than either method used alone.

In some instances, the psychiatric history of relatives may be derived from case records when a family member has received psychiatric treatment. In such cases, the information available from case records should be combined with all other available data in constructing lifetime histories of psychiatric disorders that meet either DSM or ICD criteria or the RDC. However, in general this approach rarely provides sufficient information for making lifetime diagnoses in the absence of either direct or informant report.

Another issue that has received attention in the last decade is the impact of informants' psychiatric status on their reports of psychiatric disorders in family members. Kendler et al. (1991) examined this issue in a study of twin pairs discordant for psychiatric diagnoses, derived from an epidemiological sample of adult female twin pairs. In this study, the affected twin with a history of either major depression or generalized anxiety disorder was significantly more likely to endorse the same disorder in a parent than was the unaffected cotwin. These data, however, did not allow for an inference of which report was "correct," because direct interviews with parents were not possible. That is, it was not known whether the affected twins were more accurate informants because of their familiarity with the disorder from their own experience, or whether they were biased informants who distorted family history. Along these lines, Tarullo, Richardson, Radke-Yarrow, and Martinez (1995) report that both parental agreement and mother–child agreement on childhood disorders is greater in families with an affectively ill mother than in control families, and they argue that maternal psychopathology should not be assumed to be a distorting factor in the assessment of child psychopathology.

THE BEST-ESTIMATE PROCEDURE

Once all the diagnostic data on each family member are obtained, a standard procedure is to use the best-estimate procedure to integrate the information collected on each individual (Leckman, Sholomskas, Thompson, Belanger, & Weissman, 1982). This procedure is critical, since multiple sources of data may be used (e.g., different informants, records, direct interviews), and discrepancies that require resolution will inevitably occur. The procedure is based on all available information, and the estimate is made by at least one clinician who is unaware of the diagnostic status of the proband and who has not been involved in direct interviews of any of the probands or relatives. An independent assessment is frequently obtained from a second clinician. Substantial disagreements between the two diagnosticians may be reviewed on a case-by-case basis until agreement is reached, but "blindness" with regard to the clinical status of the proband should always be maintained.

The best-estimate procedure is especially relevant for semistructured instruments such as the SADS and K-SADS, which yield clinically relevant diagnoses from different individual respondents (e.g., parent and child reports on the child). It should be noted that other instruments that may be used in family studies may have explicit algorithms for combining information from different informants, and such algorithms should be used if these instruments are employed in future family studies.

OTHER ISSUES IN ASSESSMENT

Assortative Mating

"Assortative mating," which is nonrandom mating for the disorder under study or for related disorders, is an important topic in family studies that involve children and adolescents. Several studies have documented assortative mating based on psychopathology, in which individuals with psychiatric disorders are more likely than controls to have spouses with psychiatric disorders (e.g., Colombo, Cox, & Dunner, 1990; Merikangas, Weissman, Prusoff, & John, 1988; Parnas, 1988). Assortative mating may increase the risk for psychopathology in offspring via both genetic (i.e., higher genetic loading) and environmental (i.e., increased exposure to environmental risks associated with psychopathology) mechanisms. For example, parental concordance for psychiatric illness in general poses an increased risk for offspring at risk for depression (Merikangas et al., 1988).

Family studies involving children, especially high-risk and top-down studies, should thus attempt to assess lifetime psychiatric status of both biological parents, even though only one parent is typically identified as a proband in a study. In addition, rates of disorders in offspring should be examined as a function of assortative mating, in order to compare the risks involved in having two affected parents (as opposed to one).

Assessment of Non-Nuclear Family Structures

Family studies of psychopathology involving children have usually assumed, and assessed, a conventional nuclear family structure involving a stable two-parent unit biologically related to a child, as well as full biological siblings. In general, families that have not conformed to this structure have been considered outliers in a family study and have not been included in analyses. However, fewer than 40% of children born in the 1980s in the United States will spend their entire childhood with both biological parents (Hofferth, 1985; Kazdin, 1992; National Center for Children in Poverty, 1990). Because the nuclear family structure may no longer represent the prototypical living arrangement for children (e.g., Scott, 1993), the assumptions underlying future family studies involving children and adolescents may need to be recast.

The preponderance of non-nuclear family structures presents two methodological goals for family studies of psychopathology involving children. A first goal is to develop methods for assessing such family structures in ongoing studies involving children that can be incorporated into the typical procedures used to identify pedigrees reviewed earlier in this chapter. We have developed a Rearing Parent Form (Rende, Sobin, & Weissman, 1993) to collect systematic information necessary for creating a family structure typology for each child within a family (see Haurin, 1992; Hunter & Ensminger, 1992)—namely, the child's biological parents; any adult who has lived with the child over the past 3 years and his/her precise relationship to the child (e.g., first-degree relative, spouse or partner of biological parent); and the various types of siblings (full, half-, or unrelated siblings). Preliminary data from an ongoing study of the offspring of opiate addicts revealed that only about a third of the offspring assessed had lived in a conventional nuclear family over the past 3 years, and that over a third of the siblings were half-siblings (Rende et al., 1993). Although such data need to be collected from family study designs for other forms of psychopathology, such a finding is consistent with the estimations of population trends cited earlier.

A second goal is to determine whether there are adults other than the biological parents who play a significant role in a child's life. One consideration is whether there are other adults who should be assessed when potential environmental influences on the child are being documented. Exposure to psychopathology in nonrelatives who are functioning as parents can clearly have an effect on children; therefore, in family studies such "rearing parents" should be assessed in the same manner as biological parents. In our preliminary study, we have found that over 90% of the rearing parents of offspring of opiate addicts suffer from at least one psychiatric disorder, with a majority of these individuals meeting criteria for alcohol and/or other substance abuse. The assessment of rearing parents may thus, as in this example, identify potentially salient social influences on offspring in family studies, especially in samples at high risk (Rende et al., 1998).

A related consideration involves determining who is the best informant (or source of information) about a child. Although it is common in family studies to collect information on children by interviewing one of the biological parents, the existence of non-nuclear family structures implies that the best informant on a child may not necessarily be a biological parent. This topic should receive more attention in future studies.

Proximal versus Distal Risk Factors

Research on risk and protective factors in the development of psychopathology has led to a distinction between "distal" and "proximal" risk factors, which carries implications for family studies. "Distal" factors are variables that are labeled or grouped to subsume specific environmental influences; a notable example is socioeconomic status, which is a labeled environmental factor that may reflect many specific environmental influences (Wachs & Gruen, 1982). "Proximal" factors are the actual environmental experiences nested within distal factors. With respect to psychopathology, family history of psychopathology has been classified as a distal variable, in that it is not what is experienced by individuals at risk (Baldwin, Baldwin, & Cole, 1990; Richters & Weintraub, 1990; Luthar, 1993). It has been suggested that the risk posed by such distal variables is mediated by proximal variables, such as ineffective parenting or family discord (Luthar, 1993; Richters & Weintraub, 1990).

Future studies should directly assess potential environmental risk factors and take them into account in analyses. For example, numerous studies have documented that children of depressed parents are exposed to many proximal risk factors, such as hostile, negative patterns of interactions with parents and family discord (e.g., Rutter, 1990). An explicit focus on environmental risk factors in family studies is necessary in order to reveal the specific processes by which parental psychopathology leads to negative outcomes in offspring (e.g., Rende & Plomin, 1993; Richters & Weintraub, 1990).

Phenotypic and Biological Markers

In family studies involving children and adolescents, it has been typical to assess such social and psychological traits as temperament and self-esteem in addition to psychopathology, in order to provide a more complete picture on developmental course and outcome. However, a primary advantage of assessing children at high risk for disorders is that both early manifestations of a disorder ("phenotypic markers") and biological indices of risk for a disorder ("biological markers") may be examined (Weissman et al., 1986). Hence a crucial topic for family studies involving children and adolescents is to identify such markers. They may help isolate the earliest signs of a disorder, and they may permit investigations into how these predispositions may lead, in conjunction with other risk factors, to the development of disorders.

There are a few examples of how the search for phenotypic and/or biological markers may provide some insight into the etiology of disorders in childhood. One example comes from the New York High-Risk Project, a longitudinal study of children at risk for schizophrenia or mood disorders and low-risk controls (e.g., Erlenmeyer-Kimling et al., 1993). Findings from this study indicate that childhood attentional dysfunction may be a salient index of risk for schizophrenia. Identification of phenotypic markers such as attentional dysfunction may help map out the developmental course of schizophrenia from risk in childhood to expression of symptoms in adulthood; it may also help focus the search for genetic factors involved in schizophrenia, by defining specific markers that may represent the heritable predisposition to the disorder (e.g., Gottesman, 1991).

A second example involves research on behavioral inhibition to the unfamiliar, which is a temperamental construct characterized by shy and fearful behavior. Recent studies have indicated that this temperamental construct may be an early risk factor for the development of anxiety disorders. For example, children of parents who have panic disorder with agoraphobia are at increased risk for behavioral inhibition, and children with behavioral inhibition have high rates of anxiety disorders with onsets in childhood (see Rosenbaum et al., 1993). Such work suggests that behavioral inhibition is an identifiable predictor of anxiety disorders—a predictor that may be observed in early childhood and perhaps infancy. Hence, this work demonstrates the potential of identifying specific phenotypic profiles (in the form of temperamental constructs) that may have strong associations with the development of specific forms of psychopathology.

The studies on attentional dysfunction and schizophrenia, and on behavioral inhibition and anxiety disorders, illustrate the potential utility of defining early-emerging phenotypic markers of risk for psychopathology that have a familial basis. More work of this nature may help tremendously in defining more precisely phenotypic characteristics that reflect genetic predispositions to psychopathology, and such work would undoubtedly inform research on the genetic contributions to psychiatric disorders (e.g., Rende & Plomin, 1994).

ISSUES OF DATA ANALYSIS

Issues of data analysis are crucial in the assessment of psychopathology in family studies. Several methodological concerns make the analysis of family data a complicated proposition, and proper attention to these issues is essential in drawing appropriate conclusions from family studies. In this section, analytic issues that are especially relevant to the study of childhood and adolescent psychopathology are reviewed.

Confounding Factors

Ideally, family studies match affected and control probands on potential confounding factors such as age and gender. However, such confounding factors may vary across relatives of affected and control probands (e.g., by chance, there may be more females among the relatives of affected probands than among relatives of control probands). For this reason, these potential confounding factors must be controlled for statistically while the effect of proband status on rates of disorder in relatives is estimated. A standard method is to use multivariate-regression models for survival data, such as Cox's (1972) proportional-hazards model, with the potential confounding factors included as independent variables.

Lack of Independence in Family Data

Statistical methods used to assess familial aggregation of psychiatric disorders generally make comparisons across aggregate rates of disorders based on proband status (i.e., affected vs. control). Such methods carry the assumption that the observations are independent of one another. However, this assumption is usually violated in family studies, as more than one observation per family is often made (i.e., numerous members of a given family are assessed). In general, violations of this assumption produce biased results, in that dependent data may inflate patterns of association. Although the adverse consequences of the violation of the independence assumption in family studies have not been examined empirically, this issue deserves attention because of the potential for results from family studies to be misleading. For example, one potential problem is that a small number of "highly loaded" families could suggest significant familial association in a family study, when in fact the pattern of aggregation for the remaining families in the sample may not suggest familiarity. This point is especially important because family studies often assess variable numbers of family members, thus creating the potential for methodological problems of this nature.

To date, there are no completely satisfactory methods for controlling for the dependence inherent in family data. Attempts have been made to control for such dependence by using correlated binary regression with covariates specific to each binary observation (Liang & Zeger, 1986). Another method is to include family size as a potential confounding factor in regression models such as the proportional-hazards model mentioned above; if there are highly loaded families skewing the results, then family size may make a significant contribution in the model. Similarly, an examination of the data by family may indicate whether there are a few atypical families that severely affect the pattern of familial aggregation; another approach is to calculate the number of families in which at least one relative is affected (Biederman et al., 1992).

However, these methods do not entirely handle the more general problem of dependence.

Although the dependence of family data is a fundamental problem in the calculation of familial aggregation, statistical methods geared toward the assessment of dependent data may provide clues to etiology. For example, although family studies have suggested that most psychiatric disorders in childhood and adolescence have in part a familial basis, the extent to which children within a high-risk family have similar outcomes has not been examined (Rutter et al., 1990). Although it might be thought that familial risk factors would be shared equally by all children in a family, there is much evidence documenting the extent to which siblings have very different outcomes in development (Hetherington, Reiss, & Plomin, 1994). Hence there is much interest in capitalizing on the dependence of sibling data to document the extent to which siblings with a specific risk factor in common (e.g., a depressed parent) have similar outcomes (e.g., a history of major depression), and also to attempt to identify salient environmental factors that result in similarity between siblings (shared environmental influences) as well as those that lead to differences between siblings (nonshared environmental influences).

Analytic tools to address such questions are currently available (e.g., Hetherington et al., 1994). One new approach is to capitalize on the dependence of observations in high-risk studies to model statistically the degree to which siblings at risk have similar outcomes of interest (Rende, Wickramaratne, Warner, & Weissman, 1995). In this approach, sibling resemblance is estimated via the pairwise odds ratio, which explicitly quantifies the degree of statistical resemblance between dependent observations. Using this approach in a study of offspring at high and low risk for depression, we (Rende et al., 1995) found that sibling aggregation in the high-risk cohort was more notable for anxiety than for depression, suggesting that the familial influences common to siblings at risk for depression may operate more strongly in producing anxiety.

Cohort Effects

There is increasing evidence that "cohort effects" (i.e., differences across generations) are observed for some psychiatric disorders, in that younger cohorts have higher lifetime rates of disorders than older cohorts. For example, the lifetime risk of having a major depressive disorder has increased dramatically, and the average age of onset has decreased (Weissman et al., 1993); another study, using a sibling design, documented a secular increase in childhood mood disorders (Ryan et al., 1992). Hence family studies that combine information from multiple cohorts must control for potential cohort effects by including year of birth as an independent variable in multiple-regression models (Weissman et al., 1986).

Another strategy is to focus on specific cohorts, such as same-age siblings and cousins, which are by definition subject to the same cohort or period effects (Todd et al., 1993). An example of this approach is a family study of substance misuse that found considerably higher rates of drug misuse in the siblings than in the parents of misusers (Luthar, Anton, Merikangas, & Rounsaville, 1992). Hence it has been suggested that siblings or children of addicts may constitute far more suitable groups for studying familial aggregation of drug misuse than parents may (Luthar & Rounsaville, 1993).

Age of Onset

The major outcome in a family study is usually the rate of a disorder in relatives over their lifetimes, termed "morbid risk" or "lifetime prevalence." In this sense, "lifetime risk" refers to the risk of onset of a particular disorder between birth and a particular age, such as the age of the individual when an interview is conducted. However, because age of onset varies for a given disorder and usually encompasses a rather wide range, studies must account for the fact that some individuals in a study may not yet have a disorder because they have not passed through the typical period in which first onset is usually noted. In addition, the rates of disorders in relatives must be interpreted according to the age range of the cohort under study, and not simply assessed in raw terms.

Several statistical methods have been developed to adjust for variable age of onset in relatives (see Weissman et al., 1986). One approach utilizes the general strategy of survival analysis. Survival-analytic techniques treat age of onset of disorder as a survival time, and a survival function—or lifetime risk at a given time—may be estimated by different methods (Cutler & Ederer, 1958; Kaplan & Meier, 1958). These approaches should be considered in family designs specifically focused on children and adolescents. For example, in a bottom-up study, the age range of parents may be quite wide, and hence adjustments based on age of onset should be made before determining lifetime rates of disorders in parents. In a high-risk study, if the ages of children at risk vary, adjustments may be necessary because different subjects will pass through the typical age-of-onset period at different time points in the study.

Another consideration concerning age of onset is that, in general, early-onset forms of disorders tend to be more familial than late-onset forms of disorders. As such, it is useful to consider age of onset in both probands and relatives as a factor when one is analyzing family data. One example of this approach is the demonstration that early-onset major depression is more familial than late-onset depression (Weissman et al., 1984). Considering age of onset may lead to crucial distinctions between familial and nonfamilial forms of disorders, as has been proposed, for example, by Todd et al. (1993).

NATURE, NURTURE, AND PSYCHOPATHOLOGY

Traditionally, psychiatric genetic research has followed a hierarchy in searching for genetic influences on psychiatric disorders. A first step is to conduct family studies to establish the familial nature of a disorder; a second step is to conduct behavioral genetic studies to demonstrate significant genetic influence on a disorder; and a third step is to conduct molecular genetic studies to pinpoint specific regions on the chromosome that are linked to the disorder.

Within this hierarchy, family studies represent a limited approach because they cannot disentangle genetic and environmental influences. However, as a concluding theme to this chapter, we wish to emphasize the continuing importance of family designs in the search for genetic influences on the development of psychopathology. Perhaps the most salient point to consider at this time is that molecular genetic approaches to childhood and adult psychopathology will proceed more slowly than may have been thought even a few years ago. The major obstacle is that although there are powerful methods for detecting single genes, which are necessary and sufficient causes of some disorders, most psychiatric disorders do not appear to follow simple patterns of inheritance; instead, that multiple genetic loci and environmental influences appear to contribute to phenotypic expression in a probabilistic manner. Hence, given the complex nature of psychopathology, family studies may contribute much useful information to the search for genetic underpinnings of disorders.

Three points are especially important to consider. A first point is that a given disorder may be due to various etiological influences that result in a similar phenotype. When genetic influences are considered, this situation is referred to as "genetic heterogeneity," in which specific genes may be involved in the expression of only some types of a disorder (e.g., Plomin & Rende, 1991). If genetic heterogeneity is important for a disorder, then family studies can be instrumental in identifying highly familial subtypes of the disorder that may be due to genetic influence. There is hope that such a strategy may be successful in research on disorders in childhood and adolescence, such as early-onset mood disorders (Todd et al., 1993).

A second point is that different disorders may in fact reflect common genetic etiologies. The preponderance of comorbidity in childhood and adolescent disorders (e.g., Caron & Rutter, 1991) suggests that family studies may be especially important in determining whether comorbid conditions reflect common familial influences. For example, recent studies have suggested that attention-deficit/hyperactivity disorder and mood disorders may share a common familial influence (Biederman et al., 1992), whereas panic disorder and major depression do not (Weissman et al., 1993). Such studies may be especially useful in identifying clusters of symptoms that may be due to common genetic etiologies, and others that are etiologically distinct (Wickramaratne & Weissman, 1993).

A third point is that strategies used for conducting family studies may yield some clues on the potential genetic etiology of disorders. Two approaches mentioned earlier in this chapter are relevant. One approach is to examine second- and third-degree relatives in addition to first-degree relatives in family studies; because a range of genetic relatedness is available, testing of hypotheses of genetic influence is possible (e.g., Todd et al., 1993). Another approach is to capitalize on the preponderance of non-nuclear family structures to develop behavioral genetic designs, which may sort out the effects of genes and environment on psychopathology. For example, two potential designs include quasi-adoption strategies, in which children with a history of psychopathology in biological relatives are reared by unaffected nonrelatives, and designs that compare the similarity of full siblings and half-siblings (Rende et al., 1993). All of these strategies represent ways in which prototypical family designs may help to sort out the effects of nature and nurture on psychopathology.

As a concluding comment, we wish to emphasize the importance of environment in the development of psychopathology. Because most psychiatric disorders will have complex etiologies involving both genetic and environmental sources of influence, family studies will continue to yield data on the role of environmental risk factors, as exemplified by the research on proximal risk factors for psychopathology in childhood and adolescence discussed earlier (e.g., Richters & Weintraub, 1990). The importance of these research strategies should not be minimized, given the current interest in the genetics of childhood and adolescent disorders, because it is becoming increasingly clear that both nature and nurture plays a significant role for most forms of psychopathology. In this sense, methodologies used in family studies will continue to play an essential part in the search for etiological factors involved in the expression of psychopathology in childhood and adolescence.

ACKNOWLEDGMENTS

Preparation of this chapter was supported in part by National Institute of Mental Health Grants No. MH43868, No. MH36197, and No. MH50666 to Myrna M. Weissman; a National Alliance for Research on Schizophrenia and Affective Disorder Young Investigator Award to Richard Rende; and an Aaron Diamond Foundation Fellowship in the Biomedical and Social Sciences to Richard Rende. We thank Priya Wickramaratne, PhD, for helpful comments.

REFERENCES

Adams, P. (1994). LABMAN and LINKMAN: A data management system specifically designed for genome studies of complex disease. *Genetic Epidemiology, 11,* 87–98.

Andreasen, N. C., Endicott, J., Spitzer, R. L., & Winokur, G. (1977). The family history method using diagnostic criteria: Reliability and validity. *Archives of General Psychiatry, 34,* 1229–1235.

Andrews, V. C., Garrison, C. Z., Jackson, K. L., Addy, C. L., & McKeown, R. E. (1993). Mother–adolescent agreement on the symptoms and diagnoses of adolescent depression and conduct disorders. *Journal of the American Academy of Child and Adolescent Psychiatry, 32,* 731–738.

Angold, A., Prendergast, M., Cox, A., Harrington, R., Simonoff, E., & Rutter, M. (1995). The Child and Adolescent Psychiatric Assessment (CAPA). *Psychological Medicine, 25,* 739–753.

Baldwin, A. L., Baldwin, C., & Cole, R. E. (1990). Stress-resistant families and stress-resistant children. In J. Rolf, A. S. Masten, D. Cicchetti, K. H. Nuechterlein, & S. Weintraub (Eds.), *Risk and protective factors in the development of psychopathology* (pp. 257–280). New York: Cambridge University Press.

Biederman, J., Faraone, S., Keenan, K., Benjamin, J., Krifcher, B., Moore, C., Sprich, S., Ugaglia, K., Jellineck, M. S., Steingaid, R., Spencer, T., Norman, D., Kolodny, R., Kraus, I., Perrin, J., Keller, M. B., & Tsuang, M. (1992). Further evidence for family-genetic risk factors in attention deficit hyperactivity disorder. *Archives of General Psychiatry, 49,* 728–738.

Biederman, J., Faraone, S., Milberger, S., & Doyle, A. (1993). Diagnoses of attention-deficit hyperactivity disorder from parent reports predict diagnoses based on teacher reports. *Journal of the American Academy of Child and Adolescent Psychiatry, 32,* 315–317.

Bird, H. R., Gould, M. S., & Staghezza, B. (1992). Aggregating data from multiple informants in child psychiatry epidemiological research. *Journal of the American Academy of Child and Adolescent Psychiatry, 31,* 78–85.

Caron, C., & Rutter, M. (1991). Comorbidity in child psychopathology: Concepts, issues, and research strategies. *Journal of Child Psychology and Psychiatry, 32,* 1063–1080.

Colombo, M., Cox, G., & Dunner, D. L. (1990). Assortative mating in affective and anxiety disorders: Preliminary findings. *Psychiatric Genetics, 1,* 35–44.

Cox, D. R. (1972). Regression models and life tables. *Journal of the Royal Statistical Society, 34,* 187–220.

Cutler, S. J., & Ederer, F. (1958). Maximum utilization of the life table in analyzing survival. *Journal of Chronic Diseases, 8,* 699–713.

Denny, L. (n.d.). *Genetic epidemiology core manual.* Unpublished manuscript, New York State Psychiatric Institute, Center for the Study of Youth Depression, Anxiety, and Suicide.

Erlenmeyer-Kimling, L., Cornblatt, B. A., Rock, D., Roberts, S., Bell, M., & West, A. (1993). The New York High-Risk Project: Anhedonia, attentional deviance, and psychopathology. *Schizophrenia Bulletin, 19,* 141–153.

Folstein, S. E., & Rutter, M. L. (1988). Autism: Familial aggregation and genetic implications. *Journal of Autism and Developmental Disorders, 18,* 3–30.

Gottesman, I. I. (1991). *Schizophrenia genesis: The origins of madness.* New York: Freeman.

Guze, S. B., Cloninger, C. R., Martin, R. L., & Clayton, P. J. (1983). A follow-up and family study of schizophrenia. *Archives of General Psychiatry, 40,* 1273–1276.

Hammen, C., Burge, D., Burney, E., & Adrian, C. (1990). Longitudinal study of diagnoses in children of women with unipolar and bipolar affective disorder. *Archives of General Psychiatry, 47,* 1112–1117.

Haurin, R. J. (1992). Patterns of childhood residence and the relationship to young adult outcomes. *Journal of Marriage and the Family, 54,* 846–860.

Hetherington, E. M., Reiss, D., & Plomin, R. (1994). *Separate social worlds of siblings: Impact of nonshared environment on development.* Hillsdale, NJ: Erlbaum.

Hofferth, S. L. (1985). Updating children's life course. *Journal of Marriage and the Family, 47,* 93–115.

Hunter, A. G., & Ensminger, M. E. (1992). Diversity and fluidity in children's living arrangements: Family transitions in an urban Afro-American community. *Journal of Marriage and the Family, 54,* 418–426.

Ivens, C., & Rehm, L. (1988). Assessment of childhood depression: Correspondence between reports by child, mother, and father. *Journal of the American Academy of Child and Adolescent Psychiatry, 6,* 738–741.

Kaplan, E. B., & Meier, P. (1958). Nonparametric estimation from incomplete observations. *Journal of the American Statistical Association, 53,* 457–481.

Kaufman, J., Birmaher, B., Brent, D., Rao, U., Flynn, C., Moreci, P., Williamson, D., & Ryan, N. (1997). Schedule for Affective disorders and Schizophrenia for School-Age Children—Present and Lifetime Version (K-SADS-PL). *Journal of the American Academy of Child and Adolescent Psychiatry, 36,* 980–988.

Kazdin, A. (1992). Child and adolescent dysfunction and paths toward maladjustment: Targets for intervention. *Clinical Psychology Review, 12,* 795–817.

Kendler, K. S. (1990). The super-normal control group in psychiatric genetics: Possible artifactual evidence for aggregation. *Psychiatric Genetics, 1,* 45–53.

Kendler, K. S., Gruenberg, A. M., & Tsuang, M. T. (1985). Psychiatric illness in first degree relatives of schizophrenic and surgical control patients. *Archives of General Psychiatry, 42,* 770–779.

Kendler, K. S., & Roy, M.-A. (1995). Validity of a diagnosis of lifetime major depression obtained by personal interview versus family history. *American Journal of Psychiatry, 152,* 1608–1614.

Kendler, K. S., Silberg, J. L., Neale, M. C., Kessler, R. C., Heath, A. C., & Eaves, L. J. (1991). The family history method: Whose psychiatric history is measured? *American Journal of Psychiatry, 148,* 1501–1504.

Leckman, J. F., Sholomskas, D., Thompson, W. D., Belanger, A., & Weissman, M. M. (1982). Best estimate of lifetime psychiatric diagnosis: A methodologic study. *Archives of General Psychiatry, 39,* 879–883.

Liang, K. Y., & Zeger, S. L. (1986). Longitudinal data analysis using generalized linear models. *Biometrika, 75,* 501–506.

Lish, J. D., Weissman, M. M., Adams, P. B., Hoven, C., & Bird, H. (1995). Family Psychiatric History Screen for Epidemiologic Studies (FHE): Pilot testing and validation. *Psychiatry Research, 57,* 169–180.

Luthar, S. S. (1993). Annotation: Methodological and conceptual issues in research on childhood resilience. *Journal of Child Psychology and Psychiatry, 34,* 441–453.

Luthar, S. S., Anton, S. F., Merikangas, K. R., & Rounsaville, B. J. (1992). Vulnerability to substance abuse and psychopathology among siblings of opioid abusers. *Journal of Nervous and Mental Disease, 180,* 153–161.

Luthar, S. S., & Rounsaville, B. J. (1993). Substance misuse and comorbid psychopathology in a high-risk group: A study of siblings of cocaine misusers. *International Journal of the Addictions, 28,* 415–434.

Mannuzza, S., Fyer, A. J., Endicott, J., Gallops, M. S., Martin, L. Y., Reich, T., & Klein, D. F. (1992). An extension of the acquaintanceship procedure in family studies of mental disorder. *Journal of Psychiatric Research, 26,* 45–57.

Mannuzza, S., Fyer, A. J., Endicott, J., & Klein, D. F. (1985). *Family Informant Schedule and Criteria* (FISC). New York: New York State Psychiatric Institute, Anxiety Disorders Clinic.

Mannuzza, S., Fyer, A. J., Klein, D. F., & Endicott, J. (1986). Schedule for Affective Disorders and Schizophrenia—Lifetime Version (modified for the study of anxiety disorders): Rationale and conceptual development. *Journal of Psychiatric Research, 20,* 317–325.

Merikangas, K. R., Weissman, M. M., Prusoff, B. A., & John, K. (1988). Assortative mating and affective disorders: Psychopathology in offspring. *Psychiatry, 51,* 48–57.

National Center for Children in Poverty. (1990). *Five million children: A statistical profile of our poorest young citizens.* New York: Columbia University School of Public Health.

Nurnberger, J. I., Jr., Blehar, M. C., Kaufmann, C. A., York-Cooler, C., Simpson, S. G., Harkavy-Friedman, J., Severe, J. B., Malaspina, D., & Reich, T. (1994). Diagnostic Interview for Genetic Studies: Rationale, unique features, and training. *Archives of General Psychiatry, 51,* 849–859.

Orvaschel, H., Puig-Antich, J., Chambers, W., Tabrizi, M. A., & Johnson, R. (1986). Retrospective assessment of prepubertal major depression with the Kiddie-SADS-E. *Journal of the American Academy of Child and Adolescent Psychiatry, 21,* 392–397.

Orvaschel, H., Thompson, W. D., Belanger, A., Prusoff, B. A., & Kidd, K. (1982). Comparison of the family history method to direct interview: Factors affecting the diagnosis of depression. *Journal of Affective Disorders, 4,* 49–59.

Pardes, H., Kaufmann, C. A., Pincus, H. A., & West, A. (1989). Genetics and psychiatry: Past discoveries, current dilemmas, and future directions. *American Journal of Psychiatry, 146,* 435–443.

Parnas, J. (1988). Assortative mating in schizophrenia: Results from the Copenhagen high-risk study. *Psychiatry, 51,* 58–64.

Plomin, R., & Rende, R. (1991). Human behavioral genetics. *Annual Review of Psychology, 42,* 161–190.

Puig-Antich, J. (1984). Affective disorders. In H. J. Kaplan & B. J. Sadock (Eds.), *Comprehensive textbook of psychiatry* (2nd ed., pp. 1850–1861). Baltimore: Williams & Wilkins.

Rende, R., & Plomin, R. (1993). Families at risk for psychopathology: Who becomes affected and why? *Development and Psychopathology, 5,* 529–540.

Rende, R., & Plomin, R. (1994). Genetic influences on behavioral development. In M. Rutter & D. Hay (Eds.), *Developmental principles and clinical issues in psychology and psychiatry* (pp. 26–48). Oxford: Blackwell Scientific.

Rende, R., Sobin, C., & Weissman, M. M. (1993). Assessment of non-nuclear family structures in studies of children at risk for psychopathology. *Psychiatric Genetics, 3,* 175.

Rende, R., Weissman, M. M., Nunes, E., Goldstein, R., McAvay, G., & Torres, A. (1999). *Who are "parents" in family studies of offspring at risk for psychopathology?* Manuscript submitted for publication.

Rende, R., Wickramaratne, P., Warner, V., & Weissman, M. M. (1995). Sibling resemblance for psychiatric disorders in offspring at high and low risk for depression. *Journal of Child Psychology and Psychiatry, 36,* 1353–1363.

Richters, J., & Weintraub, S. (1990). Beyond diathesis: Toward an understanding of high-risk environments. In. J. Rolf, A. S. Masten, D. Cicchetti, K. H. Nuechterlein, & S. Weintraub (Eds.), *Risk and protective factors in the development of psychopathology* (pp. 67–96). New York: Cambridge University Press.

Robins, L. N., Helzer, J., Croughan, J., & Ratcliff, K. S. (1981). The National Institute of

Mental Health Diagnostic Interview Schedule: Its history, characteristics, and validity. *Archives of General Psychiatry, 38*(4), 381–389.

Rosenbaum, J. F., Biederman, J., Bolduc-Murphy, E. A., Faraone, S. V., Chaloff, J., Hirshfeld, D. R., & Kagan, J. (1993). Behavioral inhibition in childhood: A risk factor for anxiety disorders. *Harvard Review of Psychiatry, 1,* 2–16.

Rutter, M. (1988). DSM-III-R: A postscript. In M. Rutter, A. H. Tuma, & I. S. Tann (Eds.), *Assessment and diagnosis in child psychopathology* (pp. 453–464). New York: Guilford Press.

Rutter, M. (1990). Commentary: Some focus and process considerations re: the effects on children of parental depression. *Developmental Psychology, 26,* 60–63.

Rutter, M., Macdonald, H., Le Couteur, A., Harrington, R., Bolton, P., & Bailey, A. (1990). Genetic factors in child psychiatric disorder: II. Empirical findings. *Journal of Child Psychology and Psychiatry, 31,* 39–82.

Rutter, M., Silberg, J., O'Connor, T., & Simonoff, E. (1999a). Genetics and child psychiatry: I. Advances in quantitative and molecular genetics. *Journal of Child Psychology and Psychiatry, 40,* 3–18.

Rutter, M., Silberg, J., O'Connor, T., & Simonoff, E. (1999b). Genetics and child psychiatry: II. Empirical research findings. *Journal of Child Psychology and Psychiatry, 40,* 19–55.

Ryan, N., Williamson, D. E., Iyengar, S., Orvaschel, H., Reich, T., Dahl, R., & Puig-Antich, J. (1992). A secular increase in child and adolescent onset affective disorder. *Journal of the American Academy of Child and Adolescent Psychiatry, 31,* 600–605.

Schwab-Stone, M. E., Shaffer, D., Dulcan, M. K., Jensen, P. S., Fisher, P., Bird, H., Goodman, S. H., Lahey, B. B., Lichtman, J., Canino, G., Rugio-Stipec, M., & Rae, D. D. (1996). Criterion validity of the NIMH Diagnostic Interview Schedule for Children Version 2.3 (DISC-2.3). *Journal of the American Academy of Child and Adolescent Psychiatry, 35,* 878–888.

Scott, M. M. (1993). Recent changes in family structure in the United States: A developmental–systems perspective. *Journal of Applied Developmental Psychology, 14,* 213–230.

Shapiro, S., Skinner, E. A., Kessler, L. G., Von Korff, M., German, P. S., Tischler, G. L., Leaf, P. J., Benham, L., Cottler, L., & Regier, D. A. (1984). Utilization of health and mental health services: Three Epidemiological Catchment Area Sites. *Archives of General Psychiatry, 41,* 971–978.

Sobin, T., Weissman, M. M., Goldstein, R. B., Adams, P. B., Wickramaratne, P. J., Warner, V., & Lish, J. D. (1993). Diagnostic interviewing for family studies: Comparing telephone and face-to-face methods for the diagnosis of lifetime psychiatric disorders. *Psychiatric Genetics, 3,* 227–233.

Spitzer, R. L., Williams, J. B., Gibbon, M., & First, M. B. (1992). The Structured Clinical Interview for DSM-III-R (SCID): I. History, rationale, and description. *Archives of General Psychiatry, 49,* 624–629.

Strober, M. (1984). Familial aspects of depressive disorder in early adolescence. In E. Weller (Ed.), *An update on childhood depression.* Washington, DC: American Psychiatric Press.

Strober, M., & Carlson, G. (1982). Bipolar illness in adolescents with major depression: Clinical, genetic, and psychopharmacologic predictors in a three- to four-year prospective follow-up investigation. *Archives of General Psychiatry, 39,* 549–555.

Tarullo, L. B., Richardson, D. T., Redke-Yarrow, M., & Martinez, P. E. (1995). Multiple sources in child diagnosis: Parent–child concordance in affectively ill and well families. *Journal of Clinical Child Psychology, 24,* 173–183.

Thompson, W. D., Kidd, K. K., & Weissman, M. M. (1979). A procedure for the efficient collection and processing of pedigree data suitable for genetic analysis. *Journal of Psychiatric Research, 15,* 291–303.

Todd, R. D., Neuman, R., Geller, B., Fox, L. W., & Hickok, J. (1993). Genetic studies of affective disorders: Should we be starting with childhood onset probands? *Journal of the American Academy of Child and Adolescent Psychiatry, 32,* 1164–1171.

Wachs, T. D., & Gruen, G. E. (1982). *Early experience and human development.* New York: Plenum Press.

Weissman, M. M., Gershon, E. S., Kidd, K. K., Prusoff, B. A., Leckman, J. F., Dibble, E., Hamovit, J., Thompson, W. D., Pauls, D. L., & Guroff, J. J. (1984). Psychiatric disorder in relatives of probands with affective disorders: The Yale–NIMH collaborative family study. *Archives of General Psychiatry, 41,* 13–21.

Weissman, M. M., Merikangas, K. R., John, K., Wickramaratne, P., Prusoff, B. A., & Kidd, K. K. (1986). Family-genetic studies of psychiatric disorders developing technologies. *Archives of General Psychiatry, 43,* 1104–1116.

Weissman, M. M., Wickramaratne, P., Adams, P., Lish, J., Horwath, E., Charney, D., Woods, S. W., Leeman, E., & Frosch, E. (1993). The relationship between panic disorder and major depression: A new family study. *Archives of General Psychiatry, 50,* 767–780.

Weissman, M. M., Wickramaratne, P., Merikangas, K. R., Leckman, J. F., Prusoff, B. A., Caruso, K. A., Kidd, K. K., & Gammon, G. D. (1984). Onset of major depression in early adulthood: Increased familial loading and specificity. *Archives of General Psychiatry, 41,* 1136–1143.

Weissman, M. M., Wickramaratne, P., Warner, V., John, K., Prusoff, B. A., Merikangas, K. R., & Gammon, G. D. (1987). Assessing psychiatric disorders in children: Discrepancies between mothers and children's reports. *Archives of General Psychiatry, 44,* 747–753.

Wickramaratne, P. J., & Weissman, M. M. (1993). Using family studies to understand comorbidity. *European Archives of Psychiatry and Clinical Neuroscience, 243,* 150–157.

9

Retrospective Adult Assessment of Childhood Psychopathology

✧

RONALD C. KESSLER
DANIEL K. MROCZEK
ROBERT F. BELLI

This chapter discusses methodological issues involved in obtaining accurate retrospective reports about childhood psychopathology from epidemiological surveys of adults. It is obvious that such data are subject to greater recall failure than prospective reports obtained from the same respondents by interviewing them at regular intervals during their childhood. However, a study in which a large sample of children from the general population is interviewed throughout childhood would be both enormously expensive and fraught with logistic challenges. This could explain why such a study has never been carried out. Instead, our understanding of the developmental features of childhood psychopathology is based on the results of more limited investigations, consisting for the most part of (1) small, in-depth longitudinal studies of high-risk children (e.g., Block, Gjerde, & Block, 1991; Kovacs & Paulauskas, 1984) or children in treatment (e.g., Harrington, Fudge, Rutter, Pickle, & Hill, 1990); and (2) surveys of children and adolescents in the general population (e.g., Offord, 1985; Cohen, Cohen, & Brook, 1993; Cohen, Cohen, Kasen, et al., 1993). Valid retrospective studies about childhood psychopathology obtained from adult respondents would supplement these existing studies and help identify the adult outcomes associated with childhood disorders.

Very little epidemiological research using retrospective adult reports of childhood psychopathology has been conducted, and we are unaware of any research that has attempted to validate such reports. However, a considerable body of research has used retrospective reports from adults to study the long-term effects of childhood adversities on adult psychopathology (e.g., Harris, Brown, & Bifulco, 1990; Holmes & Robins, 1988; Kessler & Magee, 1993). A review of the methodological evaluation of these studies (e.g., Christianson & Loftus, 1991; Gotlib, Mount, Cordy, & Whiffen, 1988; Robins et al., 1985) may suggest techniques for obtaining valid information about childhood psychopathology.

One of the most consistent results of these studies is that adults generally have no direct recollection of experiences that occurred during the first 5 years of their lives (Wetzler & Sweeney, 1986). This is consistent with neurophysiological studies showing that the corpus callosum is incompletely myelinized prior to age 6 (Baddeley, 1990), and with psychoanalytic studies suggesting that memories for experiences prior to that age are encoded in ways difficult to retrieve verbally (Krystal, 1990; McLaughlin, 1978). This research makes it seem unlikely that retrospective reports from adults will provide accurate information about childhood psychiatric disorders prior to age 6.

However, adult retrospective reports about childhood experiences at age 6 or later are apparently more reliable. A recent review of methodological studies concludes that "adults asked to recall salient factual details of their own childhood are generally accurate, especially concerning experiences that fulfill the criteria of being unique, consequential, and unexpected" (Brewin, Andrews, & Gotlib, 1993, p. 87). Two important caveats must be noted. First, the evidence is clear that people cannot remember the incidental detail of childhood experiences—only the central features (Sheingold & Tenney, 1982). Second, the evidence is equally clear that accurate recall requires the respondent to engage in active and extensive memory search. To ensure this precision, the respondent must understand the task and must be motivated to engage in hard work rather than to supply a superficial response (Cannell, 1985a, 1985b; Cannell, Oksenberg, & Converse, 1977; Hippler & Schwarz, 1986). Unfortunately, many respondents are prone to draw upon lay theories of childhood development based on current self-images or self-knowledge, and to *infer* their childhood attributes rather than attempt to *recall* them (Ross, 1989). Although this theory-guided self-inference requires much less work than active memory search, it usually yields less accurate retrospective reports (Ross & Conway, 1986).

Because the few extant studies of childhood psychopathology have not been validated, it is unclear whether early psychiatric symptoms can be recalled as accurately as other childhood experiences. The methodological results reviewed above suggest that researchers must (1) impress on respondents that active memory search is required, (2) motivate active memory search and honest reporting, (3) recognize the limits of autobiographical memory by limiting questions to those that can be answered accurately, and (4) develop procedures appropriate for use in general population surveys to facilitate active memory search.

A considerable amount of methodological research has been carried out by survey researchers on each of these four topics (e.g., Moss & Goldstein, 1979; Bradburn, Sudman, & Associates, 1979; Cannell, Miller, & Oksenberg, 1981). This research has advanced considerably over the past two decades as cognitive psychologists have become interested in the survey interview as a natural laboratory for studying memory processes (e.g., Biderman, 1980; Jabine, Straf, Tanur, & Tourangeau, 1984; Tanur, 1992). Several important insights that have emerged from this work suggest practical ways of improving the accuracy of retrospective reports (Sudman et al., 1996; Fowler & Cannell, 1996; Schaeffer & Maynard, 1996). We review these insights in the present chapter, and we discuss modifications that were made to a standardized psychiatric diagnostic interview for use in the National Comorbidity Survey (NCS; Kessler et al., 1994) to enhance recall of childhood psychopathology.

THE IMPORTANCE OF UNDERSTANDING THE TASK

Obviously, ambiguous questions are likely to be misconstrued. Less obvious, though, are just how ambiguous the questions posed in standard epidemiological surveys are, and how often respondents must "read between the lines." Belson (1981) investigated this issue in a set of standard survey questions and found that more than 70% of respondents interpreted at least some questions differently from the researcher, leading Belson to conclude that subtle misinterpretations are pervasive in survey situations. Oksenberg, Cannell, and Kalton (1991) came to a similar conclusion in their debriefing of a nationally representative sample of respondents who were administered standard health interview survey questions. In two-thirds of the questions in their analysis, at least one key phrase was misinterpreted by respondents. Furthermore, both Belson (1981) and Oksenberg et al. (1991) found that respondents generally believed that they understood what the investigator meant even when their interpretations of the questions were quite idiosyncratic.

How is it possible for there to be so much misunderstanding? As Oksenberg and her colleagues discovered, the answer lies partly in the fact that such terms as "physical examination," "stay in bed," and "doctor" have different meanings for different people. However, beyond these rather obvious examples of vaguely defined terms is the more fundamental fact that the survey interview situation is a special kind of interaction in which the standard rules of conversation—rules that help fill in the gaps in meaning present in most speech—do not apply. Unlike the situation in normal conversational practice, a respondent in a survey interview often has only a vague notion of whom he/she is talking to or of the purpose of the conversation (Cannell, Fowler, & Marquis, 1968). The person who asks the questions (the interviewer) is not the person who formulated the questions (the researcher), and the questioner is often unable to clarify the respondent's uncertainties about the intent of the questions. Furthermore, the flow of questions in the interview is established prior to the beginning of the conversation, which means that normal conversational rules of give and take in question-and-answer sequences do not apply. This inflexibility leads to such odd interactional moments as when the interviewer asks a question that the respondent previously answered while elaborating an earlier response, and when the interviewer answers a query about the meaning of a question by telling the respondent, "Whatever it means to you." These out-of-the-ordinary interactions occasion more misreading than do normal conversations, even when questions are seemingly straightforward (Clark & Schober, 1992).

This problem of meaning was noted many years ago by Lazarsfeld (1934), who demonstrated that a question as simple as "Why did you buy this book?" will be interpreted in vastly different ways, depending on the respondent's understanding of whether the interviewer is concerned with why *you* bought this book (as opposed to your spouse's buying it for you), why you *bought* this book (as opposed to borrowed it), why you bought *this* book (as opposed to some other book), or why you bought this *book* (as opposed to buying something else with the money). The respondent's understanding of which connotation the interviewer intends is often determined by such subtleties as voice inflection and contextual issues.

In our own pilot work for the NCS (Kessler et al., 1994), we found that misinterpretation was especially common with the inquiries about psychiatric disorder appearing in the original version of the Composite International Diagnostic Interview (CIDI; Robins, Wing, Wittchen, & Helzer, 1988), the structured diagnostic interview used in the NCS. There were various reasons for this (including ambiguous question wordings and awkward transitions), but our debriefing revealed that substantial confusion arose from respondents' failure to understand the purpose of the questions. For example, a substantial number of respondents misinterpreted the intent of such recall questions as "In your lifetime, have you ever had 2 weeks or more when nearly every day you felt sad, blue, depressed?" The misinterpretation concerned the task itself. Only about half of pilot respondents interpreted the question as it was intended by the authors of the CIDI—namely, as a request to engage in active memory search and to report episodes of the sort in the question. The other respondents interpreted the question as a request to report whether a memory of such an episode was readily accessible. These latter respondents did not believe that they were being asked to engage in active memory search and did not do so. Not surprisingly, these respondents were much less likely than those who understood the intent of the question to remember lifetime episodes.

Why did so many respondents misinterpret the intent of these questions about lifetime recall? As Marquis and Cannell (1969) discovered in their research on standard interview practice, respondents are generally ill informed and poorly motivated. Lacking clear instructions and having little grasp of research aims, they render only desultory answers. Debriefing indicates that most respondents consider being interviewed "a lark—an unimportant and uninvolving activity" (Cannell et al., 1981, p. 413). As noted by Clark and Schober (1992) in their analysis of discourse rules in survey interviews, the interaction flow in most surveys reinforces the perception that careful response is unimportant. Normal rules of conversation require a person who is asked a question to signify recognition of turn taking either by answering the question or by making some other relevant comment (e.g., "Um, let me see now . . .") within about 1 second after the question is issued (Jefferson, 1989), unless the questioner gives an explicit instruction to the contrary. When an interviewer asks a question that requires considerable thought, the respondent is likely to assume in the absence of instructions to the contrary that the interviewer is operating under normal conversational rules, and, as such, is really asking for an immediate and appropriate answer.

The work of Cannell et al. (1981) shows that this conversational artifact can be minimized by explicitly instructing respondents to answer completely and accurately. The use of such instructions can substantially improve the quality of data obtained in surveys. Our pilot work for the NCS built on this result by investigating the effect of adding clarifying statements throughout the clinical interview aimed at informing respondents that accuracy was important. For example, we experimented with the following introduction to CIDI stem questions for lifetime recall of specific psychiatric disorders: "The next question might be difficult to answer because you need to think back over your entire life. Please take your time and think carefully before answering."

The use of this introduction prompted respondents to consider longer whether they ever had such experiences as "2 weeks or more when nearly every day you felt sad, blue, depressed" or "a period of a month or more when most of the time you felt worried or anxious." Debriefing showed that this slower response time was attributed to the fact that respondents were engaging in active memory search rather than estimating. A subsequent question wording experiment showed that the use of this introduction led to a significant increase in the proportion of respondents in a national sample who endorsed lifetime diagnostic stem questions for various mood and anxiety disorders (Kessler et al., 1998).

THE IMPORTANCE OF MOTIVATION

One problem with emphasizing to respondents the need to work hard at a series of demanding and potentially embarrassing recall tasks is that more respondents than otherwise may refuse the job. Recognition of this problem by survey research methodologists has led to the development of motivational techniques intended to increase the chances that respondents will accept the job of answering completely and accurately. Three techniques that have proven to be particularly useful in this regard are the use of motivational components in instructions, the use of contingent reinforcement strategies embedded in interviewer feedback probes, and the use of respondent commitment questions.

Motivational Instructions

There is evidence that clarifying instructions and research aims can help motivate complete and accurate reporting (Cannell et al., 1981). Debriefing shows that respondents are more willing to understand laborious and possibly painful memory searches if they recognize some altruistic benefit of doing so. Even such an uncompelling rationale as "It is important for our research that you take your time and think carefully before answering" has motivational force. This is even more so when instructions include statements that have universalistic appeal, such as: "Accuracy is important, because social policy makers will be using these results to make decisions that affect the lives of all of us."

In addition, instructions that define the nature of interviewer expectations for respondent behavior help to establish a perspective on the interview that can have motivational force. The literature on cognitive factors in surveys contains many examples of the subtle ways in which perspectives established in questions influence respondents' subsequent behaviors. For example, Loftus and Palmer (1974) showed respondents a film of an automobile accident and asked them to estimate the speed at which the cars were traveling prior to the accident. Respondents estimated the rates as significantly greater if they were asked how fast the cars were traveling "when they collided" rather than "when they contacted each other." This same literature shows that perspective can have motivational force when it implies a common purpose (Clark & Schober, 1992). That is, if a question is posed in such a way that it implies that hard work will be invested in arriving at an answer, the respondent must either explicitly demur or tacitly accept the task of working hard as part of the common understanding between interviewer and respondent. By answering the question, the respondent in effect makes a commitment to honor the injunction implied in the perspective of the question, and this implied commitment in turn creates motivation to perform this task (Marlatt, 1972).

Contingent Reinforcements

Consistent with research on behavioral modification of verbal productions through reinforcement (e.g., Centers, 1964), several survey researchers have demonstrated that verbal reinforcers such as "Thanks" and "That's useful" can significantly affect the behavior of survey respondents. For example,

Marquis and Cannell (1969) showed experimentally that the use of such reinforcers resulted in a significant increase in the number of chronic conditions reported in response to an open-ended question about illnesses. However, these feedback remarks are often used in an unsystematic way—as part of general procedures to build and maintain rapport—rather than in a systematic way to reinforce good respondent performance.

On the basis of these observations, Cannell and his associates developed a method for training interviewers to use systematic feedback (both positive and negative) to reinforce respondent effort in reporting (Oksenberg, Vinokur, & Cannell, 1979a). The central feature of this method is the use of structured feedback statements coordinated with the content and timing of instructions aimed at reinforcing respondent performance. It is important to recognize that performance is what is being reinforced, rather than the content of particular answers. For example, a difficult recall question may be prefaced with the instruction "This next question may be difficult, so please take your time before answering." In contingent feedback instruction, the interviewer issues some expression of gratitude whenever the respondent seems to consider his/her answer carefully, whether he/she remembered anything or not. Alternatively, an interviewer can instruct a precipitous respondent: "You answered that awfully quickly. Was there anything [else], even something small?" Such invitations to reconsider can occur whenever the respondent gives an immediate answer, whether or not anything is reported. This structured feedback is programmed periodically throughout the interview, in order to maintain the focus on performance standards and to reinforce motivation.

Experiments carried out by Cannell and his associates (Miller & Cannell, 1977; Vinokur, Oksenberg, & Cannell, 1979) have documented that the combined use of these contingent reinforcement probes with instructions explaining the importance of careful and accurate reporting leads to substantial improvement in recall of health-related events in general population surveys, including validated dates of medical events. Importantly, their results also show that self-enhancing response biases are reduced when these strategies are used, as indicated by both a decreased tendency to underreport potentially embarrassing conditions and behaviors (e.g., gynecological problems, seeing an X-rated movie) and a decreased tendency to overreport self-enhancing behaviors (e.g., number of books read in the last 3 months, reading the editorial page of the newspaper the previous day).

Commitment Questions

We have noted above that instructions often have the effect of eliciting indirect commitment to the goal of serious and complete reporting. It is also possible to motivate a respondent to accept this goal by asking an explicit commitment question as part of the interview. We did this in the NCS by prefacing the section of the interview that asked a series of lifetime diagnostic stem questions with the following commitment question:

> This interview asks about your physical and emotional well-being and about areas of your life that could affect your physical and emotional well-being. It is important for us to get accurate information. In order to do this, you will need to think carefully before answering the following questions. Are you willing to do this?

Consistent with the results of previous studies using similar questions (Cannell et al., 1981), we found that only a small fraction of respondents answered negatively (only 35 of the 8,133 people who began the interview). These interviews were terminated, because we had decided in advance not to invest interviewer time on respondents who were not willing to work seriously at the task.

Experimental studies carried out by Cannell and his associates (Cannell et al., 1981; Oksenberg et al., 1979a; Oksenberg, Vinokur, & Cannell, 1979b) have shown that commitment questions improve accuracy of recall. Furthermore, their studies indicate that the joint use of motivating instructions, contingent feedback, and a commitment question has an interactive effect that increases the intensity of memory search and accuracy beyond the effects of any one component separately. This extends not only to the proportion of respondents in different experimental conditions who recall and report past experiences, but also to other indicators of commitment, such as amount of detail reported and use of personal records and other outside information sources as memory aids during the course of the interview.

THE LIMITS OF AUTOBIOGRAPHICAL MEMORY

Episodic and Semantic Memories

Research on basic cognitive processes has shown that memories are organized and stored in structured sets of information packages commonly called "schemas" (Markus & Zajonc, 1985). When a respondent has a history of many instances of the same experience that cannot be discriminated, the separate instances tend to blend together in memory to form a special kind of memory schema called a "semantic memory"—a general memory for a prototypical experience (Jobe et al., 1990; Means & Loftus, 1991). For example, a person may have a semantic memory of what panic attacks are like, but because the person has had many such attacks, he/she cannot specify details of any particular panic attack. In comparison, when a respondent has had only a small number of lifetime experiences of a certain sort, or when one instance stands out in memory as very different from the others, a memory can probably be recovered for that particular episode. This is called an "episodic memory."

In the case of memories of illness experiences, memory schemas tend to include not only semantic memories of prototypical symptoms, but also personal theories about causes, course, and cure (Leventhal, Nerenz, & Steele, 1984; Skelton & Croyle, 1991). Some of these theories will conceptualize the experience in illness terms, whereas others will characterize it as a moral failing, a punishment from God, or a normal reaction to stress (Gilman, 1988). These interpretations influence the extent to which different memory cues are capable of triggering the schemas.

The effects of memory schemas and the difference between semantic and episodic memories are central themes in research on autobiographical memory. Indeed, we must determine whether episodic memories can be recovered, as well as whether a respondent is answering questions by referring to episodic memories or by drawing inferences of what the past must have been like on the basis of more general semantic memories. Research shows that people are more likely to recover episodic memories for experiences that are recent, distinctive, and unique, whereas they will rely more on semantic memories for experiences that are frequent, typical, and regular (Belli, 1988; Brewer, 1986; Menon, 1994).

Asking Questions without Knowing
the Limits of Memory

When a survey question is designed to ask about a particular instance of an experience, it must be posed in such a way that the respondent knows he/she is being asked to recover an episodic memory. The researcher must have some basis for assuming that an episodic memory can be recovered for this experience. If it cannot, a question that asks for such a memory implicitly invites the respondent to infer or estimate rather than to remember, and this can have adverse effects on quality of reporting later in the interview (Pearson, Ross, & Dawes, 1992). In comparison, when a question is designed to ask a respondent to recover a semantic memory or to use semantic memories to arrive at an answer by estimation, the question should make this clear.

One difficulty with these injunctions in the case of retrospective recall questions about lifetime psychiatric disorders is uncertainty about what level of recall accuracy to expect. We confronted this problem in pilot studies for the NCS when we asked the standard CIDI questions about first onset, such as this question about panic onset: "When was the first time you had one of these sudden spells of feeling frightened or anxious and had these problems like [previously endorsed symptoms of panic]?" Debriefing of pilot respondents revealed that some people had very vivid memories of their first panic attack, while others had no such memory. The problem posed by this variation was how to develop a method of asking the question that reinforced our overall commitment to collecting complete and accurate information, while simultaneously recognizing the limits of autobiographical memory and avoiding a request for a precise answer from the subsample of respondents who were unable to recover an episodic memory for their first episode.

We resolved this problem by adapting several of the principles discussed above to a three-part question series designed to inform respondents that answers should be as precise as possible, while still acknowledging the limits of memory. The question sequence began with what has been referred to in the literature as a "prequest"—that is, a question aimed at clarifying the nature of the request for information in subsequent questions. The prequest question is as follows

> Can you remember your *exact* age the *very first time* you had a sudden spell of feeling frightened or anxious and had several of these other things ["other things" refered to a checklist of symptoms that respondents had previously reported, which was presented for visual review on a cue card] at the same time? (emphasis in original)

During the pilot work we probed positive responses to determine the basis for exact recall, and discovered that in general these respondents either were younger (i.e., the first episode was likely to have occurred more recently), had a smaller number of lifetime episodes, or had a distinctive context that allowed them to date the age of their vividly recalled first attack. On the basis of this information, the final question series simply followed this answer with the question "How old were you?" In comparison, respondents who answered the prequest negatively were asked a different follow-up question, phrased in such a way as to make it clear that we wanted an estimate, since we understood that the respondent could not provide an exact answer. This question was "*about* how old were you [the first time you had one of these attacks]?" (emphasis in original). Interviewers were instructed to accept a range response (e.g., "Sometime in my early 20s") without probing, as we were soliciting an estimate. This question was then followed by another that was designed to provide an upper bound on our uncertainty concerning age of onset and to permit the respondent to answer even when uncertain about the exact age of the first attack: "What is the earliest age you can *clearly remember* having one of these attacks?" (emphasis in original).

The latter question is much less demanding than the original question about the exact age of the very first attack; not surprisingly in light of this, virtually all respondents were able to provide an age in their answer. Interestingly, the age given in response to this question was often earlier than the lower bound of the age range given in response to the preceding question. Debriefing showed that this seemingly inconsistent result was due to the fact that estimation was typically used to arrive at the response to the question "*about* how old were you . . . ?", whereas active memory search focusing on the part of the life span implied by the answer to the preceding question was used to arrive at the response to the subsequent question. Subsequent methodological analysis shows that this age-of-onset question series yields much more plausible onset distributions than those based on standard CIDI questions (Knauper, Cannell, Schwarz, Bruce, & Kessler, 1999).

Increasing Knowledge about the Limits of Memory

As the discussion in the last few paragraphs makes clear, a major barrier to evaluating strategies for improving recall of psychiatric disorders is that we lack any clear understanding of the limits of autobiographical memory for this class of experiences. This is true, in large part, because we lack a clear validation standard. The same limitation plagues much of the research on long-term autobiographical memory in surveys. Although a few record-checking studies have been carried out to validate the accuracy of retrospective reports about such things as hospitalizations (Marquis, Cannell, & Laurent, 1972), doctor visits (Means & Loftus, 1991), voting behavior (Abelson & Loftus, 1992), and income tax returns (Withey, 1954), these are exceptions. Most methodological studies of memory in surveys are of two other sorts. One of these uses short-term test–retest designs, in which respondents' reports of attitudes or occasionally of recurring behaviors such as dietary intake (Smith, Jobe, & Mingay, 1991a, 1991b) in a baseline survey are used as the validation standard. Recall bias is then studied in a retest interview administered a few hours, a few days, or a few weeks later, often with experimental manipulations designed to assess the extent to which recall can be influenced by various types of recall cues (e.g., Pearson et al., 1992). The other type of design uses experimental manipulations such as the feedback and commitment probes described above to study changes in retrospective reports about more distant events, but without any independent source of data on the actual occurrence of these events as a validation standard (e.g., Crespi & Swinehart, 1982). Based on these two types of studies, we know that there are substantial errors in short-term retrospective reports of recurring behaviors ("What did you have to eat last Thursday?"), as well as biases in the direction of reporting more consistency than really exists in recall of attitudes after an experimental attitude change manipulation. However, these studies provide no clear evidence concerning the limits of autobiographical memory for the sort of provocative but perhaps chronologically distant experiences targeted in retrospective studies of childhood psychopathology—namely, reports about such things as recurrent depression, substance use problems, unreasonable fears, and behavior problems that occurred during one's childhood. As a result of this limitation, we are uncertain about the real limits of autobiographical memory for childhood psychopathology.

Naturalistic and experimental studies to obtain this type of data are needed. This could be done using the model of previous validation studies of health experiences (e.g., Loftus, Smith, Klinger, & Fiedler, 1992; Marquis et al., 1972; Means & Loftus, 1991). Using medical records, one could select a sample of people known to have been in treatment in the past, and could assess the extent to which they report this experience in a household survey in which they are initially unaware of the fact that their medical records are known. However, concerns could be raised that this type of study might overestimate the accuracy of long-term recall of childhood disorders, because children who were in treatment are unrepresentative of all children with psychiatric disorders: They are probably more aware of their disorders and have distinctive memory cues associated with the treatment experience that could facilitate long-term retrospective recall. Based on these concerns, a more valid type of study would be one in which data concerning childhood disorders are derived from some source other than treatment records. An obvious possibility is to reinterview a subsample of adult respondents who participated during their childhood in a general population survey of mental health, and to use the original survey data as a validation standard in evaluating the accuracy of retrospective reports.

As noted in the chapter introduction, long-term retrospective validation studies of this type have been carried out to study the accuracy of retrospective reports about other aspects of childhood. For example, Robins et al. (1985) evaluated the accuracy of retrospective reports about the childhood home environment in a sample of adults who had attended a child guidance clinic when they were children. The study compared the recollecting of respondents in their 40s with data obtained 30 years earlier. Subjects were able to provide quite good reports about major aspects of the family environment (e.g., parent work histories and family breakups), as well as to specify objective features of family life that did not involve value judgments (e.g., whether the parents fought in front of the children or hit each other). Reports were much less accurate when the questions involved judgments or interpretations rather than factual descriptions. These results allowed Robins et al. to characterize the limits of adult autobiographical memory concerning the childhood home environment, and to develop an instrument called the Home Environment Interview, which focuses on concrete descriptive questions that could be recalled with good accuracy. Precisely this sort of work is needed to extend our understanding of the limits of adult autobiographical memory for childhood psychiatric disorders, and to develop an informed strategy for stimulating adult recall of these disorders.

Ideally, such validation studies should include both a discovery and an experimental component, in addition to the investigation of variation in the accuracy of different types of recall questions. The discovery component should follow the procedures used in recent inductive cognitive-psychological studies of memory processes (e.g., Oksenberg et al., 1991; Fisher & Geiselman, 1992; Petty & Jarvis, 1996) to elicit information from respondents about the memory search strategies used, in an effort to discover whether some search strategies are superior in recovering certain types of memories. If so, this information could be used in the development of subsequent interview protocols to coach respondents in the use of effective strategies. For example, childhood psychopathology might be more easily recalled by respondents who begin thinking about their earliest memories and then move forward in time, rather than beginning with recent memories and moving backward in time (Fathi, Schooler, & Loftus, 1984; Loftus & Fathi, 1985). If this is verified, an instruction could be given to all respondents to use the "forward search" procedure. The experimental component should build on the results of the discovery component as well as on the results of the accumulated literature, to develop a series of nested experiments to evaluate the effects of various interventions on accuracy of recall.

It is important to embed experiments in recall validation studies, as most techniques that improve the accuracy of autobiographical memory are known to fail in some situations. For example, Crespi and Swinehart (1982) developed a dual-time-frame approach to improve the accuracy of reporting and dating recent (past 2 months) health-related actions (e.g., blood pressure check, eye examination). A subsequent validation study (Loftus et al., 1992) showed that this method does, in fact, improve accuracy of reports about this class of behaviors. However, other researchers (Abelson & Loftus, 1992) found that the same strategy is ineffective in improving accuracy of self-reported voting behavior. Results such as these indicate that the processes that influence accuracy of reporting vary by context, and that the effectiveness of particular strategies must be reconsidered whenever a new domain of memory is under investigation.

FACILITATING COMPLETE AND ACCURATE RECALL AND REPORTING

We have reviewed several strategies that optimize recall accuracy, including explicit instruction to respondents that complete and accurate answers are expected, as well as various techniques to motivate respondents to provide such answers. However, other techniques have been developed to improve accuracy once respondents commit themselves to active memory search. These latter techniques provide recall aids that increase the efficiency of memory work. Again, the technique used depends on the type of memory targeted. In this section, we consider how to facilitate memory in the context of four broadly conceived questions concerning recall of childhood psychiatric disorders. There are, of course, more than four questions of interest concerning such disorders, but these four are central and raise a number of important issues that have been addressed in the literature. The questions are as follows: "Did such a disorder ever occur?", "What were the associated symptoms and role impairments?", "How old were you the first time this happened?", and "What was the course of the disorder after that first occurrence?"

Remembering Whether a Disorder Ever Occurred

A good deal of evidence suggests that people who have never had certain experiences quite accurately answer "no" to "Have you ever . . . ?" questions (Glucksberg & McCloskey, 1981; Shannon, 1979). A core process used in making this judgment is the "lack-of-knowledge inference" (Genter & Collins, 1981)—that is, the conclusion a person draws from lack of knowledge of an experience that it ever happened to him/her. For example, Lessler, Salter, and Tourangeau (1989) report that survey respondents who had never heard of dental sealant felt quite confident in saying that they had never worn such sealant. The potential problem here is that the way the experience is characterized can have an important impact on the perception of lack of knowledge. This is an especially serious issue in lifetime diagnostic stem questions, which often deal with vaguely defined terms that are easily misconstrued, prompting quick and incorrect lack-of-knowledge inference. Below, we discuss several techniques that can be used to minimize this potential problem.

The Pace of the Interview

Several survey methodologists have noted that unless interviewers are carefully trained to the contrary, they will ask questions too quickly, and that this will reduce the accuracy of respondent reports (Cannell et al., 1977; Neter & Waksberg, 1964; Sudman & Bradburn, 1982). This is especially true for lifetime recall questions. At least two fairly obvious processes are involved here. First, haste on the part of the interviewer conveys the message that quick response is more important than accurate response (Clark & Shober, 1992); second, memories are more likely to be recovered when respondents are allowed to think at their own pace rather than rushed (Bradburn, Rips, & Shevell, 1987). On the basis of these observations and the analysis of interaction sequences in interviews, Cannell and his associates have recommended that interviewer reading pace should be no more than an average of two words per second (Cannell et al., 1981); that respondents should be explicitly asked to think at their own pace (Cannell & Kahn, 1968); and that critical questions should be designed to encourage periods of silence, which are explicitly defined as "thinking time" (Cannell, 1985a). Several experiments have documented that these procedures lead to more accurate recall of health-related events (Burton & Blair, 1991; Means, Swan, Jobe, & Esposito, 1994; Lessler et al., 1989).

Memory Cues

Two general types of memory cues that have been used by researchers to stimulate recall of past life events might also assist relevant recall of lifetime psychiatric disorders: concrete cues and context cues. Concrete cues consist of very explicit questions or other stimuli (pictures, smells, and sounds) that are aimed at triggering memories for particular experiences. For example, surveys about the use of medications sometimes use multicolor pill cards to stimulate memories of particular medications that the respondent has taken (Parry, Balter, & Cisin, 1970–1971). Other surveys use such recall aids as lists of products to stimulate recall of purchases or lists of life events to stimulate recall of stressful experiences. A few surveys about particularly complex topics, such as hospital visits or expenses, have even requested respondents (by means of an advance letter) to review their records and have them available as memory cues during the interview (Sudman & Bradburn, 1982). Experimental evidence shows that these strategies do, in fact, improve recall (Bradburn et al., 1987). Cues of this sort might be especially useful in asking lifetime diagnostic stem questions, because very concrete characterizations might help respondents to retrieve relevant memory schemas.

Context cues consist of broader questions about a particular life domain, which facilitate recall of events within that domain by triggering a common memory schema that can be used to structure information search (Higgins, Rholes, & Jones, 1977). For example, comparative studies show that life event reports are increased when questions about events relating to a particular area of life are embedded in a larger series of survey questions about that area (Kessler & Wethington, 1991). Context cues also appear to have a significant effect on lifetime recall of psychiatric disorders, as documented in a recently completed experiment in which we administered a series of diagnostic stem questions to a nationally representative sample of adults in a telephone survey. Half of the respondents (randomly selected) were presented with an introductory statement about the importance of careful and complete reporting. Then they were administered a commitment question prior to a series of 8 diagnostic stem questions about the lifetime occurrence of such experiences as a period of 2 weeks of feeling sad or blue, a period of 1 month or more of feeling worried or anxious, and a sudden spell or attack of panic. The remaining respondents were administered the same introduction and commitment questions, but then received 10 context questions about life "when you were a child up to the age of 12." The purpose of these questions was to provide a memory context for that part of the life span by asking such things as the following:

> During those years, did you live in just one place, move once or twice, or move around a lot?
> How do you think [staying in the same place/moving/moving around a lot] affected your childhood?

Overall, how was your relationship with your parents or the people who raised you during those years?

Did you have brothers and sisters living at home with you during those years?

(If yes) How well did you get along with them?/(If no) How did you feel about being an only child?

These questions were then followed by the same 8 diagnostic stem questions administered to the first half of the sample, except that they were confined to the time when respondents were less than 12 years of age rather than over their entire lifetimes. This same sequence—10 context questions followed by 8 diagnostic stem questions—was then repeated for each of three other periods in the life course: "during your teenage years," "during your 20s," and "from the age of 30 up to the present." The data were then aggregated and compared to determine whether this procedure led to more complete reporting. There was in fact a significant increase in the proportion of respondents who responded positively to the diagnostic stem questions when they were embedded within the stage-of-life context questions. In addition, follow-up administration of the full CIDI to all respondents who endorsed stem questions showed that not only the stem questions but also the estimated lifetime prevalence of almost all the disorders for which stem questions were included in the battery were significantly higher in the stage-of-life context subsample than in the control subsample. Furthermore, respondents in the former subsample reported their ages of onset as being earlier and were more likely to say that they could clearly remember the first episodes of their disorders than respondents in the control subsample.

Multiple Frames of Reference

We have noted above that use of a lack-of-knowledge heuristic can lead to a false conclusion that an experience never happened if the terms used are inconsistent with the schema in which memory for the experience is stored. This is a well-known phenomenon in life event research. For example, a mother who finds that her teenage son has been stealing money from her purse is unlikely to report this in response to a question about "theft," because the experience is coded in memory as something quite different, even though it fits the legal definition of theft. In order to reveal this experience, a different memory schema is required—one that asks about such things as having a major disappointment with a close friend or relative, or finding out something about a person close to you that was very upsetting, or being betrayed by a loved one. Life event researchers have shown that completeness of recall of life events can be substantially improved by using questions of the latter sort to elicit multiple frames of reference that trigger relevant memory schemas for events (Brown & Harris, 1978; Kessler & Wethington, 1991). The same insight is used in studies of eyewitness memory for the details of crimes (Fisher, Geiselman, & Amador, 1989; Fisher & Geiselman, 1992; Fisher & Quigley, 1992), where one of the core principles of stimulating accurate recall is to probe multiple representations of the situation.

This insight might be used in several ways to improve the accuracy of lifetime diagnostic stem questions regarding mental disorders. The most powerful approach might be to elaborate the descriptive details presented in the stem questions, since these questions are, in effect, vignettes intended to describe a syndrome in such a way that triggers a memory schema. In an effort to gain some insight into the ways this might be done most effectively, interviews should be conducted with children who are experiencing disorders of particular types, to elicit information about the ways they describe their experiences. Such lay representations of personal illness experiences have been shown to share a number of core features across people with the same conditions (Leventhal, Meyer, & Nerenz, 1980; Bishop, 1991; Bishop & Converse, 1986), and to vary in systematic ways across different segments of the population (Angel & Thoits, 1987; Gilman, 1988; Kleinman, 1986). Knowledge of these schemas may assist researchers in facilitating accurate recall of disorders by improving the extent to which diagnostic stem questions correspond to the schemas.

The possible utility of this approach is illustrated by recent work with black and Latino psychiatric patients to learn how they describe their disorders. This was done in an effort to refine the diagnostic stem questions for mood disorders and anxiety disorders in the CIDI. The interviews, carried out by medical anthropologists, asked respondents to describe in their own words what it was like to have their problems. After doing this, respondents were presented with the relevant diagnostic stem questions from the CIDI and asked whether they would have endorsed these descriptions if they had been administered as part of a survey. Respondents were then asked to rewrite the questions so they would more closely match their own experiences.

The results led to several important insights about ways to expand the standard CIDI questions. For example, in the case of panic disorder, the CIDI stem question is "Have you ever had a spell or attack when all of a sudden you felt frightened, anxious or very uneasy in situations when most people would not be afraid or anxious?" Yet the word "attack" was not used by respondents when describing these panic events. Nor were these words used when respondents rewrote the questions. Instead, respondents spoke of the episodes as simply occurring "all of a sudden." We asked about this failure to use the terms "spell" and "attack," and discovered that many respondents felt these words were confusing because they could be used in their cultural communities to refer to other experiences ("spell" referring to magic and "attack" to violence). As a result, respondents did not want to use these words in their own descriptions. These reports suggest that it might make sense to remove these words from any revision of the CIDI stem question and to emphasize the sudden nature of the episode instead.

We also discovered that when respondents spoke of "being frightened, anxious, or very uneasy," they did so in much more evocative terms than the CIDI, describing times when they suddenly "had a wave of terrible fear" wash over them, when they experienced a sense of terror, when they felt as if they were "going to go crazy any minute," when they "totally lost control and wanted to scream," and when they "wanted to run away or escape but had no place to go." The phrase "very uneasy" virtually never arose in the rewritten stem questions because, according to respondents' accounts, "uneasy" is too mild a word to describe their experiences. Such observations provide a number of clues about ways to write a new series of panic stem questions, each emphasizing a somewhat different cognitive–emotional dimension of panic that may tap into an illness representation more accurately than the current stem question does. The use of more evocative stem questions might plausibly lead to substantial improvement in recall, as there is evidence that emotionally charged cognitions decay more slowly in memory and can be recovered with memory cues that emphasize the content of these emotions (Reisberg & Heuer, 1992).

We also found that physiological symptoms figured much more prominently in the scripts written by people with panic than in the CIDI stem question; not being able to breathe, having one's heart beat fast, feeling faint, and a perception of impending death were commonly cited by sufferers of panic. These observations indicate that it may be wise to develop one or more variants on this panic stem question that emphasize physiological symptoms.

Related to these physiological descriptions was an objection on the part of quite a few respondents to the secondary clause in the CIDI stem question that the panic must occur "in situations when most people would not be afraid or anxious." The respondents who objected in this way reported that they would have denied the CIDI question if they had been in a survey, because their intense fears only occured at times when their hearts started suddenly pounding and they got dizzy and they thought they were going to die—a situation in which anyone would be afraid. Accordingly, panic stem questions might be revised to exclude mention of nonprovoking situations, and instead to attempt to discriminate panic (attacks occuring unexpectedly and without a precipitating cause) from phobia in a separate series of questions administered after establishing the existence of periods of suddenly feeling very frightened.

It is unclear whether children would be able to provide characterizations as rich as those obtained in these interviews with adults. Nor is it clear that the descriptions supplied by children would usefully determine diagnostic stem questions for adults recalling childhood disorders; as we know, illness representations change over time as people gain more personal experience with their symptoms (Safer, Tharps, Jackson, & Leventhal, 1979; Leventhal & Diefenbach, 1991). Nonetheless, the example above illustrates that insights into designing more evocative questions can be obtained by offering people open-ended opportunities to describe their own experiences. Although we are unaware of any work that has been done along these lines for childhood psychiatric disorders, we suspect that useful information would result from listening to children, adolescents, and young adults describe their symptoms. Special notice should be taken of changes depending on time elapsed since the childhood experiences and/or on progression of the disorder.

Remembering Symptoms and Role Impairments

After a memory for a lifetime diagnostic stem question has been elicited, it is important to query about additional criteria needed to qualify for a diagnosis. Depending on the diagnosis under consideration, the respondent must describe the existence and duration of symptoms and role impairments, as well as provide information regarding possible organicity. The demands on respondent memory imposed by these questions are quite different from those associated with answering diagnostic stem questions. In particular, symptom and impairment questions are asked in the context of a prior question that focuses memory on a specific time—an advantage over diagnostic stem questions. This focusing is known to have a positive effect on recall accuracy (Pearson et al., 1992; Hasher & Griffin, 1978), depending on whether the respondent can recall a particular instance of the disorder or can only retrieve a semantic memory.

When episodic memories cannot be readily recalled, research suggests that memories for the details of experiences can be enhanced by asking a series of context-setting questions about the distinctive circumstances associated with particular episodes. Such questions might include where the respondent lived at the time, the kind of work he/she did, whether there was a precipitating event that brought on the episode, and the like. Experimental studies of the recall of the details of validated experiences, such as doctor visits and videotaped reenactments of witnessing criminal victimizations, show that these contextual questions do, in fact, help respondents recover details for episodic memories that are otherwise not remembered (Fisher & Geiselman, 1992; Means & Loftus, 1991).

The situation is quite different when no single episode is distinguishable and the respondent has only a semantic memory of a prototypical episode. The best one can hope for in this case is to use the semantic memory as the basis for symptom reporting. Even then, there is good reason to believe that semantic memories may provide quite an accurate portrait of the consistent features of repeated experiences.

Remembering Age of Onset

There is some evidence in the literature to suggest that first experiences have a special place in autobiographical memory and that some of these memories are quite vivid (Pillemer, Goldsmith, Panter, & White, 1988; Robinson, 1992; Schuman, Belli, & Bischoping, 1997). It is likely, though, that the extent to which this is true depends on a number of factors. Our analysis of the NCS question "Can you remember your *exact* age the *very first time . . . ?*" suggests that vivid memories of first experiences are expectedly more common for acute-onset disorders (e.g., panic disorder, posttraumatic stress disorder) than for disorders with insidious onsets (e.g., dysthymic disorder, generalized anxiety disorder), and that they decrease with the total number of lifetime episodes of a disorder. It is unclear from the literature whether the use of pace, exhortations to think hard, or memory cues would be effective in recovering memories of first episodes for disorders with insidious onsets. If not, lower-bound estimates of age of onset obtained by asking about clear recall of early episodes may be the best we can hope to accomplish.

Not all respondents who can recall their first episode of a disorder can remember their age when it occurred. We were not sufficiently attentive to this in the NCS pilot studies; as a result, we combined what should have been two separate questions into a single question about clearly remembering the age of the first episode in the NCS. The two questions we should have asked are (1) "Can you remember your very first episode?" and, if so, (2) "Can you clearly remember your age at the time of this episode?"

In cases where there is a memory that an event occurred but not of when it occurred, several strategies are available to improve recall of the date. One involves the use of the same sort of contextual cues described above, where the interviewer asks a series of questions (e.g., "Where did you live at the time?", "Was there some crisis or stress that brought on the episode?", etc.) in order to assist in the recall of distinctive contexts that may be associated with when the episode occurred. A danger in using this strategy alone is that a phenomenon called "forward telescoping" can lead to underestimation of how long ago an experience occurred, due to the respondent's inferring that an event that can be vividly recalled probably did not occur as long ago as it actually did (Brown, Rips, & Shevell, 1985). Therefore, whenever contextual cues are used to improve the vividness of recall of a first episode, it is also important to use techniques that combat the potential problem of telescoping. One way this can be done is by forcing respondents to take their time and consider carefully the implications of their recollections about context for their estimation of age (Sudman & Bradburn, 1982). If a respondent can remember that the episode occurred shortly after he/she had a problem with a teacher named Mrs. Smith, and that Mrs. Smith was his/her fourth-grade teacher, the accuracy of dating age at the time will be improved substantially. The use of landmark events and a time line calendar can also help reduce telescoping (Brown & Harris, 1978; Kessler & Wethington, 1991).

Remembering Illness Course

As noted above, research shows that when people are asked difficult recall questions, they generally base their answers on estimates rather than recall. This tendency increases as the recall task becomes more difficult. For example, Bradburn et al. (1987) reported results of a study in which respondents were asked how often they had eaten at a restaurant in the past 2 months. Respondents who did not eat out very often were more likely to tally the occasions to arrive at their answer, but counting became less common when the recall period was extended to 6 months.

Empirical studies show that estimation usually proceeds with the respondent's combining whatever recall he/she may have of salient facts with semantic memories for that general class of experiences and with general knowledge to produce an answer (Bradburn et al., 1987; Brown, 1994). We have emphasized earlier in this chapter that this can lead to less accurate reports than those based on active memory search, but it is also important to recognize that estimation often yields fairly accurate responses to general questions that do not require recall of particular episodes (Pearson et al., 1992). In cases where episodic memories cannot be recovered even after extensive memory search—such as when a question is asked about the number of times respondents ate at a restaurant in the past 6 months, or when adults are asked about their drinking behavior when they were in high school—estimation may actually be more desirable (Blair & Burton, 1987; Burton & Blair, 1991). However, the precise inference strategies used to make the estimation are still unspecified. Some inference strategies may be more accurate than others, and the researcher can improve accuracy of reporting by discovering the most effective strategies and by coaching respondents to use them. However, this requires a prior program of basic research on the accuracy of alternate strategies of inferring answers to complex memory questions. No research has evaluated how respondents answer complex questions such as the following CIDI questions on the course of depression:

> In your lifetime, how many spells like that [when you felt depressed and had some of these other problems—list symptoms of depression] have you had that lasted 2 weeks or more?
> Between [any of] these spells, were you feeling OK at least for some months?
> Between [any of] these spells, were you fully able to work and enjoy being with other people?
> Did that "normal" period last at least 6 months?
> (If not) Did it last at least 2 months?

It is not clear how respondents answer these questions. If they have only had one or two episodes in their lifetimes, it is likely that they will refer to episodic memories, but estimation is more likely if the number of episodes is large (Burton & Blair, 1991). Indeed, our debriefing work for the NCS shows that this is the case. The respondents who reported a small number of episodes generally said that they counted to answer the question about number of episodes, whereas those who reported a large number said that they estimated. The work of Means and Loftus (1991) suggests that we could improve the accuracy of reports about duration and time between episodes by respondents referring to episodic memories by asking a series of concrete questions that help discriminate the episodes in the respondents' minds. If we had a better understanding of the accuracy of different estimation methods, we might also be able to improve the accuracy of the reports given by respondents who use estimation by decomposing the questions and guiding the estimation process.

OVERVIEW

Before closing, we must note that we have explicitly ignored the difficult question of whether respondents are honest either with the interviewer or with themselves in discussing their mental health. The issue of honesty is a problematic one. The methodological literature on the accuracy of respondent reports shows clearly that the perceived social desirability of responses is as important as understanding or memory in determining the accuracy of reports (Sudman & Bradburn, 1974; Kessler & Wethington, 1991). We have no way of assessing the magnitude of this problem with available data, but it clearly needs to be taken into consideration as research in this area moves forward.

Focusing only on the ability to recall rather than on willingness to disclose memories, we have reviewed a large body of research suggesting that it may be possible to recover long-term memories of salient aspects of childhood psychiatric disorders with active memory search. Other memories may be too difficult to recover, either because they were never salient or because of more active processes that might involve repression. It is important to recognize, though, that very few validation studies have been carried out concerning long-term memories of any sort, and that there have been none at all concerning reports about childhood psychiatric disorders. Studies of this sort must be conducted to advance our understanding beyond speculation.

Two considerations support our belief that validation studies are critical. First, it is quite likely that the use of careful question wording and field administration procedures could be shown by such studies to yield more valid retrospective data about childhood psychiatric disorders. Second, as the NCS revealed alarmingly high rates of untreated symptoms among the general population (Kessler et al., 1994), we must expedite the search for antecedents to these problems; interventions simply cannot wait for long-term prospective and experimental studies to advance our understanding of developmental psychopathology. Although retrospective reports have limitations, as this chapter makes amply clear, such data nonetheless constitute an invaluable supplement to more time- and cost-intensive methods. The history of epidemiological research in other substantive areas is testimony to this fact. For example, the discovery of the effects of tampon use on toxic shock syndrome and of cigarette smoking on lung cancer were both initially revealed during retrospective studies (Schlesselman, 1982). The challenge for researchers who seek to understand childhood psychiatric disorders, their causes, and their sequelae is to understand the legitimate uses and limits of retrospective data.

ACKNOWLEDGMENTS

Preparation of this chapter was supported in part by Grants No. R01 MH41135, No. K02 MH00507, and No. T32 MH16806 from the National Institute of Mental Health, and from the John D. and Catherine T. MacArthur Foundation Research Network on Psychopathology and Development.

REFERENCES

Abelson, R. D., & Loftus, E. F. (1992). Attempts to improve the accuracy of self-reports of voting. In J. M. Tanur (Ed.), *Questions about questions: Inquiries into the cognitive bases of surveys* (pp. 138–153). New York: Russell Sage Foundation.

Angel, R., & Thoits, P. (1987). The impact of culture on the cognitive structure of illness. *Culture, Medicine and Psychiatry, 11*, 465–494.

Baddeley, A. D. (1990). *Human memory: Theory and practice*. Hillsdale, NJ: Erlbaum.

Belli, R. F. (1988). Color blend retrievals: Compromise memories or deliberate compromise responses? *Memory and Cognition, 16*, 314–326.

Belson, W. A. (1981). *The design and understanding of survey questions*. Aldershot, England: Gower.

Biderman, A. (1980). *Report of a workshop on applying cognitive psychology to recall problems of the National Crime Survey*. Washington, DC: Bureau of Social Science Research.

Bishop, G. D. (1991). Understanding the understanding of illness: Lay disease representations. In J. A. Skelton & R. T. Croyle (Eds.), *Mental representation in health and illness* (pp. 32–59). New York: Springer-Verlag.

Bishop, G. D., & Converse, S. A. (1986). Illness representations: A prototype approach. *Health Psychology, 5*, 95–114.

Blair, E., & Burton, S. (1987). Cognitive processes used by survey respondents to answer behavioral frequency questions. *Journal of Consumer Research, 14*, 280–288.

Block, J., Gjerde, P. F., & Block, J. H. (1991). Personality antecedents of depressive tendencies in 18-year-olds: A prospective study. *Journal of Personality and Social Psychology, 60*, 726–738.

Bradburn, N. M., Rips, L. J., & Shevell, S. K. (1987). Answering autobiographical questions: The impact of memory and inference on surveys. *Science, 236*, 157–161.

Bradburn, N. M., Sudman, S., & Associates. (1979). *Improving interview method and questionnaire design: Response effects to threatening questions in survey research.* San Francisco: Jossey-Bass.

Brewer, W. F. (1986). What is autobiographical memory? In D. C. Rubin (Ed.), *Autobiographical memory* (pp. 25–49). New York: Cambridge University Press.

Brewin, C. R., Andrews, B., & Gotlib, I. H. (1993). Psychopathology and early experience: A reappraisal of retrospective reports. *Psychological Bulletin, 113*, 82–98.

Brown, G. W., & Harris, T. O. (1978). *Social origins of depression: A study of psychiatric disorder in women.* New York: Free Press.

Brown, N. R. (1994). Quantitative estimation: From the real world to the psychology lab. *Canadian Psychology, 35*(1), 102–103.

Brown, N. R., Rips, L. J., & Shevell, S. K. (1985). The subjective dates of natural events in very-long-term memory. *Cognitive Psychology, 17*, 139–177.

Burton, S., & Blair, E. (1991). Task conditions, response formulation processes, and response accuracy for behavioral frequency questions in surveys. *Public Opinion Quarterly, 55*, 50–79.

Cannell, C. F. (1985a). Experiments in the improvement of response accuracy. In T. W. Beed & R. J. Stimson (Eds.), *Survey interviewing: Theory and techniques* (pp. 24–62). Winchester, MA: Allen & Unwin.

Cannell, C. F. (1985b). Overview: Response bias and interviewer variability in surveys. In T. W. Beed & R. J. Stimson (Eds.), *Survey interviewing: Theory and techniques* (pp. 1–23). Winchester, MA: Allen & Unwin.

Cannell, C. F., Fowler, F. J., & Marquis, K. H. (1968). *The influence of interviewer and respondent psychological and behavioral variables on the reporting in household interviews* (Vital and Health Statistics, Series 1, *2*(26)). Washington, DC: U.S. Government Printing Office.

Cannell, C. F., & Kahn, R. (1968). Interviewing. In G. Lindzey & E. Aronson (Eds.), *The Handbook of social psychology* (Vol. 2, pp. 526–595). Reading, MA: Addison-Wesley.

Cannell, C. F., Miller, P. V., & Oksenberg, L. (1981). Research on interviewing techniques. In S. Leinhardt (Ed.), *Sociological methodology 1981* (pp. 389–437). San Francisco: Jossey-Bass.

Cannell, C. F., Oksenberg, L., & Converse, J. M. (1977). Striving for response accuracy: Experiments in new interviewing techniques. *Journal of Marketing Research, 14*(3), 306–315.

Centers, R. (1964). A laboratory adaptation of the conversational procedure for the conditioning of verbal operants. *Journal of Abnormal and Social Psychology, 67*, 334–339.

Christianson, S. A., & Loftus, E. F. (1991). Remembering emotional events: The fate of detailed information. *Cognition and Emotion, 5*, 81–108.

Clark, H. H., & Schober, M. F. (1992). Asking questions and influencing answers. In J. M. Tanur (Ed.), *Questions about questions: Inquiries into the cognitive bases of surveys* (pp. 15–48). New York: Russell Sage Foundation.

Cohen, P., Cohen, J., & Brook, J. S. (1993). An epidemiological study of disorders in late childhood and adolescence: II. Persistence of disorders. *Journal of Child Psychology and Psychiatry, 34*(6), 869–877.

Cohen, P., Cohen, J., Kasen, S., Velez, C. N., Hartmark, C., Johnson, J., Rojas, M., Brook, J., & Struening, E. L. (1993). An epidemiological study of disorders in late childhood and adolescence: I. Age- and gender-specific prevalence. *Journal of Child Psychology and Psychiatry, 34*(6), 851–867.

Crespi, I., & Swinehart, W. (1982, May). *Some effects of sequence questions using different time intervals on behavioral self-reports.* Paper presented at the meeting of the American Association for Public Opinion Research, Washington, DC.

Fathi, D., Schooler, J., & Loftus, E. F. (1984). Moving survey problems into the cognitive psychology laboratory. *Proceedings of the Survey Research Section: American Statistical Association* (pp. 19–21). Washington, DC: American Statistical Association.

Fisher, R. P., & Geiselman, R. E. (1992). *Memory-enhancement techniques for investigative interviews: Increasing eyewitness recall with the cognitive interview.* Springfield, IL: Charles C Thomas.

Fisher, R. P., Geiselman, R. E., & Amador, M. (1989). Field test of the cognitive interview: Enhancing the recollection of actual victims and witnesses of crime. *Journal of Applied Psychology, 74*, 722–727.

Fisher, R. P., & Quigley, K. L. (1992). Applying cognitive theory in public health investigations: Enhancing food recall with the cognitive interview. In J. M. Tanur (Ed.), *Questions about questions: Inquiries into the cognitive bases of surveys* (pp. 154–172). New York: Russell Sage Foundation.

Fowler, F. J., Jr., & Cannell, C. F. (1996). Using behavioral coding to identify cognitive problems with survey questions. In N. Schwarz & S. Sudman (Eds.), *Answering questions: Methodology for determining cognitive and communicative processes in survey research* (pp. 15–36). San Francisco, CA: Jossey-Bass.

Genter, D., & Collins, A. (1981). Studies of inference from lack of knowledge. *Memory and Cognition, 9*, 434–443.

Gilman, S. (1988). *Disease and representation: Images of illness from madness to AIDS.* Ithaca, NY: Cornell University Press.

Gotlib, I. H., Mount, J. H., Cordy, N. I., & Whiffen, V. E. (1988). Depression and perceptions of early parenting: A longitudinal investigation. *British Journal of Psychiatry, 152*, 24–27.

Glucksberg, S., & McCloskey, M. (1981). Decisions about ignorance: Knowing what you don't know. *Journal of Experimental Psychology: Human Learning and Memory, 7*, 311–325.

Harrington, R., Fudge, H., Rutter, M., Pickle, A., & Hill, J. (1990). Adult outcomes of childhood and adolescent depression. *Archives of General Psychiatry, 47*, 465–473.

Harris, T., Brown, G. W., & Bifulco, A. (1990). Loss of parent in childhood and adult psychiatric disorder: A tentative overall model. *Development and Psychopathology, 2*, 311–328.

Hasher, L., & Griffin, M. (1978). Reconstructive and reproductive processes in memory. *Journal of Experimental Psychology: Human Learning and Memory, 4*, 318–330.

Higgins, E. T., Rholes, W. S., & Jones, C. R. (1977). Category accessibility and impression formation. *Journal of Experimental and Social Psychology, 13*, 141–245.

Hippler, H. J., & Schwarz, N. (1986). Not forbidding isn't allowing: The cognitive basis of the forbid–allow asymmetry. *Public Opinion Quarterly, 50*, 87–96.

Holmes, S. J., & Robins, L. N. (1988). The role of parental disciplinary practices in the development of depression and alcoholism. *Psychiatry, 51*, 24–35.

Jabine, T. B., Straf, M. L., Tanur, J. M., & Tourangeau, R. (Eds.). (1984). *Cognitive aspects of survey methodology: Building a bridge between disciplines.* Washington, DC: National Academy Press.

Jefferson, G. (1989). Preliminary notes on a possible metric which provides for a "standard maximum" silence of approximately one second in conversation. In D. Roger & P. Bull (Eds.), *Conversation: An interdisciplinary perspective* (pp. 166–196). Philadelphia: Multilingual Matters.

Jobe, J. B., White, A. A., Kelley, C. L., Mingay, D. L., Sanchez, M. J., & Loftus, E. F. (1990). Recall strategies and memory for health care visits. *Milbank Quarterly, 68,* 171–189.

Kessler, R. C., & Magee, W. J. (1993). Childhood adversity and adult depression: Basic patterns of association in a U. S. national survey. *Psychological Medicine, 23,* 679–690.

Kessler, R. C., McGonagle, K. A., Zhao, S., Nelson, C. B., Hughes, M., Eshleman, S., Wittchen, H.-U., & Kendler, K. S. (1994). Lifetime and 12-month prevalence of DSM-III-R psychiatric disorders in the United States: Results from the National Comorbidity Survey. *Archives of General Psychiatry, 51,* 8–19.

Kessler, R. C., & Wethington, E. (1991). The reliability of life event reports in a community survey. *Psychological Medicine, 21,* 723–738.

Kessler, R. C., Wittchen, H.-U., Abelson, J. M., McGonagle, K. A., Schwarz, N., Kendler, K. S., Knäuper, B., & Zhao, S. (1998). Methodological studies of the Composite International Diagnostic Interview (CIDI) in the U.S. National Comorbidity Survey. *International Journal of Methods in Psychiatric Research, 7,* 33–55.

Kleinman, A. (1986). *Social origins of distress and disease: Depression, neurasthenia, and pain in modern China.* New Haven, CT: Yale University Press.

Knäuper, B., Cannell, C. F., Schwarz, N., Bruce, M. L., & Kessler, R. C. (1999). Improving accuracy of major depression age of onset reports in the U.S. National Comorbidity Survey. *International Journal of Methods in Psychiatric Research, 8,* 39–48.

Kovacs, M., & Paulauskas, S. L. (1984). Developmental stage and the expression of depressive disorders in children: An empirical analysis. *New Directions for Child Development, 26,* 59–80.

Krystal, H. (1990). An information processing view of object relations. *Psychoanalytic Inquiry, 10,* 221–251.

Lazarsfeld, P. F. (1972). The art of asking why: Three principles underlying the formulation of questionnaires. In P. F. Lazarfeld (Ed.), *Qualitative analysis: Historical and critical essays* (pp. 183–202). Boston: Allyn & Bacon. (Original work published 1934)

Lessler, J., Salter, W., & Tourangeau, R. (1989). *Questionnaire design in the cognitive research laboratory: Results of an experimental prototype* (Vital and Health Statistics, Series 6, No. 1; DHHS Publication No. PHS 89–1076). Washington, DC: U.S. Government Printing Office.

Leventhal, H., & Diefenbach, M. (1991). The active side of illness cognition. In J. A. Skelton & R. T. Croyle (Eds.), *Mental representation in health and illness* (pp. 247–272). New York: Springer-Verlag.

Leventhal, H., Meyer, D., & Nerenz, D. (1980). The common sense representation of illness danger. In S. Rachman (Ed.), *Contributions to medical psychology* (pp. 7–30). New York: Pergamon Press.

Leventhal, H., Nerenz, D., & Steele, D. J. (1984). Illness representations and coping with health threats. In A. Baum, S. E. Taylor, & J. E. Singer (Eds.), *Handbook of psychology and health* (Vol. 4, pp. 219–252). Hillsdale, NJ: Erlbaum.

Loftus, E. F., & Fathi, D. C. (1985). Retrieving multiple autobiographical memories. *Social Cognition, 3,* 280–295.

Loftus, E. F., & Palmer, J. C. (1974). Reconstruction of automobile destructions: An example of the integration between language and memory. *Journal of Verbal Language and Verbal Behavior, 13,* 585–589.

Loftus, E. F., Smith, K. D., Klinger, M. R., & Fiedler, J. (1992). Memory and mismemory for health events. In J. M. Tanur (Ed.), *Questions about questions: Inquiries into the cognitive bases of surveys* (pp. 102–137). New York: Russell Sage Foundation.

Markus, H., & Zajonc, R. B. (1985). The cognitive perspective in social psychology. In G. Lindzey & E. Aronson (Eds.), *The handbook of social psychology* (3rd ed., pp. 137–230). New York: Random House.

Marlatt, G. A. (1972). Task structure and the experimental modification of verbal behavior. *Psychological Bulletin, 78,* 335–350.

Marquis, K. H., & Cannell, C. F. (1969). *A study of interviewer–respondent interaction in the urban employment survey, final report.* Ann Arbor: Survey Research Center, University of Michigan.

Marquis, K. H., Cannell, C. F., & Laurent, A. (1972). *Reporting health events in household interviews: Effects of reinforcement, question length, and reinterviews* (Vital and Health Statistics, Series 45, No. 70). Washington, DC: U.S. Government Printing Office.

McLaughlin, J. (1978). Primary and secondary process in the context of cerebral hemispheric specialization. *Psychoanalytic Quarterly, 47,* 237–266.

Means, B., & Loftus, E. F. (1991). When personal history repeats itself: Decomposing memories for recurring events. *Applied Cognitive Psychology, 5,* 297–318.

Means, B., Swan, G. E., Jobe, J. B., & Esposito, J. L. (1994). Estimating frequencies for habitual behaviors: Reports of cigarette smoking. In N. Schwartz & S. Sudman (Eds.), *Autobiographical memory and the validity of retrospective reports* (pp. 107–120). New York: Springer-Verlag.

Menon, A. (1994). Judgments of behavioral frequencies: Memory search and retrieval strategies. In N. Schwartz & S. Sudman (Eds.), *Autobiographical memory and the validity of retrospective reports* (pp. 161–172). New York: Springer-Verlag.

Miller, P. V., & Cannell, C. F. (1977). Communicating measurement objectives in the survey interview. In D. M. Hirsch, P. V. Miller, & F. G. Kline (Eds.), *Strategies for communication research* (Vol. 6, pp. 127–151). Beverly Hills, CA: Sage.

Moss, C., & Goldstein, H. (Eds.). (1979). *The recall method in social surveys.* London: National Foundation for Educational Research.

Neter, J., & Waksberg, J. (1964). A study of response errors in the expenditures data from household interviews. *Journal of the American Statistical Association, 59,* 18–55.

Offord, D. R. (1985). Child psychiatric disorders: Prevalence and perspectives. *Psychiatric Clinics of North America, 8*(4), 637–652.

Oksenberg, L., Cannell, C. F., & Kanton, G. (1991). New strategies for pretesting survey questions. *Journal of Official Statistics, 7,* 349–365.

Oksenberg, L., Vinokur, A., & Cannell, C. F. (1979a). The effects of instructions, commitment and feedback on reporting in personal interviews. In C. F. Cannell, L. Oksenberg, & J. M. Converse (Eds.), *Experiments in interviewing techniques* (DHEW Publication No. HRA 78–3204, pp. 133–199). Hyattsville, MD: Department of Health, Education and Welfare.

Oksenberg, L., Vinokur, A., & Cannell, C. F. (1979b). Effects of commitment to being a good respondent on interview performance. In C. F. Cannell, L. Oksenberg, & J. M. Converse (Eds.), *Experiments in interviewing techniques* (DHEW Publication No. HRA 78–3204, pp. 74–108). Washington, DC: Department of Health, Education and Welfare.

Parry, H. J., Balter, M. B., & Cisin, I. H. (1970–1971). Primary levels of underreporting psychotropic drug use. *Public Opinion Quarterly, 34*(4), 582–592.

Pearson, R. W., Ross, M., & Dawes, R. M. (1992). Personal recall and the limits of retrospective questions in surveys. In J. M. Tanur (Ed.), *Questions about questions: Inquiries into the cognitive bases of surveys* (pp. 65–94). New York: Russell Sage Foundation.

Petty, R. E., & Jarvis, W. B. G. (1996). An individual differences perspective on assessing cognitive processes. In N. Schwarz & S. Sudman (Eds.), *Answering question: Methodology for determining cognitive and communicative processes in survey research* (pp. 221–257). San Francisco: Jossey-Bass.

Pillemer, D. B., Goldsmith, L. R., Panter, A. T., & White, S. H. (1988). Very long-term memories of the first year in college. *Journal of Experimental Psychology: Learning, Memory, and Cognition, 14*, 709–714.

Reisberg, D., & Heuer, F. (1992). Remembering the details of emotional events. In E. Winograd & U. Neisser (Eds.), *Affect and accuracy in recall: Studies of "flashbulb" memories* (pp. 162–211). New York: Cambridge University Press.

Robins, L. N., Schoenberg, S. P., Holmes, S. J., Ratcliff, K. S., Benham, A., & Works, J. (1985). Early home environment and retrospective recall: A test for concordance between siblings with and without psychiatric disorders. *American Journal of Orthopsychiatry, 55*, 27–41.

Robins, L. N., Wing, J., Wittchen, H.-U., & Helzer, J. E. (1988). The Composite International Diagnostic Interview: An epidemiologic instrument suitable for use in conjunction with different diagnostic systems and in different cultures. *Archives of General Psychiatry, 45*, 1069–1077.

Robinson, J. A. (1992). First experience memories: Contexts and functions in personal histories. In M. A. Conway, D. C. Rubin, H. Spinnler, & W. A. Wagennar (Eds.), *Theoretical perspectives on autobiographical memory* (pp. 223–239). Boston: Kluwer Academic.

Ross, M. (1989). Relation of implicit theories to the construction of personal histories. *Psychological Review, 96*, 341–357.

Ross, M., & Conway, M. (1986). Remembering one's past: The construction of personal histories. In R. M. Sorrentino & E. T. Higgins (Eds.), *Handbook of motivation and cognition: Foundations of social behavior* (Vol. 1, pp. 122–144). New York: Guilford Press.

Safer, M. A., Tharps, Q. J., Jackson, T. C., & Leventhal, H. (1979). Determinants of three stages of delay in seeking care at a medical clinic. *Medical Care, 12*, 11–29.

Schaeffer, N. C., & Maynard, D. W. (1996). From paradigm to prototype and back again: Interactive aspects of cognitive processing in Standardized Survey interviews. In N. Schwarz & S. Sudman (Eds.), *Answering questions: Methodology for determining cognitive and communicative processes in survey research* (pp. 65–88). San Francisco: Jossey-Bass.

Schlesselman, J. J. (1982). *Case–control studies.* Oxford: Oxford University Press.

Schuman, H., Belli, R. F., & Bischoping, K. (1997). The generational basis of historical knowledge. In J. W. Pennebaker, D. Paez, & B. Rine (Eds.), *Collective memory of political events: Social psychological perspectives* (pp. 47–77). Mahwah, NJ: Erlbaum.

Shannon, B. (1979). Have you ever been to Paris? *Acta Psychologica, 43*, 313–328.

Sheingold, K., & Tenney, Y. J. (1982). Memory for a salient childhood event. In U. Neisser (Ed.), *Memory observed* (pp. 201–212). San Francisco: Freeman.

Skelton, J. A., & Croyle, R. T. (Eds.). (1991). *Mental representation in health and illness.* New York: Springer-Verlag.

Smith, A. F., Jobe, J. B., & Mingay, D. J. (1991a). Question-induced cognitive biases in reports of dietary intake by college men and women. *Health Psychology, 10*, 244–251.

Smith, A. F., Jobe, J. B., & Mingay, D. J. (1991b). Retrieval from memory of dietary information. *Applied Cognitive Psychology, 5,* 269–296.

Sudman, S., & Bradburn, N. M. (1974). *Response effects in surveys: A review and synthesis.* Chicago: Aldine.

Sudman, S., & Bradburn, N. M. (1982). *Asking questions: A practical guide to questionnaire design.* San Francisco: Jossey-Bass.

Sudman, S., Bradburn, N. M., & Schwarz, N. (1996). *Thinking about answers: The application of cognitive processes to survey methodology.* San Francisco: Jossey-Bass.

Tanur, J. M. (Ed.). (1992). *Questions about questions: Inquiries into the cognitive bases of surveys.* New York: Russell Sage Foundation.

Vinokur, A., Oksenberg, L., & Cannell, C. F. (1979). Effects of feedback and reinforcement on the report of health information. In C. F. Cannell, L. Oksenberg, & J. M. Converse (Eds.), *Experiments in interviewing techniques: Field experiments in health reporting, 1971–1977.* Ann Arbor: Survey Research Center, University of Michigan.

Wetzler, S. E., & Sweeney, J. A. (1986). Childhood amnesia: An empirical demonstration. In D. C. Rubin (Ed.), *Autobiographical memory* (pp. 191–201). New York: Cambridge University Press.

Withey, S. B. (1954). Reliability of recall of income. *Public Opinion Quarterly, 18,* 197–204.

10

The Translation and Adaptation of Diagnostic Instruments for Cross-Cultural Use

✧

GLORISA CANINO
MILAGROS BRAVO

For several decades cross-cultural research has demonstrated that specific symptom presentations and patterns of onset, duration, risk, and outcome of mental illness, particularly in adults, vary across cultures. Symptoms reflect both a pathological and a cultural process, and an understanding of these processes is essential for both diagnosis and treatment of culturally diverse populations (Guarnaccia, Guevara-Ramos, González, Canino, & Bird, 1992). But the cross-cultural diagnostic process is affected by a number of methodological and substantive issues—namely, the definition of what constitutes a "true" case, and the use of culturally sensitive diagnostic tools in research. What follows is a discussion of these issues, which affect both research (particularly psychiatric epidemiological research) and the diagnostic process.

WHAT CONSTITUTES A CASE IN A CROSS-CULTURAL CONTEXT?

Both adult psychiatry and psychiatric epidemiology have struggled with differentiating a "case" from a "noncase." This difficulty in case definition is increased in child assessment because of a number of factors. These include the need for incorporating the perspectives of multiple informants, and the frequent disagreement among them in reports of a child's functioning; lack of knowledge among informants as to what constitutes age-appropriate functioning; and lack of agreement as to what constitutes the "right" way of classifying a child (Cantwell & Baker, 1989). This last issue concerns the question of whether psychiatric diagnoses are conceptualized as either continuous or categorical entities. The various editions of the *Diagnostic and Statistical Manual of Psychiatric Disorders* (DSM) define disorders as categorical (either present or absent); the threshold of caseness has been defined primarily by clinical tradition. However, some authors have asserted that disorders are continuous rather than discrete and have derived a topology on purely empirical grounds (Achenbach & Edelbrock, 1981).

At the core of this classification issue is the fact that normative developmental characteristics are difficult to differentiate from developmental problems or psychopathology. Many problem behaviors may be considered normal at certain ages and deviant at others. Most DSM categories in children were originally developed for adults, and only later were generalized to children. They are basically static, and their applicability for different developmental ages has been questioned by many (Radke-Yarrow, Nottelmann, Martínez, Fox, & Belmont, 1992; Costello & Angold, 1996). The lack of biological markers for many disorders, the imprecision of many measurement techniques, and the high rates of DSM disorders found in population surveys (Cantwell & Baker, 1989; Bird et al., 1988) all indicate that the issue of case ascertainment has not been resolved. The existence of this controversy indicates that the threshold at which a behavior or syndrome of behaviors is considered pathological is still uncertain in mainstream psychiatry and psychology. The implication for the diagnostic assessment of children is that it is necessary to provide estimates and correlates of childhood maladjustment, using various definitions of and instruments for assessing psychopathology.

If the state of the art in mainstream psychiatry and psychology is a lack of consensus on the definition of "caseness," deciding what constitutes a case in different cultural groups poses an even greater challenge. What follows is a cross-cultural examination of this issue of case ascertainment through the use of diagnostic instruments that may not have been designed for the culture in which they will be used.

CULTURAL SENSITIVITY OF DIAGNOSTIC TOOLS

Methodological Difficulties

Diagnostic instruments are essential for research and are good aids for clinicians, since they provide a structure and a systematic assessment procedure that increase diagnostic reliability. Yet choosing research models and diagnostic tools that are culturally sensitive is a difficult task. The more descriptive taxonomy of recent editions of the DSM has permitted the development of structured diagnostic instruments such as the Diagnostic Interview for Children and Adolescents (Herjanic & Campbell, 1977; Reich, Herjanic, Welner, & Gandhy, 1982), the Schedule for Affective Disorders and Schizophrenia for School-Age Children (Puig-Antich & Chambers, 1978; Edelbrock & Costello, 1988); the Diagnostic Interview Schedule for Children (DISC; Shaffer et al., 1996), and the Child and Adolescent Psychiatric Assessment (CAPA; Angold, Prendergast, Cox, Harrington, Simonoff, & Rutter, 1995). These instruments are based on the previously described categorical approach used in DSM. Other instruments, such as the Child Behavior Checklist (CBCL; Achenbach & Edelbrock, 1983), are based on a dimensional empirical topology. Yet most of these instruments, with the exception of the CBCL and the DISC, have not been tested for use with populations from other cultures other than mainstream U.S. culture. The CBCL has been translated and tested in several countries of the world and in at least two Hispanic cultures: Chile (Montenegro, 1983) and Puerto Rico (Rubio-Stipec, Bird, Canino, & Gould, 1990). The DISC has been translated, adapted, and tested for use among Puerto Ricans (Bravo, Woodbury, Canino, & Rubio-Stipec, 1993; Ribera et al., 1996). The latest version of the DISC (DISC-IV) and the CAPA are presently being adapted by our research team for use in many other Spanish-speaking countries and U.S. Hispanic groups, as well as in Puerto Rico.

Thus, for most researchers belonging to various cultural backgrounds and speaking languages other than English, the choice of a state-of-the-art psychiatric diagnostic interview will involve a process of translation and adaptation of the instrument. The challenge for these researchers is to assure that the translated and adapted version of the assessment tool is equivalent to the original version of the instrument. Only by achieving this equivalence will it be possible to assure any degree of comparability in studies carried out in different cultures. It is important to be able to describe similarities and differences in the results obtained in various cross-cultural studies, unconfounded by translation difficulties or other variations in instruments or their scoring.

Translation and Adaptation

The adequacy of a diagnostic instrument in a given culture does not guarantee its reliability or validity in another, even given a faithful translation. Unless an assessment tool is developed in the culture for which it is intended, the use of such an instrument requires a comprehensive translation and adaptation process. The resultant instrument must be capable of identifying the same (or very similar) phenomena as those identified by the original version, but in a dissimilar sociocultural context.

In Puerto Rico we have used a comprehensive cross-cultural model to adapt and translate a number of diagnostic instruments for children and adolescents, particularly the DISC, the CBCL, and a number of other instruments designed to measure impairment and risk for psychopathology.

This model frames the cultural adaptation of an instrument in the context of the process of establishing the measure's validity and reliability. It is based on the premise that psychopathological phenomena are universal, yet considerably influenced by the sociocultural context in which they occur. This position tends to be supported by cross-cultural research on psychological disorders (Al-Issa, 1982; Engelsman, 1982; Murphy, 1982). It has been stated that there is neither a disorder entirely free from cultural shaping nor one that can be entirely ascribed to social or cultural characteristics (Draguns, 1980; Kleinman & Good, 1985). The model involves testing an instrument for cultural equivalence in five dimensions: (1) semantic, (2) content, (3) technical, (4) conceptual, and (5) criterion (Flaherty, 1987; Bravo, Canino, Rubio-Stipec, & Woodbury-Fariña, 1991; Bravo et al., 1993; Canino & Bravo, 1994).

Semantic Equivalence

An important aspect of the translation process is to assure that the meaning of each item is similar in the language of each culture. Semantic equivalence can be achieved with a combination of translation and back-translation techniques—that is, having the instrument translated into the language desired, and then having it translated back into the original language of the instrument by someone other than the original translator (Brislin, Lonner, & Thorndike, 1973). The process is repeated until a translation is achieved that approximates the original language of the instrument. This version is then evaluated by a bilingual committee. The members of this committee must be knowledgeable about the constructs that the instruments assess, as well the population to be studied. In the case of the development of mental health instruments for children, bilingual committees must be composed of mental health researchers and clinicians who are experienced in working with children. They must make sure that the instrument's items retain their original psychiatric intent, and that the language used is appropriate for the age of targeted children.

Yet this complicated process is not sufficient to attain semantic equivalence. Field testing of the instrument is essential in order to assure that feedback from interviewers is obtained. An example of a problem encountered in seeking to attain semantic equivalence for the Spanish translation and adaptation of the DISC was the translation of the word "worry" (Bravo et al., 1993). We chose the Spanish word "*preocupación*" to translate this word. Yet the interviewers noticed that although "*preocupación*" can have a negative connotation similar to the English word, it can also have a positive one more consonant with that of the English word "concern." When parents were asked whether their children worried much about school, many answered, "Of course my child worries (*se preocupa*); he [or she] is a very responsible student," giving the interviewer the impression that such a child had shown appropriate and desirable behavior. The item was changed to "*se preocupa demasiado*" or "worries too much," in order to convey the connotation that the behavior was to be out of the normal and desirable range. This type of language equivalence cannot be achieved by a back-translation process alone.

If the instrument to be translated and adapted is to be used in several countries or with people of varied ethnicities, revision by an international or culturally varied committee is recommended. We have included this step in our development of a Spanish version of the DISC-IV. A committee composed of members from different Spanish-speaking countries (Spain, Mexico, and Venezuela) and U.S. Hispanic groups (of Mexican, Central American, and South American origin), as well as from Puerto Rico, was formed. The main goal of this committee has been to assure that the final translated version is applicable to diverse Spanish-speaking groups and comprehensible to people of varied educational levels. The initial version of the instrument was translated and adapted in Puerto Rico; it was then carefully reviewed by each committee member, and consensus was reached about the appropriate wording of items. In those cases in which a term common to all groups was not found, several ethnic variations or regionalisms were included in parentheses. For example, to translate the phrase "how often," three phrases in Spanish had to be included: "*cuán a menudo,*" "*con qué frecuencia,*" and "*qué tan seguido.*" In this way, an instrument appropriate to a wide variety of Spanish-speaking groups is being developed.

Content Equivalence

An important aspect of the process of adapting an instrument is to examine whether the content of each item is relevant to the population under study. For example, all versions of the DISC have some items designed to assess seasonal depression. Children and parents are asked whether they have ever experienced the symptoms characteristic of a dysphoric mood when days are shorter (late fall and winter) as compared to when days are longer (spring and summer). In Puerto Rico we had to change these items, since on a tropical island there are no marked differences in the length of days during the year, nor are there striking environmental differences among the various seasons. In order to convey a similar idea in a more contextually appropriate way, the item was reworded to ask about seasons: "*cuando obscurece más temprano (de octubre a marzo) y obscurece más tarde (de abril a septiembre),*" which means literally "when it grows dark sooner (from October to March) or grows dark later (from April to September)." However, even after these items were changed to make more sense in our context, we found that none of the children interviewed had experienced seasonal depression, probably because it is unlikely to occur on an island where there are no marked seasonal changes. In fact, since the DISC was tested through field trials carried out in collaboration with three North American sites (see Lahey et al., 1996), it was possible to corroborate whether the prevalence of seasonal depression was significantly lower in Puerto Rico than in the other sites. The results confirmed what was expected: The prevalence of seasonal depression was higher in two communities in the northeastern United States, lower in a Southern community, and nonexistent in Puerto Rico.

This finding was consistent with the discussions that took place in international committee meetings about these items. Although some members from the continental United States considered the concept and the original items appropriate for their sites, those coming from places nearer the equator (e.g., Venezuela) argued that it was not pertinent to their context.

Moreover, an instrument needs to be evaluated by bicultural experts prior to its use in another culture, in order to determine whether the operationalization of what constitutes normal behavior is relevant to the culture under study. For example, after careful examination of an instrument designed to measure family functioning, it became apparent that the instrument's main conceptualization of "normal" family functioning runs counter to what is considered normal in Puerto Rican families. The instrument in question, the Family Adaptability and Cohesion Evaluation Scales (Olson, Portner, & Bell, 1982), contains several items that do not reflect the cultural norms and practices of Puerto Rican culture. A respondent is asked to rate on a Likert-type scale the frequency with which, for example, children have a say in their own discipline and in solving problems, whether the children's suggestions are followed in the family, whether household responsibilities shift from person to person (or it is hard to tell who does which household chores), and whether family members consult other family members on their decisions. The typical normal Puerto Rican family is moderately authoritarian; there is a marked division of labor that conforms to sex role stereotypes, and children usually have little participation in decision making. Normal family functioning therefore cannot be measured by items that inquire about shared decision making and responsibilities and about egalitarian sex role definitions.

A similar example is given by Rogler, Malgady, and Rodríguez (1989). These authors have described how in previous research they started by trying to measure spouses' relationships through decision-making questionnaires. During the initial phase of the study, it became apparent that the items of the instrument they were considering did not apply to impoverished Puerto Rican couples, since the items inquired about decision making regarding where to go on vacation, which school the children should attend, which insurance policy to purchase, and so forth. They thought about changing the content of the items but retaining the construct of decision making. After these new items were pretested, it became clear that the construct of decision making for these families was irrelevant, since the opportunities for choice and decision making in their lives were slim. These families were at the bottom of a socially stratified system; they were struggling to meet their most basic needs.

Another instance in which examining the content validity of an instrument is crucial is the measurement of impairment and social adaptation in children from diverse cultures. Ideally, impairment measures should provide indicators of a child's psychosocial functioning and adaptation in the most important areas of the child's life—the school, the family, the community, and friends. Measures that provide objective criteria separating these important domains are necessary, since it is possible that a child may show adaptation problems in one area and not in another. Yet functional adaptation is defined in terms of the way a person's role performance conforms to the expectations of his/her reference group (Hoagwood, Jensen, Petti, & Burns, 1996). Impairment measures are thus based on behaviors or roles that are normative to a given society or context (Katsching, 1983). Given this contextual definition, one would expect definitions of "normality" to vary across different cultural and/or socioeconomic groups. Evidence from a 1985 Puerto Rican survey (Bird et al., 1988) supports the view that assessments of social adaptation must be contextually developed. Even after subjects were matched for age, sex, and socioeconomic status, differences between Puerto Rican and Anglo children and adolescents were observed, especially on the CBCL's Social Competence scores (Achenbach et al., 1990). Overall, these scores as reported by adolescent subjects themselves and by all subjects' parents and teachers were considerably lower for the Puerto Rican sample than for the Anglo sample. However, the Puerto Rican sample reported more frequent contacts with friends and got along better with family and siblings. These latter results may reflect the importance placed on close family ties and good interpersonal relations in Puerto Rican culture (Canino & Canino, 1982; Harwood, Miller, & Irizarry, 1995). Reports of involvement in sports, hobbies, organizations, or jobs were significantly lower for the Puerto Rican subjects, contributing to their lower Social Competence scores. The lack of resources in poor communities in Puerto Rico limits children's access to hobbies and formal sports programs; high unemployment rates on the island limit the availability of jobs for children and adolescents.

Although Puerto Rican children and adolescents scored considerably lower than comparable Anglo subjects on the Social Competence scale of the CBCL (i.e., as less competent), the opposite was found in studies using two other measures of impairment: the Nonclinician Children's Global Assessment Scale (CGAS) and the Columbia Impairment Scale (CIS). In the Methods for Epidemiology in Children and Adolescents study (Shaffer et al., 1996), Puerto Rican children were rated by both parents and lay interviewers on both the CGAS and the CIS as less impaired than comparable youth at the three U.S. mainland sites (Bird et al., 1996). Bird et al. (1996), in reporting the psychometric properties of both scales, noted particular site differences for the youth version of the Nonclinician CGAS; most associations with the outcome measures were found to be significantly weaker in the Puerto Rico site. Site-specific correlations between predictors of impairment and clinician validators for the Nonclinician CGAS and the CIS were all lower for the Puerto Rico site. The proportions of DISC psychiatric diagnoses accompanied by impaired functioning (as defined by a score below 70 on the parent version of the Nonclinician CGAS) were 16% for Atlanta, Georgia; 19.9% for New Haven, Connecticut; 12.8% for Westchester County, New York; and 4.1% for San Juan, Puerto Rico. Results similar to those obtained in Puerto Rico were obtained in the Great Smoky Mountains study (Costello et al., 1996). In this study the prevalence of severe emotional disturbance in children aged 9–13, defined as having a DSM-III-R diagnosis and scoring below 70 on the CGAS, was 4.2%. Higher rates of disorder were obtained when scores of 10 on the Child and Adolescent Functional Assessment Scale (7.6%) and of 2 on the CAPA impairment scale (6.8%) were used.

As these examples indicate, any measure of impairment or social adaptation must be carefully evaluated in its cultural and social context to avoid bias and misinterpretation of research results from studies using standard methods developed in a single sociocultural context. Many measures of impairment or social adaptation seem to be affected by cultural and contextual factors. Scores on the CGAS (and possibly other measures requiring the interviewer to make a judgment about the extent of functional impairment) may be influenced by the rater's experience, prior knowledge of the child, and expectations of what constitute impairment and social adaptation in a particular culture. Scores on the CIS, as well as on other measures that ask questions of a child, parent, or caregiver about the child's functioning, are likely to be influenced by that individual's perceptions of what constitutes adaptive functioning.

Technical Equivalence

Similar effects should be achieved when similar measuring techniques are used in different cultures. Sometimes differences between cultures in which the same assessment instrument has been used may be due to differences in responses caused by the assessment technique utilized; thus it is important that the technical equivalence of the instrument be assessed before the beginning of the study. For example, self-report measures of substance use that require respondents to know how to read and write are a source of unreliability in many inner-city minority populations, where functional illiteracy is a problem. The lack of appropriate reading and writing skills in the population assessed introduces a source of unreliability into the data, which may affect the results of the study. In order to maintain the anonymity of self-reports for sensitive information of this nature, and at the same time to address the problem of functional illiteracy, a number of investigators (e.g., Turner et al., 1998) have developed computerized audio systems in which subjects are not required to read items; they can answer questions posed via an audio system by pressing a key on a computer keyboard. At present there is an English version of a computerized audio DISC-IV.

Self-report instruments may not be the most appropriate assessment tools for certain populations. Ethnic minorities and other socially disadvantaged populations may be more likely to deny use of drugs, physical or sexual abuse, or other antisocial behavior that they believe will get them in trouble with the authorities. In fact, there is evidence that a significantly greater proportion of black Americans than of non-Hispanic white Americans admit that they would not be honest in reporting their illicit drug use even if they did engage in this type of behavior (Mensch & Kandel, 1988). The lower rates of drug use among African American populations reported in national surveys sponsored by the National Institute on Drug Abuse may be the results of significant underreporting in these populations.

There is also evidence that significant underreporting may occur in certain cultures when self-report measures inquire about sexual behavior. Puerto Rican adolescents reported significantly fewer problems than mainland adolescents on the Youth Self-Report version of the CBCL, particularly on such items as "I think about sex too much" (Achenbach et al., 1990). The lower scores in general could have been due to the fact that many Puerto Rican adolescents live in authoritarian family structures, in which children are expected to keep their opinions to themselves.

Thus the data suggest that the assessment of antisocial or otherwise sensitive behavior through self-reports in populations where this type of behavior is greatly censured, and/or in special populations that are at a disadvantage in the society surveyed, will need to be supplemented with other types of assessment to avoid significant underreporting. The use of key informants and of other data sources (e.g., police and medical records, or hair or urine analyses for biological detection of drug use) may be advisable. In addition, use of ethnographic methods, use of interviewers who live in the same community as the subjects being evaluated, and/or prior consistent contact of interviewers with community leaders may be necessary to avoid underreporting of sensitive information.

Conceptual Equivalence

The term "conceptual equivalence" refers to the fact that the same theoretical construct should be evaluated by an assessment instrument in the different cultures involved. Usually this type of equivalence cannot be directly assessed; instead, the relationship of the measure assessing the construct with measures of other relevant concepts is studied (e.g., the association of an instrument intended to assess psychopathology with measures of social adaptation, impairment, or school performance). In the case of the adaptation of the DISC-2.3 to Puerto Rican culture, we found that children classified by the DISC as meeting criteria for psychiatric disorders had higher levels of impairment (as measured by the CGAS; Shaffer et al., 1983), lower levels of adaptive functioning, and more school problems (dropping out, absenteeism, failure, detention, suspension, attending special classes) than children who did not meet diagnostic criteria on the DISC-2.3 (Bravo et al., 1993). The results thus suggested that the adapted instrument was evaluating phenomena related to social, psychological, and academic dysfunction in our child and adolescent population—a finding that would be expected from an instrument appropriately evaluating psychiatric disorders in our context.

Criterion Equivalence

Perhaps the most difficult part of the adaptation and translation process is achieving criterion equivalence—that is, similar interpretation of the results of the measure when these are evaluated in accordance with the established norms of each culture. This involves identifying pertinent norms in each culture and assessing when the trait or disorder evaluated is said to exist, according to these norms. When the culture for which the instrument is to be adapted is not too different from the culture for which the instrument was developed, the process of achieving criterion equivalence is not as complex.

The fact that a process of adaptation and translation has been followed does not necessarily assure complete cultural sensitivity of the instrument used. This is more apparent when the assessing instrument is based on a psychiatric categorical nosology such as the DSM, which was not developed for international use. The validation of the instrument is not the same as the validation of the nosology. Thus it is possible that in using instruments based on DSM-IV, for example, the researcher is imposing the appearance of cross-cultural homogeneity which is artifactual to the use of a constricted nosology (the "cultural fallacy"; Kleinman & Good, 1985). Only through a combination of psychometric empirical studies and ethnographic inquiry can this bias be surmounted. Researchers using this approach (see, e.g., Kinzie et al., 1982; Manson, Shore, & Bloom, 1985) have found that several culturally significant symptoms of mental distress, different from those included on questionnaires developed for English-speaking populations, appear when this issue is systematically examined. Ethnographic approaches can provide information on particular ways in which children from a different culture may express certain types of psychiatric symptomatology. These approaches can permit the assessment of culture-bound syndromes, which may not be included in the "mainstream instruments" used.

We have attempted to achieve criterion equivalence in our adaptation of the DISC by validating the instrument against the best-estimate clinical judgment of various indigenous child psychiatrists. However, this method has limitations, since the indigenous psychiatrists are using a nosology that has not been validated in their culture of origin.

CONCLUSIONS

A major undertaking for child and adolescent cross-cultural psychiatry is the comparison of symptoms and disorders across cultural boundaries. These comparisons may give clues to the etiology of childhood disorders; they can also provide evidence on whether different societal responses to mental illness affect its course, thus ultimately providing clues to the improvement of treatment in children.

However, in order for this cross-cultural comparison process to succeed, equivalence of the observations made in the different cultures is essential. If this equivalence is not obtained, it is not possible to disentangle whether the differences obtained in prevalence and risk factors associated with psychiatric disorders in children across cultures are due to differences in the methodologies employed, or are due to true cultural or contextual differences. The task of achieving equivalence requires the translation and adaptation of diagnostic instruments for identifying disorders in diverse contexts. Multiple sociocultural factors, of which linguistic equivalence is only one aspect, must be considered. We recommend the use of careful and comprehensive adaptation concepts and methods, similar to those illustrated in this chapter, for translating and adapting diagnostic instruments that are to be used in studying children whose languages and cultures differ from those of the original instrument.

REFERENCES

Achenbach, T. M., Bird, H., Canino, G., Phares, V., Gould, M., & Rubio-Stipec, M. (1990). Epidemiological comparisons of Puerto Rican and U.S. children: Parent, teacher and self-reports. *Journal of the American Academy of Child and Adolescent Psychiatry, 29*(1), 84–93.

Achenbach, T. M., & Edelbrock, C. S. (1981). Behavioral problems and competencies reported by parents of normal and disturbed children aged four through sixteen. *Monographs of the Society for Research in Child Development, 46,* 1–25.

Achenbach, T. M., & Edelbrock, C. S. (1983). *Manual for the Child Behavior Checklist and the Revised Child Behavior Profile.* Burlington: University of Vermont, Department of Psychiatry.

Al-Issa, I. (1982). Does culture make a difference in psychopathology? In I. Al-Issa (Ed.), *Culture and psychopathology* (pp. 3–29). Baltimore: University Park Press.

Angold, A., Prendergast, M., Cox, A., Harrington, R., Simonoff, E., & Rutter, M. (1995). The Child and Adolescent Psychiatric Assessment (CAPA). *Psychological Medicine, 25,* 739–753.

Bird, H. R., Canino, G., Rubio-Stipec, M., Gould, M. S., Ribera, J., Sesman, M., Woodbury, M., Huertas-Goldman, S., Pagan, A., Sanchez-Lacay, A., & Moscoso, M. (1988). Estimates of the prevalence of childhood maladjustment in a community survey in Puerto Rico. *Archives of General Psychiatry, 45,* 1120–1126.

Bird, H. R., Schwab-Stone, M., Andrews, H., Goodman, S., Dulcan, M., Rubio-Stipec, M., Moore, R. E., Chang, P. H., Canino, G., Fisher, P., Hoven, C., Gould, M. S., & Richters, J. (1996). Global measures of impairment for epidemiologic and clinical use with children and adolescents. *International Journal of Methods in Psychiatric Research, 6,* 295–307.

Bravo, M., Canino, G., Rubio-Stipec, M., & Woodbury-Fariña, M. (1991). A cross-cultural adaptation of a psychiatric epidemiologic instrument: The Diagnostic Interview Schedule's Adaptation in Puerto Rico. *Culture, Medicine and Psychiatry, 15,* 1–18.

Bravo, M., Woodbury, M. A., Canino, G. J., & Rubio-Stipec, M. (1993). The Spanish translation and cultural adaptation of the Diagnostic Interview Schedule for Children (DISC) in Puerto Rico. *Culture, Medicine and Psychiatry, 17*(3), 329–344.

Brislin, R., Lonner, W., & Thorndike, R. (1973). *Cross-cultural methods.* New York: Wiley.

Canino, G., & Bravo, M. (1994). The adaptation and testing of diagnostic and outcome measures for cross-cultural research. *International Review of Psychiatry, 6,* 281–286.

Canino, G., & Canino, I. (1982). Family therapy: A culturally syntonic approach for Hispanics. *Hospital Community Psychiatry, 33*(4), 299–303.

Cantwell, D. P., & Baker, L. (1989). Stability and natural history of DSM-III childhood diagnoses. *Journal of the American Academy of Child and Adolescent Psychiatry, 28*(5), 691–697.

Costello, E. J., & Angold, A. (1996). Developmental epidemiology. In D. Cicchetti & D. Cohen (Eds.), *Developmental psychopathology: Vol. 1. Theory and methods* (pp. 23–56). New York: Wiley.

Costello, E. J., Angold, A., Burns, B. J., Erkanli, A., Stangl, D. K., & Tweed, D. L. (1996). The Great Smoky Mountains Study of Youth: Functional impairment and severe emotional disturbance. *Archives of General Psychiatry, 53*(12), 1137–1143.

Draguns, J. G. (1980). Psychological disorder of clinical severity. In *Handbook of cross cultural psychology: Vol. 6. Psychopathology.* Boston: Allyn & Bacon.

Edelbrock, C., & Costello, A. J. (1988). Structured psychiatric interviews for children. In M. Rutter, A. H. Tuma, & I. S. Lann (Eds.), *Assessment and diagnosis in child psychopathology* (pp. 87–112). New York: Guilford Press.

Engelsman, F. (1982). Culture and depression. In I. Al-Issa (Ed.), *Culture and psychopathology* (pp. 251–274). Baltimore: University Park Press.

Flaherty, J. A. (1987). Appropriate and inappropriate research methodologies for Hispanic mental health. In M. Gaviria (Ed.), *Behavior research agenda for Hispanics* (pp. 117–186). Chicago: University of Chicago Press.

Guarnaccia, P. J., Guevara, L. M., González, G., Canino, G., & Bird, H. R. (1992). Cross cultural aspects of psychotic symptoms in Puerto Rico. *Research in Community and Mental Health, 7,* 99–110.

Harwood, R. L., Miller, J. G., & Irizarry, N. (1995). *Culture and attachment: Perceptions of the child in context.* New York: Guilford Press.

Hoagwood, K., Jensen, P., Petti, T., & Burns, B. (1996). Outcomes of mental health care for children and adolescents: I. A comprehensive conceptual model. *Journal of the American Academy of Child and Adolescent Psychiatry, 35*(8), 1055–1063.

Herjanic, B., & Campbell, W. (1977). Differentiating psychiatrically disturbed children on the basis of a structured interview. *Journal of Abnormal Child Psychology, 5,* 127–134.

Katsching, H. (1983). Methods for measuring social adjustment. In T. Helgason (Ed.), *Methodology in evaluation of psychiatric treatment* (pp. 205–218). New York: Cambridge University Press.

Kinzie, J. D., Manson, S. M., Vinh, D. T., Tolan, N. T., Anh, B., & Pho, T. N. (1982). Development and validation of a Vietnamese-language depression rating scale. *American Journal of Psychiatry, 139*, 1276–1281.

Kleinman, A., & Good, B. (Eds.). (1985). *Culture and depression: Studies in the anthropology and cross-cultural psychiatry of affect and disorder.* Berkeley: University of California Press.

Lahey, B. B., Flagg, E. W., Bird, H. R., Schwab-Stone, M., Canino, G., Dulcan, M. K., Leaf, P. J., Davies, M., Brogan, D., Bourdon, K., Horwitz, S. M., Rubio-Stipec, M., Freeman, D. H., Lichtman, J., Shaffer, D., Goodman, S. H., Narrow, W. E., Weissman, M. M., Kandel, D. B., Jensen, P. S., Richters, J. E., & Regier, D. A. (1996). NIMH Methods for Epidemiology in Children and Adolescents (MECA) study: Background and methodology. *Journal of the American Academy of Child and Adolescent Psychiatry, 35*(7), 855–864.

Manson, S. M., Shore, J. H., & Bloom, J. D. (1985). The depressive experience in American Indian communities: A challenge for psychiatric theory and diagnosis. In A. Kleinman & B. Good (Eds.), *Culture and depression: Studies in the anthropology and cross-cultural psychiatry of affect and disorder* (pp. 331–368). Berkeley: University of California Press.

Mensch, B. S., & Kandel, D. B. (1988). Underreporting of substance use in a national longitudinal youth cohort. *Public Opinion Quarterly, 52*, 100–124.

Montenegro, H. A. (1983). *Salud mental del escolar: Estandarización del inventario de problemas conductuales y destrezas sociales de T. Achenbach en niños de 6 a 11 años.* Santiago, Chile: CIDE.

Murphy, H. B. M. (1982). Culture and schizophrenia. In I. Al-Issa (Ed.), *Culture and psychopathology* (pp. 221–249). Baltimore: University Park Press.

Olson, D. H., Portner, J., & Bell, R. O. (1982). *FACES II: Family Adaptability and Cohesion Evaluation Scales.* Minneapolis: University of Minnesota, Department of Family Social Science.

Puig-Antich, J., & Chambers, W. (1978). *The Schedule for Affective Disorders and Schizophrenia for School-Aged Children.* New York: New York State Psychiatric Institute.

Radke-Yarrow, M., Nottelmann, E., Martínez, P., Fox, M. B., & Belmont, B. (1992). Young children of affectively ill parents: A longitudinal study of psychosocial development. *Journal of the American Academy of Child and Adolescent Psychiatry, 31*(1), 68–77.

Reich, W., Herjanic, B., Welner, Z., & Gandhy, P. R. (1982). Development of a structured psychiatric interview for children: Agreement on diagnosis comparing child and parent interviews. *Journal of Abnormal Child Psychology, 10*(4), 325–336.

Ribera, J. C., Canino, G. J., Rubio-Stipec, M., Bravo, M., Bird, H. R., Freeman, D., Shrout, P., Bauermeister, J., Alegría, M., Woodbury, M., Huertas, S., & Guevara, L. M. (1996). The Diagnostic Interview Schedule for Children (DISC 2.1) in Spanish: Reliability in a Hispanic population. *Journal of Child Psychology and Psychiatry, 37*(2), 195–204.

Rogler, L. H., Malgady, R. G., & Rodríguez, O. (1989). *Hispanics and mental health: A framework for research.* Malabar, FL: Robert E. Kriger.

Rubio-Stipec, M., Bird, H., Canino, G., & Gould, M. (1990). The internal consistency and concurrent validity of a Spanish translation of the Child Behavior Checklist. *Journal of Abnormal Child Psychology, 18*(4), 393–406.

Shaffer, D., Fisher, P., Dulcan, M., Davis, D., Piacentini, J., Schwab-Stone, M., Lahey, B., Bourdon, K., Jensen, P., Bird, H., Canino, G., & Regier, D. (1996). The NIMH Diagnostic Interview Schedule for Children (DISC 2. 3): Description, acceptability, prevalences, and performance in the MECA study. *Journal of the American Academy of Child and Adolescent Psychiatry, 35*(7), 865–877.

Shaffer, D., Gould, M. S., Brasic, J., Ambrosini, P. J., Fisher, P., Bird, H. R., & Aluwahlia, S. (1983). A Children's Global Assessment Scale (CGAS). *Archives of General Psychiatry, 40*, 1228–1231.

Turner, C., Ku, L., Rogers, S. M., Lindberg, L. D., Pleck, J. H., & Sonenstein, F. L. (1998). Adolescent sexual behavior, drug use and violence: Increased reporting with computer survey technology. *Science, 280*, 867–873.

11

The Context of Assessment: Culture, Race, and Socioeconomic Status as Influences on the Assessment of Children

✦

PATRICIA COHEN
STEPHANIE KASEN

In this chapter we address the question of how race, ethnicity, socioeconomic status (SES), and culture may influence the emotional or behavioral assessment of a child. These influences may come about because those providing the basic information and judgments exhibit biases in attributing problems to a child of a given ethnicity, SES, or culture in comparison to other children, or because bias exists in the assessment instruments that are employed. Or they may come about because of differences in the way informants behave, or because interviewers with different characteristics have differing success rates in eliciting cooperation from children from different groups and in objectively evaluating the information obtained. Many of these issues are translated into good practice in the *Guidelines for Providers of Psychological Services to Ethnic, Linguistic, and Culturally Diverse Populations*, published by the American Psychological Association (APA) Office of Ethnic Minority Affairs (1991). In what follows we review these issues as they relate to children, and we present the currently available empirical evidence. We focus first on influences that may be attributable to characteristics of the child, and then examine the influences due to methods of assessment and to those obtaining and evaluating the information.

Because the empirical information is so sparse, it may be useful to think of this discussion as a guide to the issues and potential biases that need to be taken into account in planning child assessments and in selecting, training, and monitoring the assessors. In particular, we have very little evidence regarding the potentially important influence of a child's SES on the quality and validity of these assessments, although it is likely that the effects are pervasive. Furthermore, there is no reason to think that racial, ethnic, or cultural influences are stable over time or geographical space. For example, the effect of a white examiner on the performance of black children in the South in the 1960s may not be closely reflected by effects on black children in an urban Northern setting in the 1990s. Thus there will be an ongoing need for assessors to be sensitive to local conditions, and perhaps particularly for them to be sensitive to the influence that they themselves may have on the responses of the children they assess (Rosnow & Rosenthal, 1996).

INFLUENCES OF CHILD CHARACTERISTICS ON RESPONSES TO ASSESSMENT MATERIALS

Many differences among children in test performance and other assessment outcomes have been found to be associated with membership in cultural and demographic subgroups (Moran, 1990; Raadal, Milgrom, Cauce, & Mancl, 1994; Reynolds & Brown, 1984; Reynolds, 1982). These differences may stem from real variation in the children's behavior or other relevant characteristics, or from factors in the assessment procedure or setting. However, it is not always possible to ascertain which of these mechanisms is operating in a given testing situation.

Despite the long recognition of the potential influence of cultural factors (Chess, Clark, & Thomas, 1953), very little empirical evidence of such influence is available in the assessment of child psychopathology. More empirical evidence is available from the area of cognitive testing. For over two decades, a body of research has addressed the issue of cultural bias within the domain of intellectual and ability testing (e.g., Clarizio, 1982; Jenson, 1980; Oakland & Feigenbaum, 1979; Reynolds & Kaiser, 1990; Reynolds & Piersel, 1983). The impetus for these studies was strengthened by concern about the placement of minority children into remedial and special education classes. In a class action suit, it was alleged that a disproportionate number of minority children were in special classes because of unfair testing practices (*Larry P. v. Riles,* 1979). The ruling in favor of the plaintiffs labeled IQ tests as biased, and enjoined the state of California against using IQ test results as the sole criteria for placing minority children in special classes (Bersoff, 1982).

In contrast, examination of bias in tests measuring the emotional, motivational, attitudinal, and interpersonal characteristics of children has been minimal, although critiques of adult instruments would suggest that problems may well exist (López & Nuñez, 1987; Vega & Rumbaut, 1991). Where evidence of group differences has been documented, minority children and lower-SES children have often been found to respond in ways that have been interpreted as more deviant (Moran, 1990). Unfortunately, many of the studies addressing this issue have been characterized by small samples and a lack of control for variables relevant to the emotional and social development of children, such as poverty and inadequate environmental supports.

Performance differences between ethnic groups of children have been reported on personality and symptom measures. Perhaps the most well-established findings are with regard to anxiety. Employing meta-analytic techniques, Hembree (1988) demonstrated higher test anxiety in African American than in European American second- through fourth-graders. Clawson, Firmont, and Trower (1980) reported higher scores for African American students than for European American students with similar educational backgrounds on trait, state, and test anxiety. Likewise, Reynolds, Plake, and Harding (1983) reported higher anxiety scores among African American children on the Revised Children's Manifest Anxiety scale, as well as ethnic differences that varied by age and sex. Children of parents with an anxiety disorder are more likely to be anxious themselves (Turner, Beidel, & Costello, 1987; Weissman, Leckman, Merikangas, Gammon, & Prusoff, 1984). Because higher rates of certain anxiety disorders are reported in African American adults compared to other cultural groups (Robins et al., 1984; Neal & Turner, 1991), African American children may be more at risk for anxiety problems than are mainstream European American children. Other findings have indicated different rates of psychiatric diagnoses across cultural groups, as well as variations across classification systems developed in separate cultures. Kim and Chun (1993) reported higher rates of depression among Asian American adolescent girls and lower rates of affective disorders among Asian American adolescent boys compared to their European American peers. Minde and Minde (1995) found that although 51% of clinically referred Cree children did not qualify for a DSM-III-R diagnosis, their severe behavioral symptoms could be categorized in terms of five types of sociocultural disturbances. Tao (1992) used *Diagnostic and Statistical Manual of Mental Disorders*, third edition (DSM-III) criteria to rediagnose attention deficit disorder with hyperactivity in an outpatient sample originally diagnosed by Nanjing criteria, and reported a 63% rate of concordance; this finding suggested that the Chinese system defined a broader concept of the disorder.

Findings regarding demographic group differences on other assessment measures vary. Green and Kelley (1988) found ethnic differences on Minnesota Multiphasic Personality Inventory scores within a delinquent population. In a large clinical sample tested with the Personality Inventory for Children (PIC), African American children had higher scores than European American children on scales indicative of somatic complaints, and lower scores on scales reflecting internalizing disorders and social skills (Lachar & Gdowski, 1979). In addition, variations in the relationship between self-esteem and delinquency (Leung & Drasgow, 1986) and in rates of hyperactivity (Spring, Blundern, Greenberg, & Yellin, 1977) have been attributed to ethnic and racial differences. However, Ward and McFall (1986) failed to find differences in mean social problem-solving skills between disparate racial groups of adolescent girls. And, in the same vein, standardization data on the Child Behavior Checklist (CBCL) indicate that race and SES differences on the Teacher's Report Form and the Youth Self-Report are too small to warrant separate norms (Achenbach & Edelbrock, 1983). On the other hand, Raadal et al. (1994), using a random sample of 890 low-income public elementary school children and their mothers, reported that CBCL total and subscale scores were significantly higher than the norms, and that a greater proportion of these children scored in the clinical/borderline range. Many other popular instruments used in the assessment of children do not have standardization information on population subgroups other than those based on age or sex.

Some data suggest that SES differences may underlie the findings in studies where more deviant outcomes in measured behaviors have been attributed to the influence of ethnic or racial group membership. In some instances these interpretive pitfalls stem from methodological issues. Generalizations about drug use and other deviant behaviors among black youth are frequently based on samples drawn from nonrepresentative, captive, often low-income populations (e.g., clinical populations, incarcerated youth, and urban student populations); consequently, poor minority youth are contrasted with their more advantaged white peers (Bell-Scott, 1987; McKenry, 1987; McKenry, Everett, Ramseur, & Carter 1989). Even when SES is controlled for, the comparison may be inadequate because SES is typically more normally distributed in white samples (Engram, 1982) or may be nonlinearly related to the measures of psychopathology. Furthermore, whereas the independent effects of ethnic status and SES are tested, the combined deleterious effects of minority status and lower SES in race–SES interactions are rarely examined (McKenry et al., 1989).

DIFFERENTIAL RELIABILITY OR VALIDITY OF ASSESSMENT INSTRUMENTS

As noted, in most studies where race or ethnic mean differences are shown, there is no clear evidence whether they reflect bias in assessment or real group differences. Such evidence would consist of differential stability or course of the problem, differential relationships to risk factors or outcomes, or differential relationships with presumably more objective indicators of the problem. In one of the few available studies, Kline and Lachar (1992) administered the PIC to mothers of over 1,300 children and adolescents referred for mental health services, and collected symptom ratings from teachers and clinicians. They found no evidence that race or sex moderated the relationship of the PIC scales with teacher and clinician symptom ratings. Similarly, analyses by subgroup on the Reynolds Adolescent Depression Scale showed no differential validity by race. On the other hand, the Center for Epidemiologic Studies Depression Scale (CES-D) used with conventional cutoffs may produce more false positives among Native American adolescents than are produced with normative samples (Manson, Ackerson, Dick, Baron, & Fleming, 1990).

In some cases it has been suggested that subgroup differences in factor structure of a measure may be an indication of bias or differential validity. Using data from a national survey of 12- to 17-year-olds, Roberts (1992) found similar factor structures represented by positive affect, negative affect, and psychosomatic symptoms in European American and African American youths on a 12-item version of the CES-D. However, among Mexican American and other Hispanic American youths, negative affect and psychosomatic symptoms clustered together, suggesting that somatic complaints may play a more prominent role in the presentation of depression among these two groups. Politano, Nelson, Evans, Sorenson, and Zemen (1986) found that the factor structure of the Children's Depression Inventory differed for African American and European American psychiatric inpatients aged 6 to 18. On the other hand, Reynolds and Paget (1981), using a national normative sample of 4,972 children aged 6 to 19, reported very high coefficients of congruence across African American and European American children, as well as by sex, on a five-factor solution of the Revised Children's Manifest Anxiety Scale.

Differences found between demographic groups in the correlates of assessments are sometimes taken as evidence of bias (Moran, 1990). However, such differences in group traits may very well exist; thus variations in construct validity may reveal true differences between groups. Circumventing the biased use of such measures may require alterations in the interpretation of results based on group membership. For example, Leung and Dragow (1986) examined the relationship between self-esteem and delinquent behavior in three ethnic groups of adolescents: blacks, whites, and Hispanics. A negative relationship held only for whites, suggesting either that the self-esteem scale was not equivalent across groups, that other relevant factors may not have been held constant, or that there are true ethnic differences in the meaning of those variables.

ETHNICITY AND PROJECTIVE/ABILITY-RELATED TESTS

In the review above, we have focused on findings with very structured assessment instruments designed to measure psychopathology. However, many of those who currently assess children for emotional or behavioral problems use either projective tests (such as the Rorschach or the Children's Apperception Test) or ability-related tests (such as the Bender–Gestalt, the Goodenough Draw-a-Person, or an IQ test) (Hutton, Dubes, & Muir, 1992). The validity of these tests when they are used for the purpose of measuring affective problems has long been in doubt (e.g., Gittelman, 1985), despite their popularity with clinicians. Because children of disadvantaged SES often demonstrate low verbal fluency when tested with standard instruments, one major concern is the degree to which language is salient to performance on some of these tests. Perhaps the most important issue in the context of this chapter is that projective techniques and ability-related tests provide great latitude for assessors to exercise their general attitudes and potential biases to influence the assessment. Thus, these assessment methods need to be used with even more caution than is the case for measures that are more objective. A thematic apperception test designed for Hispanic and black respondents, the Thematic Apperception Test for Urban Hispanic Children, "Tell Me a Story" (TEMAS), appears to mitigate the problem of verbal fluency (at least for Hispanics) and to have some validity in discriminating outpatients from a general population of children (Constantino, Malgady, Rogler, & Tsui, 1988; Malgady, Constantino, & Rogler, 1984). Of course, the one set of procedures that allows even wider latitude for potential assessor bias is the use of idiosyncratic clinical interviews.

ETHNIC DIFFERENCES IN PROBLEM DISCLOSURE

There is good evidence of probable ethnic differences in willingness to admit problems or misbehaviors. One area in which research has been conducted is in the willingness to report use and abuse of alcohol and various illicit drugs to researchers. It is virtually universally found that African American and Hispanic adolescents report lower rates of ever having tried drugs and of current drug use than do other American youth. Large concentrations of minority children are found in the major urban centers of the United States, where youth are more likely to be apprehended for drug involvement. It is, however, also possible that children in high-drug-use areas who are not involved in a major way with drugs are in fact less likely to try them than are children in other areas, because of their higher exposure to some of the consequences. Despite a number of efforts to resolve this question, the evidence remains subject to alternative interpretations. Benson and Donahue (1989) examined reports of at-risk behaviors in a large representative sample of high school seniors, and found that black seniors reported significantly fewer at-risk behaviors (particularly drug-related ones) than white seniors. Black high school seniors in another study reported less drug use than did white seniors, and were also more likely to refuse to answer questions about negative behaviors (Johnston, Bachman, & O'Malley, 1986). Although these samples were random ones, they were confined to those youth who were still in high school in their senior year; thus confounds of SES, race, and school dropout rates may be in effect. Nevertheless, it is likely that findings about self-disclosure in adults of different ethnic groups may generalize to children and adolescents. Lower self-disclosure has been consistently found among black adults than among white adults when both are responding to a white therapist (Ridley, 1984), even after SES and education have been controlled for.

Other attitudinal or behavioral characteristics of cultural and other demographic groups that affect informants' reports may also be interpreted incorrectly by an unknowing assessor (Koss-Chioino & Vargas, 1992). For example, Asian informants are often more reluctant to discuss personal matters than are informants from other ethnic groups for fear of shame, and may make only veiled references to problems of a personal or familial nature. On the other hand, Chinese parents, who usually have very high academic expectations for their children, may be overconcerned when their children's characteristics appear to be suggestive of attention deficit and hyperactivity syndromes, particularly in China, where government policies promoting "one couple, one child" families have enhanced the importance of each child's achievement (Tao, 1992).

Poor language proficiency and variations in first language among participants in the assessment process may present substantial barriers to adequate assessment. It may be very difficult to find an adequate translation for some concepts and words when one is moving from one language to another; consequently, it is reasonable to expect that inaccurate interpretations of culturally relevant concepts may occur. Furthermore, when researchers are devising a translated form of a standard assessment instrument, there may be no exact equivalent terminology for some of the concepts used in the original (Geisinger, 1994; Okazaki & Sue, 1995). A number of these issues are discussed by Malgady, Rogler, and Costantino (1987) with regard to the assessment of Hispanic children, as well as by Canino and Bravo in Chapter 10 of the present volume. The overall recommendation is that, until the utility of using standard assessment instruments with Hispanic clients has undergone extensive study, it may be necessary to avoid using those instruments with those who are not acculturated into the mainstream culture.

Age and sex differences in mean symptom scores and diagnostic prevalences among children are of course very commonly found. In general, we fail to acknowledge that these may be attributable in part to bias in question wording, although it is probably the case that wording effects often do operate differentially in age and sex subgroups. There is some evidence that boys tend to compare themselves with boys, whereas girls may compare themselves to both girls and boys. Measures that compare a child to peers may not indicate whether the referent peer group is meant to include boys and girls or same-sex peers only, thus altering at least some responses to behaviors in which the prevalence differs for boys and girls. Furthermore, no clear evidence about the probable age differences in those tendencies is available. These potential problems suggest that it may be pertinent to describe the membership of the intended reference group when one is devising or administering an instrument that includes such comparisons.

It has also been suggested that diagnostic criteria may themselves be biased with regard to ethnicity (Rogler, 1992) and sex (Frick et al., 1994). In addition to potential problems with several adult DSM diagnoses, the DSM conduct disorder criteria may be biased toward male as compared to female misbehaviors. The establishment of objective criteria for diagnoses has not prevented race and sex biases in the *de facto* assignment of diagnostic categories to adults (Loring & Powell, 1988), and there is every reason to believe that such biases will also appear for children.

INFLUENCES OF ASSESSOR CHARACTERISTICS

Assessor Attitudes

As Geller (1988) has pointed out in regard to studies of adults, therapeutic resources are nearly always scarce. Outcome research has emphasized exclusion and failure criteria; consequently, "the determination of which applicants are best qualified for admission to a particular form of therapy often has the character of a qualifying examination or a selective admissions procedure" (p. 115). As such, assessments may be expected to have the same SES and ethnic biases that have been found in treatment studies, where attractiveness, success, and verbal ability have been found to be so influential.

Higher prevalences of mental health problems and compromised functioning—including depression and anxiety disorders, delinquency, substance abuse, suicide, and school failure—have been been documented in indigenous youth compared to their majority peers in North America (Beiser & Attneave, 1982; Costello, Farmer, Angold, Burns, & Erkanli, 1997; Davis, Hoffman, & Nelson, 1990; Kirmayer, 1994; Manson et al., 1990; Oneil, 1995), in New Zealand (Mellsop, Taumoepeau, & Smith, 1993), in Scandinavia (Kvernmo & Heyerdahl, 1998), and in Australia (Brady, 1993). However, in a recent comparison of teacher-, parent-, and self-reported symptoms of conduct disorder and depression among Native and non-Native children in the Flower of Two Soils longitudinal study, non-Native teachers reported elevated conduct disorder and depressive symptom levels among Native students, whereas parents and children reported more depressive symptoms in non-Native students and no group difference in conduct disorder symptoms (Dion, Gotowiec, & Beiser, 1998). The authors concluded that cultural distance may contribute to a negative bias among non-Native teachers in their evaluation of the mental health of Native students, and may influence patterns of referral. Other investigative findings from the Flower of Two Soils data suggest that self-concept, which is in part a product of interactions with teachers, becomes increasingly negative over time among Native children, and may contribute to the difficulties they experience in the majority culture's schools (Beiser, Sack, Manson, Redshirt, & Dion, 1998).

Perhaps one of the most blatant opportunities for biased assessment arises in the consideration of whether identified problems are indicative of psychopathology at all. Several provocative studies by Lewis and colleagues have demonstrated inequitable social consequences for African American and European American delinquents based on psychiatric assessment. Clinical observations indicated that many African American delinquents referred for psychiatric evaluation were dismissed as characterologically impaired despite clear evidence of psychotic or organic disorder, whereas European American delinquents exhibiting similar behaviors were diagnosed and referred for psychiatric services (Lewis, Balla, & Shanok, 1979). This served as an impetus to review medical histories of African American and European American delinquents known to the juvenile court (Lewis & Shanok, 1977). African American delinquents had more frequent histories of trauma that might lead to behavioral problems, yet African American delinquents and their parents were less likely than European American delinquents and their parents to be referred for and to receive psychiatric services (Lewis et al., 1979). Following that up, Lewis, Shanok, Cohen, Kligfeld, and Frisone (1980) compared psychiatric symptoms, violent behaviors, and medical histories of a 1-year sample of adolescents from the same community who were sent to correctional school or were cared for in the state psychiatric unit serving the area. Violence and psychiatric symptomatology were equally prominent in both groups. Race was the best predictor of setting: Delinquents sent to correctional school were more likely to be African American, to be male, and to have a history of trauma. Westendorp, Brink, Roberson, and Ortiz (1986) also found black adolescents to be underrepresented among the psychiatrically hospitalized and overrepresented among the incarcerated. In contrast, Kaplan and Busner (1992) examined ethnicity, age, and sex of children admitted during a 1-year period for psychiatric services and for correctional services in one New York State county and found no effect of ethnicity on population-corrected admission rates to the mental health system; however, more black than white children were admitted to the correctional facility. The fact that hospitalization rates were equivalent does not, of course, indicate that children who were hospitalized were equivalent with regard to problem level.

Biases in the gatekeepers to clinical services may account for differential treatment recommendations and subsequent differences in clinical populations. Harrison, McDermott, Wilson, and Schrager (1965) showed that recommendations for treatment following assessment were related to SES of the family, with children in higher-SES families being recommended more frequently for psychotherapy. Lower-SES children also may be referred as frequently but are seldom actually treated (Cohen & Hesselbart, 1993). Others have reported that ethnic minority children, although referred for therapeutic intervention more frequently than the dominant population, have higher rates of premature termination of therapy (Takeuchi, Bui, & Kim, 1993). After controlling for SES, Fabrega, Ulrich, and Mezzich (1993) found that black adolescents referred for psychiatric treatment had lower levels of standard clinical psychopathology but higher levels of social oppositional behavior than did white adolescents referred for treatment.

Previous research has found African American and other ethnic minority youths to be overrepresented in community mental health clinics, relative to their presence in the community (Cheung & Snowden, 1990; Snowden & Cheung, 1990; Sue, Fujino, & Takeuchi, 1991). On the other hand, ethnic minority parents and other family members are reported to be more reluctant to seek out formal professional help for their children than their ethnic majority counterparts, due in part to financial limitations and availability of nonprofessional (i.e., family and community) sources of help (Briones, Heller, & Chalfant, 1990), in part to lower perceptions of problem severity (Brione et al., 1990; McMiller & Weisz, 1996), and in part to wary attitudes toward professionals and agencies (Broman, 1987; Neighbors, 1985; Hall & Tucker, 1985; Staggers, 1987). Takeuchi et al. (1993) suggested that an overrepresentation of African American and other ethnic minority youth in mental health clinics results largely from coercive referrals related to contact with social and legal agencies. When coercive referrals are eliminated, voluntary contact with mental health professionals among African American and Hispanic American families seeking advice for problems with their children is less than that of European American families in similar circumstances (McMiller & Weisz, 1996).

Despite the general paucity of strong empirical evidence regarding the effects of ethnicity or race on the psychological assessment of the child, it is worth reviewing the theoretically likely kinds of problems that may arise. In an excellent review of the evidence for clinical judgment bias with regard to adult assessments, López (1989) notes that "in addition to overpathologizing actual symptoms, practitioners may also minimize symptoms of actual pathology: that is, they may judge actual symptoms as representing normative behavior, when in fact the symptoms represent abnormal behavior" (p. 186). He notes that the kinds of biases that are theoretically likely include biased attributions (as when symptoms are attributed to patient-internal causes for one group but external causes for another, or to motivation in one group and ability in another) and biased views of base rates (as when symptoms or disorders are believed to typify one group more than another). Other forms of bias may arise from clinicians' memory or recall for certain symptoms (where expectation-incongruent symptoms may be recalled less readily than expectation-congruent symptoms), and from hypothesis testing (where clinicians use strategies that tend to confirm prior expectations and devalue inconsistent information). At another extreme are the assessors who, in an attempt to avoid cultural bias, often miss pathology when it is identified as a cultural trait. Alternatively, pathology may not be recognized because specific cultural norms are not considered or known. For example, Asian American children are often underdiagnosed with hyperactivity because they are measured against European American cultural norms (Sata, 1990).

Demographic Characteristics of Assessors

There are several probable reasons for the paucity of information on effects of assessors' ethnicity, age, or sex on the assessment of psychopathology. Although some researchers attempt to match the race of interviewers and subjects (see below), lay assessors in the United States are typically white women. In clinical settings several factors combine to make evaluation of these issues difficult and unlikely, including nonrandom assignment of children to assessment staffers, relatively small numbers of total staff members, and (in particular) small numbers of staffers in demographic subgroups. If one adds to these the problems in determining unambiguously whether an assessment is biased or otherwise inadequate on the basis of empirical relationships to validators, it becomes clear why such information is hardly ever more than a suggestive (and often unreported) side finding in any clinical research program. However, Sue and Zane (1987) have noted that cultural or racial differences may have profound effects on the credibility ascribed to a mental health professional by a client. Credibility may be undermined by culturally based discrepancies between the professional and client in any of three areas: conceptualization of the problem, formulation of the means for problem resolution, or definition of the goals for treatment. Without adequate credibility, there is little likelihood that the assessor will obtain the necessary cooperation from both parent and child to ensure accurate assessment.

Assessor–Child Demographic Congruity

It is often considered to be good practice to match the ethnicity of an assessor with that of a child. The underlying assumption of this preference is presumably that the child and parent will feel more at ease and thus will be more willing to reveal problems and cooperate with the assessment. Research on adults has suggested that racially similar patient–therapist pairs generate more self-exploration (Carkhuff & Pierce, 1967), at least in the initial interview. In fact, we were not able to identify published reports examining this issue for the assessment of children, and conclusions from the literature on adult clients are conflicting (Sue, 1988). Although at least some members of minority groups indicate that they would prefer to speak to mental health professionals of their own cultural or racial group, empirical work comes primarily from analogue studies rather than from real investigations involving random assignment. The fact is that so few available mental health professionals come from minority groups that adequate empirical study of the effects of client–professional ethnic correspondence is extremely difficult. Furthermore, even when race and ethnicity are "matched," there tends to be a residual SES difference when families are from low-SES areas. And low SES may well be more influential on assessor bias than is ethnicity or race per se.

It is, however, very likely that minority children may be influenced by the status differences that they perceive between assessors and themselves (Katz, Robinson, Epps, & Waly, 1964). Although objective evidence is sparse, it seems likely that children may react with the same negative mood effects that can result from activated negative racial attitudes in adults (Hass, Katz, Rizzo, Bailey, & Moore, 1992). Parents may also react negatively to the assessment of their children, and some professionals see the involvement of same-ethnic-group professionals as a key component of successful data gathering (Rogler, Barreras, & Satana-Cooney, 1981). On the other hand, studies of the effects of ethnic matching on the responses of adults to a psychiatric interview have not shown systematic improvement (Dohrenwend & Dohrenwend, 1969). Nor has research based on responses to national surveys shown unambiguous positive effects of racial matching (Schuman et al., 1989).

There is, however, some evidence to suggest that assessors may respond differentially to demographic similarity in making judgments about children. Lethermon, Williamson, Moody, and Wozniak (1986) used African American and European American female raters to rate videotapes of African American and European American children on the Social Skills Test for Children. Despite training, there were rater group differences in some ratings, as well as interactions between rater race and child race in the direction of higher prosocial ratings for same-racial-group children. Using videotaped vignettes, Mann et al. (1993) found that Chinese and Indonesian clinicians gave significantly higher scores for hyperactive and disruptive behaviors than did Japanese and American clinicians.

The notion that behaviors that are more common in some assessors' cultural backgrounds than in others' might well be evaluated differently is theoretically compelling, if not actually empirically well tested. For example, we have heard of cases in which certain maternal behaviors such as yelling at children, hitting children, or "affectionate" denigrating were discounted as risky behaviors because they were culturally congruent. Because there are no current empirical data showing that these behaviors are less risky in one group than in another, we really have little evidence for deciding definitively that this is false discounting. Older biases based on assessors' cultural or theoretical backgrounds, such as a view that a child who sleeps in the same room as his/her parents is necessarily psychiatrically ill, may have been mitigated by the introduction of clear criteria for diagnostic ascription. In any case, potential biases based on unfamiliarity with cultural norms are readily removed by appropriate training and monitoring of assessors (although they may

creep back in during the course of clinical practice). However, cultural variations in the interpretation of the meaning of particular behaviors are harder
to eliminate, because evidence regarding their validity or lack of validity is
generally lacking.

Gender and Age of Assessors

Research on the effects of assessors' age has also generally not been done, although it is widely believed that adolescents, and perhaps younger children as
well, feel more comfortable with and confiding in a younger person than in
an older one. Similarly, we have little reason to assume that assessments will
be differentially successful when conducted by males or females. However,
the evaluation of the meaning of specific behaviors may, in theory, vary as a
function of the sex of the evaluator. For example, Horn and Haynes (1981)
found that male and female raters rated the same videotapes of disruptive
child behavior differently on the dimension of normality. There were no differential effects attributable to the sex of the behaving child.

On the whole, differences between assessors, especially in working clinical contexts, are likely to be substantial, but not particularly related to their
demographic group membership. Interviewer or observer bias increases as
the requirements for subjectivity in scoring increase. This is most likely to occur in instances where overall ratings or diagnoses are based only in part
upon standard and objective data. As overall ratings are most likely to receive
the greatest weight in the interpretation of test results and in the ensuing decisions regarding children, the importance of assessment bias increases. Such
judgments have generally not been the object of research.

DIFFERENTIAL IMPACT
OF VULNERABILITY FACTORS

Various risk factors for childhood psychopathology are more common in ethnic minority and poor families. There is a link between stressful life events or
less positive life experiences on the one hand, and minority group membership and lower SES on the other (Coddington, 1972; Ladner, 1971; Newcomb, Huba, & Bentler, 1981). Given the association between adverse events
and problematic adjustment (e.g., Gad & Johnson, 1980; Pryor Brown, Powell, & Earls, 1989; Sterling, Cowen, Weissberg, Lotyczewski, & Boike, 1985;
Vaux & Ruggerio, 1983), children in minority and low-income families are
more likely to suffer the effects of multiple simultaneous risk factors. Such
risks have been shown to have a more than cumulative effect on psychopathology. Nevertheless, any given assessment may identify only a fraction of the operating risk factors. For example, an area in which such an ef-

fect can be seen is the developmental outcome of pre- and perinatal problems, which are more frequent in poor and minority populations. The deleterious effects of the resulting infant vulnerability is much greater in children whose families are of lower-SES backgrounds, whereas children in middle-SES families typically outgrow all but the most severe of these problems (Kopp & Kaler, 1989; Sameroff & Chandler, 1975). In general, vulnerabilities can be expected to be more consequential in families with fewer personal, social, or economic resources upon which they can draw. Therefore one area of importance in assessment, especially of children from the lowest-SES families (regardless of ethnic status), is the identification of particular risks and vulnerabilities.

SUMMARY

An assessment is more than a procedure. It is a process whose products precipitate decision making, action taking, and policy formulation. In the assessment of psychopathology in children, such data are used on individual children to provide the justification for service delivery and collectively to determine the need for services. Consequently, the impact of group membership on assessment results can have far-reaching effects on children's lives. It behooves us to examine critically whether cultural and other demographic influences on assessment and case dispositions are consistent with effective use of assessment for the mental well-being of children. Mental health professionals who are engaged in the assessment of children should familiarize themselves with the special issues that may arise with the families they may encounter. As noted earlier, many of these issues are reflected in the standards for practice published as *Guidelines for Providers of Psychological Services to Ethnic, Linguistic, and Culturally Diverse Populations* (APA Office of Ethnic Minority Affairs, 1991). Some more specific guidelines are available for Native American children (Everett, Proctor, & Cartmell, 1983), Hispanic children (Rosado, 1986; Zuniga, 1988), and Asian Americans (Sue & Sue, 1987).

In addition to issues affecting the direct assessment of a child's psychopathology, it is important to assess the risks presented by the child's context. When populations are poor, a multiplicity of risks will tend to co-occur, compounding the clinical picture and often enhancing the need for intervention.

REFERENCES

Achenbach, T., & Edelbrock, C. (1978). The classification of child psychopathology. *Psychological Bulletin, 85,* 1275–1301.

Achenbach, T., & Edelbrock, C. (1983). *Manual for the Child Behavior Checklist and Revised Child Behavior Profile.* Burlington, VT: Department of Psychiatry, Unversity of Vermont.

American Psychologic Association (APA) Office of Ethnic Minority Affairs. (1991). *Guidelines for providers of psychological service to ethnic, linguistic, and culturally diverse populations.* Washington, DC: American Psychological Association.

Beiser, M., & Attneave, C. L. (1982). Mental disorders among Native American children: Rates and risk periods for entering treatment. *American Journal of Psychiatry, 139,* 193–198.

Beiser, M., Sack, W., Manson, S., Redshirt, R., & Dion, R. (1998). Mental health and the academic performance of First Nations and majority-culture children. *American Journal of Orthopsychiatry, 68,* 455–467.

Bell-Scott, P. (1987). Introduction. In Consortium for Research on Black Adolescence (Ed.), *Black adolescence: Topical summaries and annotated bibliographies of research* (pp. 5–9). Storrs: University of Connecticut, School of Family Studies. (ERIC Document Reproduction Service No. ED 285 924)

Benson, P. L., & Donahue, M. J. (1989). Ten-year trends in at-risk behaviors: A national study of black adolescents. *Journal of Adolescent Research, 4,* 125–139.

Bersoff, D. N. (1982). The legal regulation of school psychology. In C. R. Reynolds & T. B. Gutkin (Eds.), *The handbook of school psychology* (pp. 1043–1074). New York: Wiley.

Brady, M. A. (1993). Health issues for Aboriginal youth: Social and cultural factors associated with resilience. *Journal of Pediatric Child Health, 2,* 56–59.

Briones, D., Heller, P., & Chalfant, H. (1990). Socioeconomic status, ethnicity, psychological distress, and readiness to utilize a mental health facility. *American Journal of Psychiatry, 147,* 1333–1340.

Broman, C. (1987). Race differences in professional help seeking. *American Journal of Community Psychology, 15,* 473–489.

Carkhuff, R., & Pierce, R. (1967). Differential effects of therapist race and social class upon patient depth of self-exploration in the initial interview. *Journal of Consulting Psychology, 31,* 632–634.

Chess, S., Clark, K. B., & Thomas, A. (1953). The importance of cultural evaluation in psychiatric diagnosis and treatment. *Psychiatric Quarterly, 27,* 102–114.

Cheung, F., & Snowden, L. (1990). Community mental health and ethnic minority populations. *Community Mental Health Journal, 26,* 277–291.

Clarizio, H. F. (1982). Intellectual assessment of Hispanic children. *Psychology in the Schools, 19,* 61–71.

Clawson, T. W., Firmont, C. K., & Trower, L. L. (1980). Test anxiety: Another origin for racial bias in standardized testing. *Measurement and Evaluation in Guidance, 13,* 210–215.

Coddington, R. D. (1972). The significance of life events as etiologic factors in the diseases of children: II. A study of a normal population. *Journal of Psychosomatic Research, 21,* 237–242.

Cohen, P., & Hesselbart, C. (1993). Children's mental health services: Demographic distortions in delivery. *Journal of the American Public Health Association, 83,* 49–52.

Constantino, G., Malgady, R. G., Rogler, L. H., & Tsui, E. C. (1988). Discriminant analysis of clinical outpatients and public school children by TEMAS: A thematic apperception test for Hispanics and blacks. *Journal of Personality Assessment, 52,* 670–678.

Costello, E., Farmer, E., Angold, A., Burns, B., & Erkanli, A. (1997). Psychiatric disorders among American Indian and white youth in Appalachia: The Great Smoky Mountains study. *American Journal of Public Health, 87,* 827–832.

Davis, G. L., Hoffman, R. G., & Nelson, K. S. (1990). Differences between Native Americans and whites on the California Psychological Inventory. *Psychological Assessment, 2,* 238–242.

Dion, R., Gotowiec, A., & Beiser, M. (1998). Depression and conduct disorder in Native and non-Native children. *Journal of the American Academy of Child and Adolescent Psychiatry, 37,* 736–742.

Dohrenwend, B. P., & Dohrenwend, B. S. (1969). *Social status and psychological disorder.* New York: Wiley.

Engram, E. (1982). *Science, myth, reality: The black family in one-half century of research.* Westport, CT: Greenwood.

Everett, F., Proctor, N., & Cartmell, B. (1983). Providing psychological services to American Indian children and families. *Professional Psychology: Research and Practice, 14,* 588–603.

Fabrega, H., Ulrich, R., & Mezzich, J. E. (1993). Do Caucasian and black adolescents differ at psychiatric intake? *Journal of the American Academy of Child and Adolescent Psychiatry, 32,* 407–413.

Frick, P. J., Lahey, B. B., Applegate, B., Kerdyke, L., Ollendick, T., Hynd, G. W., Garfinkel, B., Greenhill, L., Beiderman, J., Barkley, R. A., McBurnett, K., Newcorn, J., & Waldman, I. (1994). DSM-IV field trials for the disruptive behavior disorders: Symptom utility estimates. *Journal of the American Academy of Child and Adolescent Psychiatry, 33,* 529–539.

Gad, M., & Johnson, J. (1980). Correlates of adolescent life stress as related to race, SES, and levels of perceived social support. *Journal of Clinical Psychology, 9,* 13–16.

Geisinger, K. F. (1994). Cross-cultural normative assessment: Translation and adaptation issues influencing the normative interpretation of assessment instruments. *Psychological Assessment, 6,* 304–312.

Geller, J. D. (1988). Racial bias in the evaluation of patients for psychotherapy. In L. Comas-Diaz & E. E. H. Griffith (Eds.), *Clinical guidelines in cross-cultural mental health* (pp. 112–134). New York: Wiley.

Gittelman, R. (1985). The use of psychological tests in clinical practice with children. In D. Shaffer, A. A. Ehrhardt, & L. L. Greenhill (Eds.), *The clinical guide to child psychiatry* (pp. 447–474). New York: Free Press.

Green, S. B., & Kelley, C. K. (1988). Racial bias in prediction with the MMPI for a juvenile delinquent population. *Journal of Personality Assessment, 52,* 263–275.

Hall, L., & Tucker, C. (1985). Relationships between ethnicity, conceptions of mental illness, and attitudes associated with seeking psychological help. *Psychological Reports, 57,* 907–916.

Harrison, S. I., McDermott, J. F., Wilson, P. T., & Schrager, J. (1965). Social class and mental illness in children. *Archives of General Psychiatry, 13,* 411–417.

Hass, R. G., Katz, I., Rizzo, N., Bailey, J., & Moore, L. (1992). When racial ambivalence evokes negative affects, using a disguised measure of mood. *Personality and Social Psychology Bulletin, 18,* 786–797.

Hembree, R. (1988). Correlates, causes, effects, and treatment of test anxiety. *Review of Educational Research, 58,* 47–77.

Horn, W. F., & Haynes, S. N. (1981). An investigation of sex bias in behavioral observations and ratings. *Behavioral Assessment, 3,* 173–183.

Hutton, J. B., Dubes, R., & Muir, S. (1992). Assessment practices of school psychologists: Ten years later. *School Psychology Review, 21,* 271–284.

Jenson, A. R. (1980). *Bias in mental testing.* New York: Free Press.

Johnston, L. D., Bachman, J. G., & O'Malley, P. M. (1986). *Monitoring the future: Questionnaire responses for the nation's high school seniors, 1985.* Ann Arbor: University of Michigan, Institute for Social Research.

Kaplan, S. L., & Busner, J. (1992). A note on racial bias in the admission of children and adolescents to state mental health facilities versus correctional facilities in New York. *American Journal of Psychiatry, 149,* 768–772.

Katz, I., Robinson, J. M., Epps, E. G., & Waly, P. (1964). The influence of the experimenter and instructions upon the expression of hostility by Negro boys. *Journal of Social Issues, 20,* 339–347.

Kim, L. S., & Chun, C. A. (1993). Ethnic differences in psychiatric diagnosis among Asian American adolescents. *Journal of Nervous and Mental Disease, 181,* 612–617.

Kirmayer, L. J. (1994). Suicide among Canadian aboriginal peoples. *Transcultural Psychiatric Research Review, 31,* 3–58.

Kline, R. B., & Lachar, D. (1992). Evaluation of age, sex, and race bias in the Personality Inventory for Children (PIC). *Psychological Assessment, 4,* 333–339.

Kopp, C. B., & Kaler, S. R. (1989). Risk in infancy: Origins and implications. *American Psychologist, 44,* 224–230.

Koss-Chioino, J. D., & Vargas, L. A. (1992). Through the cultural looking glass: A model for understanding culturally responsive psychotherapies. In L. A. Vargas & J. D. Koss-Chioino (Eds.), *Working with culture: Psychotherapeutic interventions with ethnic minority children and adolescents* (pp. 1–22). San Francisco: Jossey-Bass.

Kvernmo, S., & Heyerdahl, S. (1998). Influence of ethnic factors on behavior problems in indigenous Sami and majority Norwegian adolescents. *Journal of the American Academy of Child and Adolescent Psychiatry, 37,* 743–751.

Lachar, D., & Gdowski, C. L. (1979). *Actuarial assessment of child and adolescent personality: An alternative guide for the Personality Inventory for Children.* Los Angeles: Western Psychological Services.

Ladner, J. A. (1971). Growing up black. In J. H. Williams (Ed.), *Psychology of women: Selected readings* (pp. 2123–2124). New York: Norton.

Larry P. v. Riles, 343 F. Supp. 1306 (N. D. Cal. 1979).

Lethermon, V. R., Williamson, D. A., Moody, S. C., & Wozniak, P. (1986). Racial bias in behavioral assessment of children's social skills. *Journal of Psychopathology and Behavioral Assessment, 8,* 329–337.

Leung, K., & Drasgow, F. (1986). Relation between self esteem and delinquent behavior in three ethnic groups. *Journal of Cross-Cultural Psychology, 17,* 151–167.

Lewis, D. O., Balla, D. A., & Shanok, S. S. (1979). Some evidence of race bias in the diagnosis and treatment of the juvenile offender. *American Journal of Orthopsychiatry, 49,* 53–61.

Lewis, D. O., & Shanok, S. S. (1977). Medical histories of delinquent and nondelinquent children: An epidemiological study. *American Journal of Psychiatry, 134,* 1020–1025.

Lewis, D. O., Shanok, S. S., Cohen, R. J., Kligfeld, M., & Frisone, G. (1980). Race bias in the diagnosis and disposition of violent adolescents. *American Journal of Psychiatry, 137,* 1211–1216.

López, S. R. (1989). Patient variable biases in clinical judgment: Conceptual overview and methodological considerations. *Psychological Bulletin, 106,* 184–203.

López, S. R., & Nuñez, J. A. (1987). The consideration of cultural factors in selected diagnostic criteria and interview schedules. *Journal of Abnormal Psychology, 96,* 270–272.

Loring, M., & Powell, B. (1988). Gender, race, and DSM-III: A study of the objectivity of psychiatric diagnostic behavior. *Journal of Health and Social Behavior, 29,* 1–22.

Malgady, R. G., Costantino, G., & Rogler, L. H. (1984). Development of a Thematic Apperception Test (TEMAS) for urban Hispanic children. *Journal of Consulting and Clinical Psychology, 52,* 986–996.

Malgady, R. G., Rogler, L. H., & Costantino, G. (1987). Ethnocultural and linguistic bias in mental health evaluation of Hispanics. *American Psychologist, 42,* 228–234.

Mann, E. M., Ikeda, Y., Mueller, C. W., Takahashi, A., Tao, K. T., Humris, E., Li, B. L., & Chin, D. (1993). Cross-cultural differences in rating hyperactive–disruptive behaviors in children. *American Journal of Psychiatry, 149,* 1539–1542.

Manson, S. M., Ackerson, L. M., Dick, R. W., Baron, A. E., & Fleming, C. M. (1990). Depressive symptoms among American Indian adolescents: Psychometric characteristics of the Center for Epidemiologic Studies Depression Scale (CES-D). *Psychological Assessment, 2,* 231–237.

McKenry, P. (1987). Drug abuse. In Consortium for Research on Black Adolescence (Ed.), *Black adolescence: Topical summaries and annotated bibliographies of research* (pp. 37–49). Storrs: University of Connecticut, School of Family Studies. (ERIC Document Reproduction Service No. ED 285 924)

McKenry, P., Everett, J. E., Ramseur, H. P., & Carter, C. J. (1989). Research on black adolescents: A legacy of cultural bias. *Journal of Adolescent Research, 4,* 254–264.

McMiller, W. P., & Weisz, J. R. (1996). Help-seeking preceding mental health clinic intake among African-American, Latino, and Caucasian youths. *Journal of the American Academy of Child and Adolescent Psychiatry, 35,* 1086–1094.

Mellsop, G. W., Taumoepeau, B., & Smith, D. A. R. (1993). Mental health services in New Zealand. *International Journal of Mental Health, 22,* 87–100.

Minde, R., & Minde, K. (1995). Socio-cultural determinants of psychiatric symptomatology in James Bay Cree children and adolescents. *Canadian Journal of Psychiatry, 40,* 304–312.

Moran, M. P. (1990). The problem of cultural bias in personality assessment. In C. R. Reynolds & R. W. Kamphaus (Eds.), *Handbook of psychological and educational assessment of children: Personality, behavior, and context* (pp. 524–545). New York: Guilford Press.

Neal, A. M., & Turner, S. M. (1991). Anxiety disorders research with African Americans: Current status. *Psychological Bulletin, 109,* 400–410.

Neighbors, H. (1985). Seeking professional help for personal problems: Black Americans' use of health and mental health services. *Community Mental Health Journal, 21,* 156–166.

Newcomb, M., Huba, G., & Bentler, P. (1981). A multidimensional assessment of stressful life events among adolescents: Derivation and correlates. *Journal of Health and Social Behavior, 22,* 400–414.

Oakland, T., & Feigenbaum, D. (1979). Multiple sources of test bias on the WISC-R and Bender Gestalt test. *Journal of Consulting and Clinical Psychology, 47,* 968–974.

Okazaki, S., & Sue, S. (1995). Methodological issues in assessment research with ethnic minorities. *Psychological Assessment, 7,* 367–375.

Oneil, J. D. (1995). Issues in health-policy for indigenous peoples in Canada. *Australian Journal of Public Health, 19,* 559–566.

Politano, P. M., Nelson, W. M., Evans, H. E., Sorenson, S. B., & Zeman, D. J. (1986). Factor analytic evaluation of differences between black and Caucasian emotionally disturbed children on the Children's Depression Inventory. *Journal of Psychopathology and Behavioral Assessment, 8,* 1–7.

Pryor Brown, L. J., Powell, J., & Earls, F. (1989). Stressful life events and psychiatric symptoms in black adolescent females. *Journal of Adolescent Research, 4,* 140–151.

Raadal, M., Milgrom, P., Cauce, A. M., & Mancl, L. (1994). Behavior problems in 5- to 11-year-old children from low-income families. *Journal of the American Academy of Child and Adolescent Psychiatry, 33*, 1017–1035.

Reynolds, C. R. (1982). The problem of bias in psychological assessment. In C. R. Reynolds & T. B. Gutkin (Eds.), *The handbook of school psychology* (pp. 178–208). New York: Wiley.

Reynolds, C. R., & Brown, R. T. (1984). Bias in mental testing: An introduction to the issues. In C. R. Reynolds & R. T. Brown (Eds.), *Perspectives in bias on mental testing* (pp. 1–40). New York: Plenum Press.

Reynolds, C. R., & Kaiser, S. M. (1990). Test bias in psychological assessment. In T. B. Gutkin & C. R. Reynolds (Eds.), *The handbook of school psychology* (2nd ed., pp. 487–525). New York: Wiley.

Reynolds, C. R., & Paget, K. D. (1981). Factor analysis of the Revised Children's Manifest Anxiety Scale for blacks, whites, males, and females with a national normative sample. *Journal of Consulting and Clinical Psychology, 49*, 352–359.

Reynolds, C. R., & Piersel, W. C. (1983). Multiple aspects of bias on the Boehm Test of Basic Concepts (Forms A & B) for white and Mexican-American children. *Journal of Psychoeducational Assessment, 1*, 17–24.

Reynolds, C. R., Plake, B. S., & Harding, R. E. (1983). Item bias in the assessment of children's anxiety: Race and sex interaction on items on the Revised Children's Manifest Anxiety Scale. *Journal of Psychological Assessment, 1*, 17–24.

Ridley, C. R. (1984). Clinical treatment of the nondisclosing Black client: A therapeutic paradox. *American Psychologist, 39*, 1234–1244.

Roberts, R. E. (1992). Manifestations of depressive symptoms among adolescents: A comparison of Mexican-Americans with the majority and other minority populations. *Journal of Nervous and Mental Disease, 180*, 627–633.

Robins, L. N., Helzer, J. E., Weissman, M. M., Orvaschel, H., Greunberg, E., Burke, J. D., & Regier, D. A. (1984). Lifetime prevalence of specific psychiatric disorders in three sites. *Archives of General Psychiatry, 41*, 949–958.

Rogler, L. H. (1992). The role of culture in mental health diagnosis: The need for programmatic research. *Journal of Nervous and Mental Disease, 180*, 745–747.

Rogler, L. H., Barreras, O., & Satana-Cooney, R. (1981). Coping with distrust in a study of intergenerational Puerto Rican families in New York City. *Hispanic Journal of Behavioral Sciences, 3*, 1–17.

Rosado, J. W. (1986). Toward an interfacing of Hispanic cultural variables with school psychology service delivery systems. *Professional Psychology: Research and Practice, 17*, 191–199.

Rosnow, R. L., & Rosenthal, R. (1996). *Beginning behavioral research: A conceptual primer* (2nd ed.). Englewood Cliffs, NJ: Prentice-Hall.

Sameroff, A., & Chandler, M. (1975). Reproductive risk and the continuum of caretaking casualty. In F. Horowitz (Ed.), *Review of child development research* (Vol. 4, pp. 187–244). Chicago: University of Chicago Press.

Sata, L. (1990, April). *Working with persons with Asian backgrounds.* Paper presented at the Cross-Cultural Psychotherapy Conference, Hahnemann University, Philadelphia.

Schuman, H., Converse, J. M., Singer, E., Frankel, M. R., Glassman, M. B., Groves, R. M., Magilavy, L. J., Miller, P. V., & Cannell, C. F. (1989). The interviewer. In E. Singer & S. Presser (Eds.), *Survey research methods: A reader* (pp. 247–323). Chicago: University of Chicago Press.

Snowden, L., & Cheung, F. (1990). Use of inpatient mental health services by members of ethnic minority groups. *American Psychologist, 45,* 347–355.

Spring, C., Blundern, D., Greenberg, L. M., & Yellin, A. M. (1977). Validity and norms of a hyperactivity rating scale. *Journal of Special Education, 2,* 313–321.

Staggers, B. (1987). Health care issues of black adolescents. In R. Jones (Ed.), *Black adolescents* (pp. 99–122). Berkeley, CA: Cobb & Henry.

Sterling, S., Cowen, E. L., Weissberg, R. P., Lotyczewski, B. S., & Boike, M. (1985). Recent stressful life events and young children's school adjustment. *American Journal of Community Psychology, 31,* 87–98.

Sue, D., & Sue, S. (1987). Cultural factors in the clinical assessment of Asian Americans. *Journal of Consulting and Clinical Psychology, 55,* 479–487.

Sue, S. (1988). Psychotherapeutic services for ethnic minorities. *American Psychologist, 43,* 301–308.

Sue, S., Fujino, H., & Takeuchi, D. (1991). Community mental health services for ethnic minority groups: A test of the cultural responsiveness hypothesis. *Journal of Community and Clinical Psychology, 59,* 533–538.

Sue, S., & Zane, N. (1987). The role of culture and cultural techniques in psychotherapy: A critique and reformulation. *American Psychologist, 42,* 37–45.

Takeuchi, D., Bui, K., & Kim, L. (1993). The referral of minority adolescents to community mental health centers. *Journal of Health and Social Behavior, 34,* 153–164.

Tao, K. T. (1992). Hyperactivity and attention deficit disorder syndromes in China. *Journal of the American Academy of Child and Adolescent Psychiatry, 31,* 1165–1166.

Turner, S. M., Beidel, D., & Costello, A. (1987). Psychopathology in the offspring of anxiety disorder patients. *Journal of Consulting and Clinical Psychology, 55,* 229–235.

Vaux, A., & Ruggerio, M. (1983). Stressful life change and delinquent behavior. *American Journal of Community Psychology, 11,* 169–183.

Vega, W. A., & Rumbaut, R. G. (1991). Ethnic minorities and mental health. *Annual Review of Sociology, 17,* 351–383.

Ward, C. I., & McFall, R. M. (1986). Further validation of the Problem Inventory for Adolescent Girls: Comparing Caucasian and black delinquents and nondelinquents. *Journal of Consulting and Clinical Psychology, 54,* 732–733.

Weissman, M. M., Leckman, J. F., Merikangas, K. R., Gammon, C. D., & Prusoff, B. A. (1984). Depression and anxiety disorders in parents and children. *Archives of General Psychiatry, 41,* 845–852.

Westendorp, F., Brink, K. L., Roberson, M. K., & Ortiz, I. E. (1986). Variables which differentiate placement of adolescents into juvenile justice or mental health systems. *Adolescence, 21,* 23–37.

Zuniga, M. E. (1988). Assessment issues with Chicanas: Practical implications. *Psychotherapy, 25,* 288–293.

IV

BIOLOGICAL MEASURES

✧

12

Sleep and Neuroendocrine Measures

✧

RONALD E. DAHL
LORAH DORN
NEAL D. RYAN

Ideally, measures of sleep and neuroendocrine function can provide windows on the developing brain and opportunities to investigate the neurobiological underpinnings of developmental psychopathology. However, the process of obtaining such psychobiological measures in children can be a methodological quagmire. Our research group, initially under the direction of the late Joaquim Puig-Antich, MD, has performed sleep and neuroendocrine studies in hundreds of children and adolescents over the past decade. The methodologies utilized in our studies have evolved over time, and numerous pragmatic and conceptual issues have proven critical in the performance and interpretation of these studies. This chapter reviews a range of general and specific issues relevant to carrying out and interpreting such investigations.

GENERAL CONCEPTUAL AND METHODOLOGICAL ISSUES

Stress and Adaptation

Sleep and neuroendocrine measures are sensitive to both physiological and psychological stressors. In many situations, however, the process of obtaining these stress-sensitive measures can *produce* stress responses in the children and adolescents being tested. For example, the process of adapting to a new environment, the presence of unfamiliar people who may be perceived as threatening, separation from parents, application of scalp electrodes for electroencephalographic (EEG) measures, the insertion of needles or catheters, or even the collection of saliva or urine can be stressful for children and can directly influence sleep and neuroendocrine measures. Furthermore, there may be complex interactions between perceived stress and psychopathology. For example, a child with an anxiety disorder may experience a threatening procedure quite differently than a child with conduct disorder may. Adaptation effects and inpatient status can further complicate these issues. That is, outpatients and normal controls undergo different adaptational sequences (coming from their home environments), compared to inpatients who have already adjusted to a hospital setting over days to weeks. Finally, maturational influences can also show complex interactions in the domain of adaptation effects and subjective stressors. Even 1 to 2 years of maturation can result in a significant change in a child's subjective experience of procedures and setting. Thus these studies require careful attention to psychological experiences of perceived threat including adaptation to place, people, and procedures; separation from families; anticipatory anxiety; previous experience; individual behaviors related to the procedures; and maturational influences.

Age and Pubertal Effects

Normal maturation results in rapid changes in both subjective and physiological domains, and these affect sleep and neuroendocrine function across childhood and adolescence. EEG sleep measures can change 40% across adolescence, while neuroendocrine axes regulating growth and reproductive function also undergo dramatic and categorical changes over these ages. Children are growing rapidly in physical size, with significant alteration of metabolic rate, body mass index, and distribution of fluid spaces. Furthermore, brain changes involved in pubertal maturation can precede (by years) the physical changes of puberty. Therefore, biological measures must be carefully controlled with respect to age and pubertal maturation. The effects of age and maturation may be as large as or larger than those of diagnostic category; thus inclusion of the former effects in the data-analytic model is crucial.

Sleep–Wake Schedules

Sleep–wake schedules represent complex and important methodological issues for studies of sleep and neuroendocrine function. Many children and adolescents follow erratic schedules, which can shift dramatically on weekends and vacations compared to school nights. Furthermore, many adolescents appear to be relatively sleep-deprived because of their social schedules (Carskadon, 1990), independent of their biological needs for sleep. A basic methodological question is whether to use a child's or adolescent's "usual home sleep schedule" or to impose a uniform schedule across subjects. Either choice creates methodological difficulties: If the investigator imposes the same schedule across all subjects, then this must be done for at least 1–2 weeks to permit adaptation to the new schedule and realignment of sleep and neurobiological rhythms. Moreover, this method does not take into account possible individual differences in total sleep requirements. The alternative strategy of the "usual home sleep schedule" results in subjects' being studied while sleeping at different clock times, and creates the possibility of studying children and adolescents who are obtaining suboptimal total sleep or following nonoptimal schedules. This methodology also creates the opportunity for erroneous group differences when inpatient samples are being studied. That is, inpatients have adapted to a uniform ward schedule that often includes earlier bedtimes and wake-up times (and possibly longer total sleep times) than children and adolescents may follow at home.

For all of the statements above regarding sleep, similar problems exist for neuroendocrine studies, since both sleep and circadian influences are critical to the regulation of (HPA) axis, growth hormone (GH), prolactin, and many others. Although the best methodological approach to this complex issue continues to be debated among researchers, the critical factor is that the investigator specify the methodological details used in a particular protocol and include analyses to address these issues (e.g., including important covariates in the statistical analyses, aligning data by sleep onset as well as clock time).

Catheters and Blood Sampling

For the large majority of children undergoing psychobiological studies, the most difficult aspect of these studies is the insertion of needles to obtain blood samples. Since repeated blood samples are invariably necessary to profile neuroendocrine status, there are two strategies: repeated venipunctures or an indwelling intravenous (IV) catheter. In our experience, even three venipunctures are considerably more stressful than the indwelling catheter (Dahl, Kaufman, et al., 1992). A major difficulty with repeated venipunctures is *anticipatory anxiety*. That is, children have one painful procedure and then know that more are coming; as a result, anxiety often escalates before each subsequent venipuncture. On the other hand, if an indwelling catheter is placed at the beginning (or *before* the psychobiological studies are performed), children can adapt to the painless IV catheter if it permits free range of motion and normal activities. Such an approach is usually not physically or psychologically distressing.

Thus our strategy for most psychobiological protocols is to place the indwelling catheter in an antecubital vein as carefully and painlessly as possible, prior to the *initiation* of the studies. The procedure requires patience and flexibility (talking to children, reassuring them, giving them a sense of control, letting them know that they can stop the procedure at any point) so as not to overwhelm the children. Specifically, (1) we explain each step before it is performed; (2) we explain that in our experience, most children tell us that the worst part of the procedure is not the needle insertion but the "worrying about it before it happens," and that by the time it hurts, the procedure is over; and (3) we explain as soon as the needle breaks the skin, the plastic tubing is advanced and the needle is withdrawn, leaving only the plastic catheter in place. In over 90% of the cases, the children agree that the anticipatory fear was worse than the actual pain.

Once the catheter is in place, there are a number of methodological issues concerning the maintenance of the catheter, including flow and patency through the catheter, safety with regard to infection and leakage, and the methodology of withdrawing blood for samples. Although adult studies often use continuous (slow) pump withdrawal, it has been our experience that in children and adolescents (who require the utilization of relatively small-bore catheters because of smaller vein size), a continuous-withdrawal pump is unsatisfactory because of frequent clotting of the IV catheter (and because of the stress effects concomitant with reinserting a failed IV). We utilize a continuous slow infusion of heparinized saline with a three-way stop-cock system that permits the easy infusion of medications and withdrawal of individual timed blood samples (Puig-Antich, 1984). We also utilize fairly long tubing (8 feet), with a small blood volume connected to a mobile system (on wheels) that the children can move about during activities, games, and so on. This long tubing permits us to sample from outside the bedroom during sleep as well.

Another critical methodological issue is the "dead space" within the catheter. The standard methodology for dealing with the dead space is to withdraw a larger volume than is in the line through one port on the three-way stop-cock (until the return shows undiluted blood), and then to obtain the blood sample from a proximal port. Recently we evaluated the issue of blood volume draw compared to dead space in a controlled study. We found that it was necessary to draw double the volume of the dead space in order to eliminate dilution of the blood by the infusing solution. Thus, with 4-cc tubing, it was necessary to withdraw 8 cc to be certain that the blood sample did not have some dilution. These results conform to other published findings (Preusser et al., 1989).

Total Blood Volume

Another issue regarding blood sampling in small children concerns guidelines of a reasonable amount of blood volume to be withdrawn without causing health consequences. Often this forces investigative teams to set priorities and use creative strategies to obtain sufficient blood volumes for 24-hour blood levels of multiple hormones and for poststimulation tests. In addition, it becomes crucial to have assay procedures that can be performed reliably with extremely small blood volumes, to balance the needs for the previous constraints.

Assays and Blood Samples

A review of assay procedures to measure hormone levels is beyond the scope of this chapter. There are various techniques to measure substances in small amounts in blood and serum; each requires specific methodologies and sample handling, such as coating tubes with proper substances and preservatives, keeping tubes at a certain temperature, centrifuging, pipetting techniques, and super-freezing to permit multiple samples to be run in the same assay. The specific methodologies must be outlined in complete detail, in conjunction with the laboratory performing the actual assays.

Salivary Methods

An alternative to indwelling catheters and blood handling is to measure hormones in saliva. For at least two reasons, salivary sampling has been a particularly appealing methodology for researchers interested in biology and behavior. First, it provides a noninvasive method of sampling that can be used in the field (outside specialized clinical facilities) and without highly trained technicians to collect the samples. Second, particularly when stress-sensitive hormones are being studied, saliva sampling presumably provides a better "baseline" or prestress measure than does venipuncture. This latter point may be important when investigators are examining reactivity to various stress paradigms, such as mental challenges (Bohnen, Nicolson, Sulon, & Jolles, 1991); conflict tasks (Granger, Weisz, & Kauneckis, 1994); novelty and challenge (Dorn, Susman, & Petersen, 1993); and combined social and cognitive challenges, such as those involved in the Trier Social Stress Test for both adults and children (Buske-Kirschbaum et al., 1997; Kirschbaum, Pirke, & Hellhammer, 1993). Whether or not salivary cortisol reflects the same trajectory as serum cortisol in all stress paradigms is less clear. For example, in our laboratory, significant rises in serum cortisol in response to a stressor were generally reflected in salivary cortisol measures; however, the cortisol nadir (often of greatest interest in relation to psychopathology; Dahl, 1991) was not reflected accurately by salivary measures.

Collection and measurement of salivary hormones can be challenging. Various methodologies are utilized to gather saliva, including spitting directly in a tube, soaking cotton rolls inserted in the side of the mouth, or inserting a sialistic capsule into the mouth. Each has its own limitation. Additional concerns in saliva sample collection include the consideration of activities prior to collection. For example, teething in infants (Hertsgaard, Gunnar, Carson, Brodersen, & Lehman, 1992) or toothbrushing can alter the saliva cortisol concentration, as blood may then appear in the collection. Blood and/or food contaminants can alter the assay results (Ellison, 1988). In addition, breast milk or infant formula can affect the assay (Magnano, Diamond, & Gardner, 1989), along with such oral stimulants as drink mix crystals (Schwartz, Granger, Susman, Gunnar, & Laird, 1998). Other methodological issues in the collection of saliva have been reviewed elsewhere (Ellison, 1988; Gunnar, 1992; Schwartz et al., 1998).

Unfortunately, not all hormones can be measured in saliva because of properties of the hormones themselves (e.g., lower concentrations in saliva) and/or properties of saliva or the assay. Because a saliva hormone concentration represents the free concentration of the hormone compared to the total concentration (bound plus free) in serum, the quantities are lower in saliva (Ellison, 1988). For example, the concentration of cortisol in saliva represents about one-fifth the concentration of the serum concentration. With these lower concentrations in saliva, some assays are not sensitive enough to measure some hormones in saliva. This, however, is not the case for cortisol, as saliva cortisol measurement has received the most attention in the literature (see Kirschbaum, Read, & Hellhammer, 1992, and Kirschbaum & Hellhammer, 1994, for multiple references). In addition, some hormones cannot be measured in saliva because acidic properties of saliva interfere with the assay. Modifications of the radioimmunoassay kit also may require larger quantities of the saliva sample, which may not be feasible in some subjects (e.g., infants). New methods such as enzyme immunoassay have addressed the problem and use smaller sample sizes and detect lower concentrations, hence providing a useful methodology for future research (http://www.salvmetrics.com).

Hormones other than cortisol can be measured in saliva (for a summary, see Kirschbaum et al., 1992). For example, measurement of testosterone in saliva has been shown to be reliable, and its use in the research arena has been extensive (Dabbs, Jurkovic, & Frady, 1991; Dabbs, 1991; Schaal, Tremblay, Soussignan, & Susman, 1996; Scerbo & Kolko, 1994). Other hormones that have been measured in saliva (but infrequently) include dehydroepiandrosterone (Swinkels, Ross, Smals, & Benraad, 1990), androstenedione (Baxendale & James, 1984; Swinkels, van Hoff, Ross, Smals, & Benraad, 1992), estradiol (Lipson & Ellison, 1996; Worthman, Stallings, & Hofman, 1990), progesterone (Evans, 1986; Lipson & Ellison, 1996), and melatonin (Clemons, Geffen, Otto, Pratt, & Harker, 1996). The key to initially determining the validity of measurement in saliva is comparing the serum and saliva concentrations of the hormone. Again, in this regard, corticol has received the most attention in the literature. Correlations range from high to modest.

Sample collection must be carefully thought out, and the research laboratory must have significant expertise in salivary assays. Clearly, additional methodological studies are necessary to test whether salivary measure can reliably capture the small differences in hormone secretion patterns that are necessary for research paradigms.

Urine Measures

An additional approach to blood and serum sampling has been the measurement of urine metabolites. This is a complex methodology for at least three reasons. First, in children and even adolescents, it can be quite difficult to collect all urine samples reliably. Although it may seem surprising compared to the already described difficulties with obtaining blood and saliva, both we and other investigators have found that it is often more difficult to obtain complete urine collection. The reasons include loss of samples secondary to bedwetting, missing samples, and the difficulties of storing and handling large volumes of urine. Second, although urine measures provide relatively inexpensive integrated measures of hormone production, they generally lack temporal precision. Third, there are often complexities regarding metabolites in the urine and how accurately they reflect serum levels of particular hormonal substances.

Child Management

As mentioned above in regard to dealing with stress and adaptation, the particular environment, staff, and procedures have a large effect on these measures. Similarly, there are complex methodological decisions regarding limit setting, selection of activities, dealing with conflicts and difficulties, family visitation, and oppositional behavior. The way the staff handles bedtime, bedtime struggles, children's anxiety, child–child interactions, and child–family interactions will have direct effects on sleep and hormone measures. A delicate balance must be reached between setting consistent and firm limits on the one hand, and permitting sufficient flexibility, freedom to select activities, encouraging family visitation, and permitting some social interaction on the other. Key factors in our experience include specific and detailed protocols; enthusiastic, well-trained staff members who are experienced in dealing with children with psychopathology; and carefully documented logs describing individual behaviors and unusual events.

SPECIFIC MEASURES AND TESTS

EEG Measures of Sleep

The traditional measures of sleep utilize three sets of electrophysiological channels: EEG, electro-oculographic (for eye movements), and electromyographic (for muscle tone). The patternings of these three sets of channels are used to designate specific stages of sleep according to consensus conventions (Rechtschaffen & Kales, 1968). Night recordings are scored in 30- or 60-second intervals, and the following are noted: sleep latency (time to official sleep onset), rapid-eye-movement (REM) latency (time from sleep onset to the beginning of the first REM period), and the amounts and percentages of individual sleep stages (1, 2, 3, and 4 and REM). Stages 3 and 4 are often combined under the heading of delta or slow wave sleep. The amount of wakefulness after sleep onset is also calculated and contributes to the calculation of such variables as sleep efficiency or sleep maintenance, which indicates the percentage of the recording period (from lights out to wake-up time) or of sleep time (from sleep onset to wake-up time) that was spent asleep.

One critical issue influencing many of these variables is the process of falling asleep. In particular, the many details of handling a child at bedtime in a sleep laboratory—sleeping with wires, sleeping in an unfamiliar environment, the presence or absence of parents, the use of transitional objects, and the need for a sense of safety—are critical factors in the physiological process of sleep (since sleep is in essence a "turning off" of the vigilance system). Children's protest behaviors, oppositional behaviors, and fears can all directly influence the timing of lights out and onset of sleep. Thus many of the most important dependent variables require consistency in the behavioral realm in dealing with children at bedtime. On the other hand, inflexibility can also cause significant problems interfering with bedtime and sleep latency. Furthermore, as discussed in earlier sections, the particular issues change across the maturational dimension and are quite different for a 6-year-old, 12-year-old, and an 18-year-old.

So, as described earlier, issues of adaptation can also be major sources of variance. One strategy is to record for two or more nights, while children become accustomed to the wires, environment, staff members, and so forth. A typical strategy is to use a second or third, in the laboratory to calculate baseline summary sleep variables. It is difficult to generalize about the best strategy for obtaining "baseline" measures. An important conceptual issue is to obtain sufficient data for actively examining adaptation effects relevant to the specific sample of subjects with a particular laboratory and procedure, as there appears to be considerable individual variance in adaptation (Dahl et al., 1990).

Another issue our research group has examined specifically is adaptation of EEG sleep measures in children and adolescents sleeping with a indwelling catheter (Dahl et al., 1996). In a controlled study using a within-subject design of five young adolescents studied for five consecutive nights with and without an IV catheter in place, we found that the catheter's effects on sleep were negligible by the second night. That is, the adaptation to sleeping with EEG wires and an IV catheter is exactly parallel to adapting to the EEG wires alone. These data supported our present approach—that is, inserting the IV catheter at the beginning of the study, to permit subjects to adapt to the laboratory conditions completely in the knowledge that the threatening, "painful" procedure is over—rather than an earlier design of introducing the catheter on the last day and night of the study.

Sleep Challenge Tests

A different approach to sleep measures is to challenge the sleep system. One such strategy is the use of cholinergic agonists, which have been used in many adult studies; IV infusion of arecoline has been used in one study of depressed and control children (Dahl et al., 1994). A similar strategy is the use of scopolamine, an anticholinergic agent (Poland, Tondo, Rubin, Trelease, & Lesser, 1989). Another alternative strategy is to challenge the sleep system with sleep deprivation or restriction protocols, and subsequently to measure recovery sleep (Dahl et al., 1996; Naylor et al., 1993). Yet another strategy is to measure threshold of arousal during sleep as a challenge technique (Busby & Pivik, 1983).

Although a thorough review and critique of these approaches is beyond the scope of this chapter, the main issue is the need for a well-formulated question regarding sleep physiology or sleep measures. The particular question being asked about the regulation of sleep will then drive methodological decisions concerning the particular type of protocol that will best address the question.

Baseline Neuroendocrine Measures

Baseline measures of hormone secretion patterns have been used in numerous adult studies in attempts to quantify neuroendocrine regulation. This strategy employs frequent sampling across the circadian cycle to characterize the details of hormone secretion. A typical example is obtaining 24-hour patterns of cortisol or adrenocorticotropic hormone (ACTH) to characterize the HPA axis. There are critical decisions concerning the frequency and the timing of sampling that will best characterize the underlying hormone pattern. The secretory (pulse frequency) and half-life of the substance being measured will influence the decision concerning optimal frequency of measurement. On the other hand, in children and adolescents, the total permissible blood volume that may be withdrawn limits the total number of samples that may be used to characterize the hormonal pattern.

Furthermore, there are often times of particular interest that should be examined (sleep onset, sleep offset, meals, etc.). For example, cortisol and ACTH appear to have a physiologically quiescent period preceding and following sleep onset. The interaction between sleep onset and the HPA axis is of particular interest with respect to child and adolescent depression (Dahl, Ryan, et al., 1992); thus we have made careful efforts to measure hormone secretion patterns over shorter intervals of time in this period.

Summary variables to characterize the hormone profile have also been a subject of considerable discussion. Standard programs (Veldhuis et al., 1994) have been used to calculate pulse frequency, pulse amplitude, mean levels, peak levels, nadirs, and so forth. However, relatively simpler approaches—including 24-hour mean, peak, time of maximal rise, length of quiescent period, and mean nadir during the quiescent period—appear to capture the between-group differences seen in many studies.

Neuroendocrine Challenge Tests

As we have discussed above in regard to sleep, an alternative to simply measuring baseline levels is to challenge neuroendocrine regulatory systems to address potential differences in these systems.

A well known strategy is to suppress the axis (e.g., to use dexamethasone to suppress the HPA axis) and then to measure the recovery from suppression. Alternatively, challenge agents such as corticotropin-releasing hormone or GH-releasing hormone (GHRH) can be used to stimulate the axis, and the subsequent output can then be measured.

In the mathematical analysis of hormonal stimulation secondary to a stimuli, the area under the curve (or occasionally this area divided by unit time) is frequently used. Because there are measurement errors in the measurement of physiological data, it is important to use the trapezoidal rule to calculate the area under the curve (which weights the two bounding samples with half the weight as all the interior samples, which are weighted the same) rather than Simpson's approximation (which gives differing weights to adjacent interior samples).

Growth Hormone

There has been considerable interest in the regulation of GH secretion in child and adolescent psychopathology. Dysregulation of GH appears to represent an area of psychobiological continuity between child and adult forms of depressive disorders. Various pharmacological challenge agents that stimulate the release of GH have been used, including GHRH, clonidine, and in older studies insulin-induced hypoglycemia, with the primary outcome measure being the amount of GH secretion in response (Ryan et al., 1994). However, the control of GH secretion is complicated; adequate assessment of this axis may require more than just measuring GH secretion, including examination of GHRH release and basal somatomedin-C levels. In addition, growth velocity in children should be assessed to obtain a longer-term integrated view of this system. Figure 12.1 is a schematic outline of the control and feedback loops involved in this system.

Serotonergic Probes

Specific studies of serotonin in mood disorders are particularly interesting, because of the very strong and well-replicated link between decreased sero-

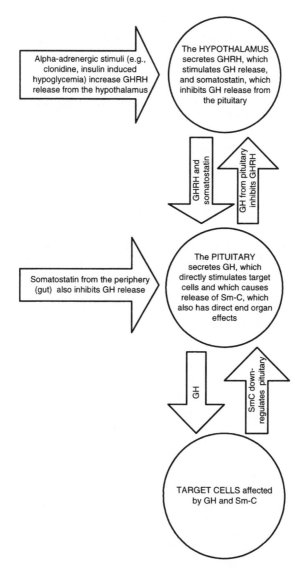

FIGURE 12.1. Control and feedback loops involved in growth hormone (GH) secretion. GHRH, GH-releasing hormone; SmC, somatomedin-C.

tonin turnover and suicide. In addition, serotonin appears to be strongly involved in the control of multiple somatic functions that are dysregulated during depression (e.g., sleep, feeding, locomotor activity, and aggression). Pharmacological agents that stimulate central serotonergic systems cause a release
of prolactin and/or cortisol. Pharmacological agents that have been studied

in adults with major depressive disorder include precursors of serotonin, such as tryptophan and 5-hydroxytryptophan; direct agonists, such as quipazine, meta-chlorophenylpiperazine (MCPP), and ipsapirone; reuptake blockers; and, best studied, the indirect agonist fenfluramine. As discussed elsewhere (Ryan et al., 1992), all currently available agents present compromises. One study thus far has used L–5-hydroxytryptophan as a pharmacological challenge in children with major depressive disorder (Ryan et al., 1992), and that study found abnormalities in cortisol and prolactin stimulation exactly paralleling those seen in adults.

CONCLUSIONS

Measures of sleep and neuroendocrine function have, over the past two decades, shed considerable light on mood and other disorders throughout the life span. Obtaining such measures in children and adolescents presents special methodological problems, which must be given careful consideration and attention if accurate and reliable data area to be obtained and if the experience is to be a positive one for the young subjects.

REFERENCES

Baxendale, P. M., & James, V. H. T. (1984). Specificity of androgen measurements in saliva. In G. F. Read, D. Fiad-Fahmy, R. F. Walker, & K. Griffiths (Eds.), *Immunoassays of steroids in saliva* (pp. 228–237). Cardiff, UK: Alpha Omega.

Bohnen, N., Nicolson, N., Sulon, J., & Jolles, J. (1991). Coping style, trait anxiety and cortisol reactivity during mental stress. *Journal of Psychosomatic Research, 35,* 141–147.

Busby, K., & Pivik, R. T. (1983). Failure of high intensity auditory stimuli to affect behavioral arousal in children during the first sleep cycle. *Pediatric Research, 17*(10), 802–805.

Buske-Kirschbaum, A., Jobst, S., Wustmans, A., Kirschbaum, C., Raugh, W., & Hellhammer, D. (1997). Attenuated free cortisol response to psychosocial stress in children with atopic dermatitis. *Psychosomatic Medicine, 59,* 419–426.

Carskadon, M. A. (1990). Patterns of sleep and sleepiness in adolescents. *Pediatrician, 17,* 5–12.

Clemons, A. A., Geffen, J. F., Otto, J. M., Pratt, K. L., & Harker, C. T. (1996). Dithiothreitol treatment permits measurement of melatonin in otherwise unusable saliva samples. *Journal of Pineal Research, 10,* 21–23.

Dabbs, J. M., Jr. (1991). Salivary testosterone measurements: Collecting, storing, and mailing saliva samples. *Physiology and Behavior, 49,* 815–817.

Dabbs, J. M., Jr., Jurkovic, G. J., & Frady, R. L. (1991). Salivary testosterone and cortisol among late adolescent male offenders. *Journal of Abnormal Child Psychiatry, 19,* 469–478.

Dahl, R. E., Kaufman, J., Ryan, N. D., Perel, J., Al-Shabbout, M., Birmaher, B., Nelson,

B., & Puig-Antich, J. (1992). The dexamethasone suppression test in children and adolescents: A review and a controlled study. *Biological Psychiatry, 32,* 109–126.

Dahl, R. E., Puig-Antich, J., Ryan, N. D., Nelson, B., Dachille, S., Cunningham, S., Trubnick, L., & Klepper, T. (1990). EEG sleep in adolescents with major depression: The role of suicidality and inpatient status. *Journal of Affective Disorders, 19,* 63–75.

Dahl, R. E., Ryan, N. D., Matty, M., Birmaher, B., Al-Shabbout, M., Williamson, D. E., & Kupfer, D. J. (1996). Sleep onset abnormalities in depressed adolescents. *Biological Psychiatry, 39*(6), 400–410.

Dahl, R. E., Ryan, N. D., Perel, J., Birmaher, B., Al-Shabbout, M., Nelson, B., & Puig-Antich, J. (1994). Cholinergic REM induction test with arecoline in depressed children. *Psychiatry Research, 51,* 269–282.

Dahl, R. E., Ryan, N. D., Puig-Antich, J., Nguyen, N. A., Al-Shabbout, M., Meyer, V. A., & Perel, J. (1991). 24-hour cortisol measures in adolescents with major depression: A controlled study. *Biological Psychiatry, 30,* 25–36.

Dahl, R. E., Ryan, N. D., Williamson, D. E., Ambrosini, P. J., Rabinovich, H., Novacenko, H., Nelson, B., & Puig-Antich, J. (1992). The regulation of sleep and growth hormone in adolescent depression. *Journal of the American Academy of Child and Adolescent Psychiatry, 31*(4), 615–621.

Dorn, L. D., Susman, E. J., & Petersen, A. C. (1993). Cortisol reactivity and anxiety and depression in pregnant adolescents: A longitudinal perspective. *Journal of Psychoneuroendocrinology, 18,* 219–239.

Ellison, P. T. (1988). Human salivary steroids: Methodological considerations and applications in physical anthropology. *Yearbook of Physical Anthropology, 31,* 115–142.

Evans, J. J. (1986). Progesterone in saliva does not parallel unbound progesterone in plasma. *Clinical Chemistry, 31,* 542–544.

Granger, D. A., Weisz, J. R., & Kauneckis, D. (1994). Neuroendocrine reactivity to parent–child conflict, internalizing behavior problems, and control-related beliefs in clinic-referred youngsters. *Journal of Abnormal Psychology, 103,* 267–276.

Gunnar, M. R. (1992). Reactivity of the hypothalamic–pituitary–adrenocortical system to stressors in normal infants and children. *Pediatrics, 90*(3), 491–497.

Hertsgaard, L., Gunnar, M. R., Larson, M., Brodersen, L., & Lehman, H. (1992). First time experiences in infancy: When they appear to be pleasant, do they activate the adrenocorticl stress response? *Developmental Psychobiology, 25,* 319–333.

Kirschbaum, C., & Hellhammer, D. H. (1994). Salivary cortisol in psychoneuroendocrine research: Recent developments and applications. *Psychoneuroendocrinology, 19,* 313–333.

Kirschbaum, C., Pirke, K. M., & Hellhammer, D. H. (1993). The "Tier Social Stress Test": A tool for investigating psychobiological stress responses in a laboratory setting. *Neuropsychobiology, 28,* 76–81.

Kirschbaum, C., Read, G. F., & Hellhammer, D. H. (1992). *Assessment of hormones and drugs in saliva in biobehavioral research.* Seattle: Hogrefe & Huber.

Lipson, S. F., & Ellison, P. T. (1996). Comparison of salivary steroid profiles in naturally occurring conception and non-conception cycles. *Human Reproduction, 11,* 2090–2096.

Magnano, C. L., Diamond, E. J., & Gardner, J. M. (1989). Use of salivary cortisol measurements in young infants: A note of caution. *Child Development, 60,* 1099–1101.

Naylor, M. W., King, C. A., Lindsay, K. A., Evans, T., Armelagos, J., Shain, B. N., & Greden, J. F. (1993). Sleep deprivation in depressed adolescents and psychiatric controls. *Journal of the American Academy of Child and Adolescent Psychiatry, 32*(4), 753–759.

Poland, R. E., Tondo, L., Rubin, R. T., Trelease, R. B., & Lesser, I. M. (1989). Differential effects of scopolamine on nocturnal cortisol secretion, sleep architecture, and REM latency in normal volunteers: Relation to sleep and cortisol abnormalities in depression. *Biological Psychiatry, 25*(4), 403–412.

Preusser, B. A., Lash, J., Stone, K. S., Winningham, M. L., Gonyon, D., & Nickel, J. T. (1989). Quantifying the minimum discard sample required for accurate arterial blood gasses. *Nursing Research, 38*(5), 276–279.

Puig-Antich, J., Goetz, R., Davies, M., Fein, M., Hanlon, C., Chambers, W. J., Tabrizi, M. A., Sachar, E. J., & Weitzman, E. D. (1984). Growth hormone secretion in prepubertal major depressive children. II. Sleep related plasma concentrations during a depressive episode. *Archives of General Psychiatry, 5,* 463–466.

Rechtschaffen, A., & Kales, A. (Eds.). (1968). *A manual of standardized terminology, techniques and scoring system for sleep stages of human subjects.* Los Angeles: UCLA.

Ryan, N. D., Birmaher, B., Perel, J. M., Dahl, R. E., Meyer, V., Al-Shabbout, M., Iyengar, S., & Puig-Antich, J. (1992). Neuroendocrine response to L–5-hydroxytryptophan challenge in prepubertal major depression: Depressed versus normal children. *Archives of General Psychiatry, 49,* 843–851.

Ryan, N. D., Dahl, R. E., Birmaher, B., Williamson, D. E., Iyengar, S., Nelson, B., Puig-Antich, J., & Perel, J. M. (1994). Stimulatory tests of growth hormone secretion in prepubertal major depression: Depressed versus normal children. *Journal of the American Academy of Child and Adolescent Psychiatry, 33,* 824–833.

Scerbo, A. S., & Kolko, D. J. (1994). Salivary testosterone and cortisol in disruptive children: Relationship to aggressive, hyperactive, and internalizing behaviors. *Journal of the American Academy of Child and Adolescent Psychiatry, 33,* 1174–1184.

Schaal, B., Tremblay, R., Soussignan, B., & Susman, E. J. (1996). Male pubertal testosterone linked to high social dominance but low physical aggression: A 7 year longitudinal study. *Journal of the American Academy of Child and Adolescent Psychiatry, 35,* 1322–1330.

Schwartz, E. B., Granger, D. A., Susman, E. J., Gunnar, M. R., & Laird, B. (1998). Assessing salivary cortisol in studies of child development. *Child Development, 69,* 1503–1513.

Swinkels, M. J. W., Ross, H. A., Smals, A. G. H., & Benraad, T. J. (1990). Concentrations of total and free dehydroepiandrosterone in plasma and dehydroepiandrosterone in saliva of normal and hirsute women under basal conditions and during administration of dexamethasone/synthetic corticotropin. *Clinical Chemistry, 36,* 2042–2046.

Swinkels, M. J. W., van Hoff, H. J. C., Ross, H. A., Smals, A. G. H., & Benraad, T. J. (1992). Low ratio of androstenedione to testosterone in plasma and saliva of hirsute women. *Clinical Chemistry, 38,* 1819–1823.

Veldhuis, J. D., & Johnson, M. L. (1994). Analytical methods for evaluating episodic secretory activity within neuroendocrine axes. *Neurosci-Biobehav, 18*(4), 605–612.

Worthman, C. M., Stallings, J. F., & Hofman, L. F. (1990). Sensitive salivary estradiol assay for monitoring ovarian function. *Clinical Chemistry, 36,* 1769–1773.

13

Neurochemical Measures

✧

EDWIN H. COOK, JR.
MARKUS J. P. KRUESI

The first question that one may reasonably ask about the role of neurochemical measures in the assessment of child and adolescent psychopathology is this: What is the relevance of studying molecules when the primary goal of assessment in psychopathology is the study of child and adolescent mental function and behavior? The first reason is that neurochemicals are used in every mental process and behavior. Although normal neurochemical function doesn't guarantee the absence of psychopathology, severely disrupted neurochemical function is certainly a major risk factor for the development of psychopathology. Phenylketonuria (PKU) may be one of the best examples of the application of neurochemistry to identification of an etiologically homogeneous psychopathological syndrome and development of a specific preventative neurochemical intervention (dietary restriction of phenylalanine). All psychopharmacological agents act by modulating neurochemistry. In addition to aiding in the development of preventative and therapeutic strategies for psychopathological syndromes, neurochemical knowledge can inform the study of psychopathology. For example, delineation of the metabolic basis of fragile X syndrome by cytogenetic and, more recently, molecular tools has allowed study of the relatively specific psychopathology associated with this syndrome not only in mentally retarded probands, but in "carriers" (Reiss, Freund, Baumgardner, Abrams, & Denckla, 1995).

When one is thinking about the relationship of neurochemistry to child and adolescent psychopathology, it is important to note whether a neurochemical finding represents a "trait" (a persistent response), a "state" (a response only under certain environmental conditions), or a "scar" (a response that appears only after onset of illness or trauma and then persists). Although answering this question may require study of patients affected with a psychopathological condition and in remission, determining whether a neurochemical finding represents a trait or state may usually be done by examining whether normal children and adolescents vary in the measure over time. For example, whole-blood serotonin (5-hydroxytryptamine, or 5-HT) is a relatively stable measure over time after puberty (McBride et al., 1998), but plasma norepinephrine (NE) levels may double during the performance of mental arithmetic (Mefford et al., 1981). "State" and "trait" are concepts related to "nature" and "nurture." It follows that neurochemical measures may represent effects of nature or nurture, depending on the measure and the conditions of measurement. Therefore, although most people associate neurochemistry with studies of "nature," many neurochemical measures are as responsive to the environment as are self-reports of anxiety and mood. In addition, long-term changes in neurochemical measures representing "scar" may occur after disturbances ranging from metabolic "trauma" (e.g., congenital hypothyroidism) to emotional trauma (e.g., sexual abuse).

SYNAPTIC ORGANIZATION

Any discussion of neurochemistry is premature without a review of basic principles of organization of the nervous system. Although full reviews of this topic are available in several monographs (Jessell, Kandel, Lewin, & Reid, 1993; Siegel, Agranoff, & Albers, 1998), a brief summary is included here, with an emphasis on features relevant to child and adolescent psychopathology. Developmental neurobiology is a broader field of relevance to child and adolescent psychopathology (Purves & Lichtman, 1985; Cook & Leventhal, 1992).

The functional unit of the nervous system is the synapse. Although the cellular unit is the nerve cell, nerve cells have no function in isolation from other nerve cells. The most familiar interaction between nerve cells at a synapse is short-term and anterograde. A neurotransmitter—for example, dopamine—is released from synaptic vesicles after presynaptic neuron excitation. After release, dopamine diffuses through a short distance and binds to a receptor at the postsynaptic neuron—for instance, the D_1 receptor. After dopamine binds to the D_1 receptor, the receptor changes shape and, through interaction with a "heterotrimeric" (composed of three different subunits— α, β, γ) G protein, causes an increase in the activity of the enzyme adenylyl cyclase. Adenylyl cyclase catalyzes the conversion of adenosine trisphosphate (ATP) to the second messenger, cyclic adenosine monophosphate (cAMP). Several cAMP-dependent protein kinases are up-regulated by increased levels of cAMP. These protein kinases (third messengers) phosphorylate several proteins at specific serine and threonine amino acid residues within the postsynaptic neuron, causing an acute (seconds to minutes) change in the activity of the postsynaptic neuron.

In addition to the rapid changes described above, caused by phosphorylation of proteins already present near the neuronal membrane, ligands may cause longer-term (minutes to days) changes in the activity of the cell by altering the synthesis of new proteins. Therefore, one of the most exciting areas of molecular biology of neurons is an understanding of the mechanisms by which binding of ligands on the outside of the cell regulate the expression of genes within the cell. Although only an oversimplified view is within the scope of this chapter, a rudimentary awareness of the two basic mechanisms is necessary. One mechanism is closely related to second-messenger systems, such as cAMP stimulation by D_1 receptors. One of the proteins phosphorylated by a cAMP-dependent protein kinase is cAMP-response-element-binding protein (CREB). CREB, like many proteins, is activated by phosphorylation (Sheng, Thompson, & Greenberg, 1991). It then is able to be translocated from the cytoplasm to the nucleus where it binds to cAMP response element (CRE), a consensus sequence of deoxyribonucleic acid (DNA) found in the regulatory sequences of many genes. After CREB binds to DNA, it activates or represses the transcription of genes such as tyrosine hydroxylase and somatostatin, which are also transcription factor proteins capable of activating or repressing transcription of other genes in the cell (Armstrong & Montminy, 1993). Transcription results in production from DNA code of messenger ribonucleic acid (mRNA), which then serves as a template for the production of proteins (translation) in the postsynaptic neuron.

The two examples above illustrate anterograde neurotransmission from the presynaptic to the postsynaptic neuron. However, there are important retrograde influences of postsynaptic neurons on presynaptic neurons. For example, long-term potentiation (LTP) is a neural phenomenon linked to memory in the hippocampus, in which a stimulus leads to greater postsynaptic output because of changes in both the presynaptic and postsynaptic neurons. The presynaptic neuron releases glutamate, which affects both Na^+ and Ca^{++} ion channels in the postsynaptic neuron (Jessell & Kandel, 1993). Elevation in Ca^{++} ion concentration within the postsynaptic neuron activates calcium-calmodulin-dependent protein kinase, which may increase the activity of nitric oxide synthase. This leads to an increase in nitric oxide, which diffuses back to the presynaptic neuron and increases the likelihood that a stimulus to the presynaptic terminal will result in glutamate release (Snyder, 1992). LTP is felt to be important in development and learning. For example, mice have been bred that do not have calcium-calmodulin-dependent protein kinase, or that have specific mutations altering its regulation. These mice are unable to learn spatial cues and do not have normal hippocampal LTP (Silva, Paylor, Wehner, & Tonegawa, 1992; Silva, Stevens, Tonegawa, & Wang, 1992; Giese, Fedorov, Filipkowski, & Silva, 1998).

The longest-term (days to years) retrograde influence is the effect of protein trophic factors such as nerve growth factor, released by target neurons that bind to receptors in the presynaptic neuron and support the survival of the presynaptic neuron. After several trophic or growth factors bind to their receptors, the receptors often double up to form "homodimers" (proteins composed of two identical subunits) and autophosphorylate on their own tyrosine residues. Subsequently, growth-receptor-factor-binding protein 2 binds to the homodimerized protein and then binds to a protein called "son of sevenless." Son of sevenless then binds to Ras, leading to phosphorylation of Ras within the membrane (Egan et al., 1993; Rozakis-Adcock, Fernley, Wade, Pawson, & Bowtell, 1993). Ras-guanosine triphosphate then phosphorylates Raf (Dickson, Sprenger, Morrison, & Hafen, 1992). Phosphorylated Raf then phosphorylates mitogen-activated protein (MAP) kinase kinase. MAP kinase kinase subsequently phosphorylates MAP kinase, which phosphorylates c-fos, c-myc, and/or c-jun, which regulate transcription of genes (Crews & Erikson, 1993). This transduction system is known to interact with the adenylyl cyclase system mentioned above.

Many current neurochemical researchers remember the recent dogma that there was one neurotransmitter for each neuron. However, cotransmission of more than one neurotransmitter has been demonstrated for several neurons; for example, glutamatergic neurons in the hippocampus often also secrete opiate peptides, such as dynorphin (Wagner, Terman, & Chavkin, 1993). In this example, it appears that glutamate functions as the classic neurotransmitter and induces LTP, whereas dynorphin serves the function of decreasing the activity of neighboring nerve cells (heterosynaptic depression), perhaps to increase the specificity of signaling in a specific pair of neurons.

In addition to neuron–neuron communication, neuron–glial cell relationships may be as or more important to central nervous system (CNS) function, particularly during development. Oligodendrocytes (one type of glial cell) play the vital role of insulating axons so that transmission across large distances is efficient. Multiple sclerosis provides a pathological illustration of the role of the oligodendrocytes. In multiple sclerosis, myelin within oligodendrocytes is lost, with concomitant changes in motor, sensory, and affective function. Astrocytes have been shown to have more neuron-like effects. For example, astrocytes are similar to neurons in that they can take up neurotransmitters, perhaps assisting in the termination of signals between neurons (Kimelberg & Katz, 1985). The most elegant relationship between neurons and glial cells has been demonstrated in the hippocampus, which is a recurrent topic of this chapter because of its role in explicit memory. Some 5-HT neurons originating in the raphé nuclei within the brainstem terminate in the hippocampus adjacent to glial cells. The glial cells have 5-HT_{1A} receptors, which mediate release of a trophic factor, $S\text{-}100\beta$, that supports the survival of the 5-HT neurons in a retrograde manner (Whitaker-Azmitia, Murphy, & Azmitia, 1990; Azmitia, Griffin, Marshak, Van Eldik, & Whitaker-Azmitia, 1992; Mazer et al., 1997).

BASIC NEUROCHEMISTRY

The complete number and function of neurochemicals involved in brain development are currently unknown. Thousands of genes are expressed in each neuronal cell. This underestimates the number of neurochemicals, because many receptors are composed of a large number of possible combinations of subunits. For example, the γ-aminobutyric acid$_A$ (GABA$_A$) receptor has been implicated in anxiety and memory. It is composed of at least five different classes of subunits (α, β, γ, δ, and ρ). The first class of subunits, α, has six members that can combine with four different β subunits, although it is likely that all possible combinations do not exist functionally. When one considers the complexity of the psychological demands placed on children and adolescents, the diversity of neurochemicals is not surprising.

Much of neurochemical investigation has focused on monoamines and their receptors. These include the catecholamines (dopamine, NE, and epinephrine) and the indoleamine 5-HT. Catecholamines have received the most investigation in studies of neurochemistry, because two of the most commonly used psychopharmacological agents (stimulants and neuroleptics) have effects on dopamine, although their effects on dopamine are not necessary or sufficient for treatment of any child and adolescent psychopathological condition.

Understanding of neurochemistry of catecholamines requires knowledge of the metabolism of catecholamines. (See Figure 13.1.) Cate-

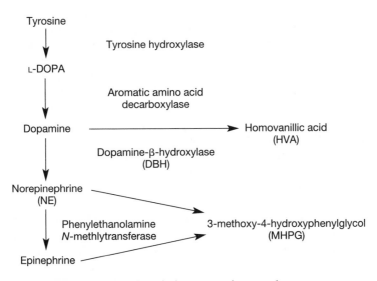

FIGURE 13.1   Catecholamine synthesis pathway.

cholamines are derived from the essential amino acid phenylalanine. Phenylalanine is hydroxylated to tyrosine by phenylalanine hydroxylase in catecholamine-containing neurons. A loss of function of this enzyme leads to the disorder PKU. Phenylalanine hydroxylase activity is dependent on the enzyme dihydropteridine reductase. Mutations of this enzyme can also lead to the phenotype of PKU. Tyrosine is hydroxylated to dihydroxyphenylalanine (L-DOPA) by tyrosine hydroxylase in catecholamine-containing neurons. Interestingly, this same reaction is catalyzed by tyrosinase in melanin-containing cells. L-DOPA is decarboxylated to dopamine by aromatic amino acid decarboxylase. Dopamine may be stored and released in dopamine-containing cells, or it may be hydroxylated to NE by dopamine-β-hydroxylase (DBH).

Metabolism of catecholamines may best be divided into intraneuronal metabolism and extraneuronal metabolism. Intraneuronal metabolism occurs in the mitochondria at the nerve terminal. The enzymes monoamine oxidase A (MAO-A) and monoamine oxidase B (MAO-B) lead to oxidative deamination of monoamines, with MAO-A metabolizing NE, 5-HT, and dopamine, and MAO-B metabolizing phenylethylamine and dopamine (Youdim & Riederer, 1993). Extraneuronally, catechol-O-methyltransferase deactivates catecholamines. Although these enzymes are responsible for degradation of catecholamines, the most significant means of termination of signaling at catecholamine neurons is uptake of catecholamines by transporters in the presynaptic nerve terminal, thereby removing the neurotransmitter from the synapse. Table 13.1 lists the receptors that mediate the effects of catecholamines.

5-HT has a similar synthetic and metabolic pathway. An amino acid precursor, L-tryptophan, is hydoxylated to 5-hydroxytryptophan by tryptophan hydroxylase. After 5-hydroxytryptophan is formed, it is rapidly decarboxylated to 5-HT. Because the pathway is limited by the hydroxylation step and the hydroxylation is limited by the availability of L-tryptophan (the substrate), an increase in tryptophan concentration in the nerve cell may lead to an increase in neuronal 5-HT synthesis. 5-HT is principally metabolized to 5-hydroxyindoleacetic acid (5-HIAA), although the primary method of inactivation at the synapse is through uptake back into the presynaptic neuron. Figure 13.2 illustrates the metabolic pathway from tryptophan to 5-HIAA and an alternate tryptophan pathway through kynurenine. Table 13.2 lists the receptors to which 5-HT binds at both presynaptic and postsynaptic nerve terminals.

The monoamine neurotransmitters are only the most studied neurotransmitters in relationship to psychopathology. More recently, the more abundant excitatory amino acids glutamate and aspartate, and the inhibitory neurotransmitter GABA, have been studied more frequently in basic neurochemistry; however, assessment of these neurotransmitters in association with child and adolescent psychopathology has been very limited. In addi-

TABLE 13.1. Catecholamine Receptors

	Signal transduction	Notes	References
		Dopamine	
D_1	↑ AC	= D_{1A}; association with hyperactivity in knockout mice	Dearry et al. (1990); Monsma et al. (1990); Sunahara et al. (1990); Zhou et al. (1990)
D_2	↓ AC		Bunzow et al. (1988); Grandy et al. (1989)
D_3	↓ AC		Giros et al. (1990); Sokoloff et al. (1990)
D_4	↓ AC	Replicated family-based association with ADHD and repeat in coding region	Van Tol et al. (1991); Smalley et al. (1998); Swanson et al. (1998)
D_5	↑ AC	= D_{1B} = $D_{1\beta}$	Grandy et al. (1991); Sunahara et al. (1991); Tiberi et al. (1991); Weinshank et al. (1991)
Dopamine transporter		= DAT1; replicated family-based association with ADHD; hyperactivity in knockout mouse	Shimada et al. (1991); Vandenbergh et al. (1992); Cook et al. (1995); Gill et al. (1997); Waldman et al. (1998)
		Norepineprhine and epinephrine	
α_{1A}	↑ PLC		Lomasney et al. (1991)
α_{1B}	↑ PLC		Cotecchia et al. (1988)
α_{1C}	↑ PLC		Schwinn et al. (1990)
α_2C10	↓ AC	= α_{2A}; found on platelets	Kobilka et al. (1987)
α_2C4	↓ AC	= α_{2C}	Regan et al. (1988)
α_2C2	↓ AC	= α_{2B}	Weinshank et al. (1990)
β_1	↑ AC		Frielle et al. (1987)
β_2	↑ AC		Dixon et al. (1986)
β_3	↑ AC		Emorine et al. (1989)
NE transporter		= NET	Pacholczyk et al. (1991)

Note. AC, adenylyl cyclase; PLC, phospholipase C.

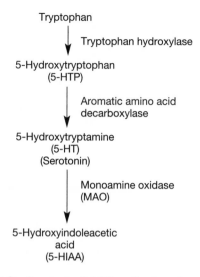

Tryptophan

↓ Tryptophan hydroxylase

5-Hydroxytryptophan
(5-HTP)

↓ Aromatic amino acid
decarboxylase

5-Hydroxytryptamine
(5-HT)
(Serotonin)

↓ Monoamine oxidase
(MAO)

5-Hydroxyindoleacetic
acid
(5-HIAA)

FIGURE 13.2   Serotonin (5-HT) synthesis and metabolism pathway.

tion, peptide neuromodulators such as endogenous opiate compounds are likely to be important in child and adolescent psychopathology research.

NEUROCHEMICAL REGULATION

Synthesis, metabolism, release, and uptake of neurotransmitters, as well as signaling through receptors, are dependent on the production of proteins. These proteins are all encoded by genes. Each cell in the brain has an identical set of roughly 3 billion base pairs of DNA. The presence of functional neurotransmitter-related proteins is determined by genetic regulation. DNA must first be *transcribed* to RNA and spliced to mRNA to begin the process of protein production. An example of the relevance of this step of regulation to psychopathology is the recent finding of a variant in the "promoter" (the area of DNA that regulates transcription rate) of the serotonin transporter, which regulates amount of expressed protein and may be associated with anxiety-related traits or disorders (Lesch et al., 1996). Neuron-specific production of neurotransmitter-related proteins occurs because of tissue-specific transcription factors, which "turn on" transcription of RNA from genes. Once mRNA is produced, it may be *translated* into protein. Once the primary structure of proteins is formed by translation, proteins must be folded into their three-dimensional secondary structure. In the case of many neurotransmitter receptors, proteins are formed as subunits that must be combined with other subunits to form the functional tertiary structure of the receptor. An-

TABLE 13.2. Serotonin (5-HT) Receptors

	Signal transduction	Notes	Variants	Chromosome	References
5-HT$_{1A}$	↓ AC	= HTR1A	I28V (Nakhai et al., 1995), G22S (Nakhai et al., 1995), N417K (Lam et al., 1996)	5	Fargin et al. (1988); Goldman et al. (1994); Erdmann et al. (1995)
5-HT$_{1B}$	↓ AC	= 5-HT$_{1D\beta}$; association with aggression in knockout mice	F124C (Nöthen et al., 1994)	6q13	Hartig et al. (1992); Goldman et al. (1994); Saudou et al. (1994)
5-HT$_{1D}$	↓ AC	= 5-HT$_{1D\alpha}$; found in trigeminal ganglia		1p35	Hartig et al. (1992); Goldman et al. (1994)
5-HT$_{1E}$	↓ AC	= S31		6q14–6q15	McAllister et al. (1992); Goldman et al. (1994); Levy et al. (1994)
5-HT$_{1F}$	↓ AC	= 5-HT$_{1E\beta}$ = MR77		3p	Lovenberg et al. (1993)
5-HT$_{2A}$	↑ PLC	Formerly 5-HT$_2$; sequence identical in brain and platelets Cook et al. (1994)	A439V (Ozaki et al., 1996), H444Y (Erdmann et al., 1996; Ozaki et al., 1996), T25N (Erdmann et al., 1996)	3q14.1–13q14.2	Julius et al. (1990); Chen et al. (1992)
5-HT$_{2B}$	↑ PLC	= 5-HT$_{2F}$		2q36.3–2q37.1	Foguet et al. (1992); Kursar et al. (1992); Schmuck et al. (1994); Le Coniat et al. (1996)
5-HT$_{2C}$	↑ PLC, ↑ GC	= 5-HT$_{1C}$; sudden death in knockout mice; choroid plexus, splice variant, RNA editing	C23S (Lappalainen et al., 1995)	Xq21	Julius et al. (1988); Goldman et al. (1994); Kaufman et al. (1995); Tecott et al. (1995)
5-HT$_3$	Ion channel	Ondansetron; splice variants, 2 adjacent genes (5-HT$_{3A}$ & 5-HT$_{3B}$)		11q23.1–11q23.2	Maricq et al. (1991); Uetz et al. (1994); Miyake et al. (1995); Weiss et al. (1995)

(continued)

TABLE 13.2. (continued)

	Signal transduction	Notes	Variants	Chromosome	References
5-HT₄	↓ AC	Zacopride; two splice variants, 5-HT₄ₗ and 5-HT₄ₛ		5q	Adham et al. (1994); Gerald et al. (1995)
5-HT₅A	?	colocalized with mouse reeler mutant and human holoprosencephaly 3		7q36.1	Erlander et al. (1993); Matthes et al. (1993); Schanen et al. (1996)
5-HT₅B	?	? pseudogene in humans		2q11–2q13	Erlander et al. (1993); Matthes et al. (1993); Grailhe et al. (1994)
5-HT₆	↑ AC	= St-B17; clozapine, clomipramine, splice variant		1p35–1p36	Monsma et al. (1993); Ruat et al. (1993); Kohen et al. (1996)
5-HT₇	↑ AC	Clozapine, risperidone, splice variant, and pseudogene	P279L	10q	Bard et al. (1993); Meyerhof et al. (1993); Plassat et al. (1993); Gelernter et al. (1995); Goldman et al. (1996)
5-HTT	Transporter	= SLC 6A4		17q11.1–17q12	Gelernter & Freimer (1994)

Note. AC, adenylyl cyclase; PLC, phospholipase C; GC, guanylyl cyclase.

other critical step is the proper cellular localization of each protein. Addition of carbohydrates (especially to the N-terminal portion of proteins such as transporters) and lipids (especially through palmitoylation and farnesylation) is often an essential step in determining functional localization and interaction of neurotransmitter-related proteins.

One of the more exciting areas of basic neurochemical research of relevance to research in child and adolescent psychopathology is the study of the determination of neuronal phenotype. In other words, how does a dopaminergic nerve cell develop into a dopaminergic nerve cell? Although the specific steps are beyond the scope of this chapter and current knowledge, the generalization is that influences from the outside of the cell regulate which genes will originally be activated and which will be repressed. In addition to outside cells turning on specific transcription factors, a less well-known process is how some of the DNA structure is changed from inactive to active chromatin. In the development of a specific nerve cell, the interaction is complex and epigenetic, involving sequential interaction with many different types of neurons and glial cells before stable expression of gene products (e.g., choline acetyltransferase) heralds the "birth" of a specific neuronal type (e.g., acetylcholinergic). In addition to the role of neighboring cells in determining which genes will be stably expressed, interaction with neighboring cells will determine the complex geometry of a given nerve cell. These interactions are examples of long-term effects of neurotransmission. In addition to classic neurotransmission as described above, many of the interactions leading to localization of nerve cells occur through interaction of integral membrane proteins (integrins) in the nerve cell with proteins such as laminin on the surface of other neurons or glial cells.

GENERAL METHODOLOGY

Many of the methodological considerations for neurochemical studies in child and adolescent psychiatric research are derived or extrapolated from precedents established in studies of adults or nonhumans. Assumptions equating the biological properties of children and adults are not always correct (Kruesi & Rapoport, 1992), just as cross-species generalizations may be problematic. Moreover, developmental considerations in pediatric samples require additional methodological appraisal.

Each biological parameter has methodological considerations of its own. Thus a truly comprehensive, detailed review of all neurochemical methods in psychiatric research exceeds the limits of this chapter. We will review methodological considerations for cerebrospinal fluid (CSF) monoamine metabolite studies as illustrative examples for a subject that could fill volumes on its own.

Methods for CSF monoamine metabolite studies in child psychiatry (and most other neurochemical investigations) necessitate an exacting obsessiveness if meaningful results are to be obtained. The history of such studies in adults provides evidence for this. Initial optimism about CSF amine metabolite studies in psychiatric illness were followed by mixed results, which then led investigators to reexamine methodological problems (Jimerson & Berrettini, 1985). As of 1985, Jimerson and Berrettini listed 20 methodological variables needing to be controlled in CSF monoamine metabolite studies. Table 13.3 presents an updated version.

Representativeness of Samples

Critical questions about samples are "Who are you measuring?" and "What are the measures?" Diagnostic, inclusion, and exclusion criteria for the pathological group are often debated and discussed. Are the patients in research studies truly representative of those from clinical samples? This question plagues neurobiological investigation, just as it appears to confound psychotherapy research with children and adolescents (Weisz, Weiss, & Donenberg, 1992). A more recent development is scrutiny of the "normal controls" used as contrast subjects.

Control Groups

The use of "normal controls" has been an integral part of psychiatric research for decades. The assumption inherent in this practice is that such controls represent a "healthy" baseline or standard against which abnormal subjects or patients are compared. Conclusions based on the significant differences between these groups are then drawn as to the nature of the patients'

TABLE 13.3. Methodological Variables in Cerebrospinal Fluid (CSF) Studies

1. Diagnostic criteria	14. Sex effects
2. Phase of illness	15. Age effects
3. Control group	16. Height effects
4. Medication status	17. Body weight
5. Other physical illness	18. Probenecid level
6. Diet	19. State anxiety
7. Motor activity	20. Personality variables
8. Time of day	21. Needle angle
9. Lumbar puncture position	22. Atmospheric pressure
10. Site of lumbar puncture	23. Pubertal status
11. CSF aliquot	24. Rearing conditions
12. CSF storage conditions	25. Social competence/position in
13. Assay methodology	dominance hierarchy
	26. Blood cell contamination

pathology, as well as the health of the normal population (which the controls are thought to represent).

Normal controls are usually volunteers obtained in a variety of ways who agree to participate in the research protocol. CSF from contrast individuals without a psychiatric diagnosis is most apt to be collected when lumbar puncture is done for clinical reasons. These normal or "healthy" subjects are selected while the investigators control for dependent variables that they seek to hold constant between all groups. A definition of "health" is necessary for meaningful reference values (Winkel & Statland, 1984). Although "health" and "normality" are difficult concepts to define (Vacha, 1978), the most practical approach is to define health by excluding pathology. Even such a straightforward aim, however, is far from simple. Researchers and theorists of reference values caution that a subject's claim to be healthy should be regarded with skepticism (Grasbeck, 1981). An often implicit assumption is that the control group is in other ways equivalent to a randomly selected sample from the normal population. The question of whether those who volunteer themselves as participants deviate in any way from the healthy population they are thought to represent was raised in the late 1950s and early 1960s. These studies found that half of the adults volunteering as psychiatrically "normal controls" had significant psychopathology (Lasagna & von Felsinger, 1954; Pollin & Perlin, 1958; Escover, Malitz, & Wilkins, 1961).

The first psychiatric study of children who volunteered as "normal control" subjects for biological psychiatric research found that 44% of 152 applicants (aged 6 to 18) for participation as paid normal controls were ineligible, and that at least 31.8% of the child volunteers had probable or certain psychiatric disorders (Kruesi, Lenane, Hibbs, & Major, 1990). Successive screenings, including rating scales and structured interviews, were necessary to obtain controls meeting a defined standard of psychiatric health. Thus careful scrutiny of child volunteers in biological psychiatric research is needed to assure meaningful comparisons.

The importance of stringent scrutiny of controls is seen in a report by Gibbons, Davis, and Hedeker (1990). A comparison of most of the world's data on CSF biogenic amines (5-HIAA, homovanillic acid [HVA], and 3-methoxy-4-hydroxyphenylglycol [MHPG]) from adults revealed that the variability attributable to between-center differences was on the order of two to four times larger for "healthy" controls than for the psychiatric patient samples. For example, the variance attributable to academic center differences in 5-HIAA was only 9.8% for the patient sample but 24.6% for controls. The authors concluded that the care taken in screening normal controls is not commensurate with that taken in screening patients.

Because of the small sample sizes used in most biological psychiatry research, substantial differences between controls and index cases are essential. Otherwise, significant findings may be missed (Rothpearl, Mohs, & Davis, 1981; Pulver, Bartko, & McGrath, 1988).

Diagnostic Criteria

CSF concentrations of a variety of neurotransmitters, metabolites, and neurochemical markers have been shown to differ between diagnostic groups. For example, CSF 5-HIAA concentrations were lower in children and adolescents with disruptive behavior disorders than in age-, sex-, and race-matched persons with obsessive–compulsive disorder (Kruesi, Rapoport, et al., 1990). Recently, CSF concentrations of glial fibrillary acidic protein were found to be lower in autistic than in normal children (Rosengren et al., 1992). Children with Tourette's disorder have lower CSF HVA concentrations than contrast patients do (Cohen, Shaywitz, Caparulo, Young, & Bowers, 1978; Butler, Koslow, Seifert, Caprioli, & Singer, 1979; Singer, Butler, Tune, Seifert, & Coyle, 1982).

Phase of Illness

Mood disorders in adults provide evidence for state-dependent neurochemistry. For example, in adults CSF somatostatin concentrations are lower in depression and higher in more euthymic states (see Rubinow, 1986, for review). In contrast to studies with adults, pediatric patients in a depressed state did not have lower CSF somatostatin concentrations (Kruesi, Swedo, Leonard, Rubinow, & Rapoport, 1990). Nonetheless, the possibility of state-dependent neurochemistry warrants methodological consideration.

Medication Status/Pharmacological Exposure

Alteration of CSF neurotransmitter/metabolite concentrations by pharmacological agents is a logical expectation. For example, lithium treatment of adults with bipolar disorders increases CSF 5-HIAA (Bowers, Heninger, & Gerbode, 1969; Berrettini et al., 1985). Extrapolation from adult studies has led us to use a 3-week "washout" (drug-free) period in an effort to minimize any effect of prior medication exposure. Information about changes in CSF with drug treatment in pediatric patients is limited. In one study, amphetamine resulted in a significant decrease in CSF HVA in hyperkinetic children (Shetty & Chase, 1976). Studies also need to consider *in utero* drug exposure, which can alter neurochemical metabolite levels. Neonates with cocaine exposure documented by positive meconium or urine assays had CSF HVA concentrations lower than those of controls (Needlman, Zuckerman, Anderson, Mirochnick, & Cohen, 1993).

Other Physical Illness

Medical/neurological illnesses other than primary psychiatric disorders have been associated with altered CSF neurochemical values. For example, decreased 5-HIAA concentrations have been reported with febrile convulsions in children (Giroud et al., 1990).

Diet

Diet is often considered a methodological variable, because concentrations of some neurotransmitters or metabolites may be influenced by diet. Dietary amino acids are known precursors for monoamines. Effects of diet (or lack thereof) on metabolite concentrations may differ by diagnostic group. For example, 3 weeks of a low-monoamine diet resulted in decreased CSF MHPG in depressed adults, but had no effect upon normal controls (Muscettola, Wehr, & Goodman, 1977). However, dietary intake of tyrosine and tyramine did not alter plasma MHPG, HVA, or vanillylmandelic acid (Cox, Baker, & Spielman, 1988). Although oral loading with up to 100 mg/kg of tryptophan increased plasma tryptophan levels, whole-blood 5-HT levels were unaffected (Cook et al., 1992).

Motor Activity

Repeatedly, studies indicate that motor activity changes CSF monoamine concentrations (Post, Kotin, Goodwin, & Gordon, 1973; Bertilsson & Asberg, 1984; Guthrie et al., 1986). However, hyperactive individuals do not differ from controls in CSF 5-HIAA concentration (Shetty & Chase, 1976; Cohen, Caparulo, Shaywitz, & Bowers, 1977; Shaywitz, Cohen, & Bowers, 1977). Hyperactivity ratings of boys with attention-deficit/hyperactivity disorder (ADHD) correlated with their CSF HVA concentrations (Castellanos et al., 1994, 1996).

Time of Day

For many biological measures, time of day is a necessary methodological variable to control. For example, serum calcium–magnesium ratios in children varied by time of day (Schmidt et al., 1994). Studies in adults have shown that blood-based 5-HT levels vary at different times of the day (Yuwiler, Ritvo, Bald, Kipper, & Koper, 1971; Wirz-Justice, Lichtensteiner, & Feer, 1977; Pietraszek et al., 1992). Plasma MHPG and HVA each showed a time-of-day effect in adults, with significant differences in concentration between 8 A.M. and noon (Cox et al., 1988). Circadian variation in CSF 5-HIAA has been reported (Nicoletti, Raffaele, Falsaperla, & Paci, 1981). Studies of 24-hour CSF monitoring have provided further evidence for diurnal variation (Kling et al., 1994; Kirwin et al., 1997).

Position and Site of Lumbar Puncture

Studies of adults have suggested the possibility that the position of the patient for lumbar puncture (e.g., sitting vs. lateral decubitus) may make a difference in the concentration of metabolites (Siever et al., 1975). A study of seven adults found lower HVA and 5-HIAA concentrations at more caudal lumbar puncture sites (Nordin, 1991), which is quite plausible, given the well-known cranial–caudal concentration gradient (Moir, Ashcroft, Crawford, Eccleston, & Guldberg, 1970; see just below).

CSF Aliquot

Concentration gradients for CSF 5-HIAA and HVA clearly exist in children and adolescents, based upon measurements of 195 aliquots from 26 patients (Kruesi, Swedo, Hamburger, Potter, & Rapoport, 1988). The finding of concentration gradients of monoamine metabolites versus aliquots of lumbar CSF in children and adolescents is consistent with reports in adults. That is, higher concentrations of these substances are seen with each successive aliquot collected. For monoamine metabolite studies in the CSF of children and adolescents, we have used a 5-ml pool from the third to the eighth successive milliliters collected.

Needle Angle

The angle of needle insertion for lumbar puncture also influences acidic monoamine metabolite concentrations in CSF (Nordin, 1989). This is likely to be another reflection of the cranial–caudal concentration gradient.

Sex Effects

Some adult studies have found gender differences in CSF neurochemistry. One early pediatric study using a less specific fluorometric assay method found greater CSF HVA concentrations in girls than in boys (Habel, Yates, McQueen, Blackwood, & Elton,1981). However, a later pediatric study did not confirm the finding (Riddle, Anderson, et al., 1986). Nonetheless, the practice of checking for gender differences is wise.

Age, Height, and Weight

Studies have examined age, weight, and/or height as intervening variables in measurements of bioactive compounds. Consistent decreases in CSF concentration for HVA and 5-HIAA with age during childhood have been reported (Seifert, Foxx, & Butler, 1980; Riddle, Anderson, et al., 1986; Kruesi, Swedo, Hamburger, et al., 1988). Most pediatric CSF studies cover relatively large age spans and have small n's. Thus potential influences of weight or height, if present, are apt to escape detection.

Probenecid

The technique of probenecid administration to block egress of acidic metabolites out of the CSF space has largely disappeared from child psychiatry research practice. Interpretation of results of the probenecid technique are complicated by relationships between monoamine metabolite concentrations and probenecid (Sjostrom, 1972), probenecid–metabolite correlations seen across diagnostic groups (Cowdry, Ebert, van Kammen, Post, & Goodwin, 1983), probenecid-induced release of transmitters (Lake, Wood, Ziegler, Ebert, & Kopin, 1978), and the nausea and emotional upset experienced by patients (Cohen et al., 1977).

State Anxiety

A significant positive correlation between global anxiety in pediatric patients with obsessive–compulsive disorder and CSF MHPG concentrations has been reported (Swedo et al., 1992). A similar relationship between anxiety and plasma MHPG was seen in another study (Pliszka, Rogeness, Renner, Sherman, & Broussard, 1988).

Personality Variables

Personality variables, such as impulsivity, have been found to relate to CSF monoamine concentrations in adults (Asberg, Schalling, Traskman-Bendz, & Wagner, 1987; Coccaro et al., 1989). Impulsivity as assessed by the child version of the Eysenck Personality Questionnaire (Eysenck, Easting, & Pearson, 1984) did not correlate with CSF monoamine levels in children with either disruptive behavior disorders or obsessive–compulsive disorder (Kruesi, Rapoport, et al., 1990).

Atmospheric Pressure

Significant inverse correlations between atmospheric pressure and CSF concentrations of HVA and 5-HIAA have been reported in some (Garelis, Young, Lal, & Sourkes, 1974; Nordin, Swedin, & Zachau, 1992), but not all (Faustman, Elliott, Ringo, & Faull, 1993), studies.

Puberty

Pediatric studies warrant examination of pubertal status in addition to age for a number of reasons. The substances in question may be related to puberty. For example, the catecholamines NE and dopamine play important roles in regulating the reproductive system, and perhaps in the timing of puberty. Change in a neurochemical concentration with puberty may be disproportionate to change in age. For example, the slope of the concentration gradients for CSF 5-HIAA and HVA differed significantly for prepubertal children versus adolescents (Kruesi, Swedo, Hamburger, et al., 1988). Similarly, the variance seen in whole-blood 5-HT was most pronounced before and after puberty (McBride et al., 1998).

Rearing Conditions/Social Competence

Whether variance due to environment (such as rearing conditions) or due to genetic influences is greater for CSF monoamine metabolite concentrations is open to question, and the more interesting issues relate to gene–environment interaction (Kruesi & Jacobsen, 1998). Social influences and 5-HT have been related in a number of studies. Dominant vervet monkeys were found to have higher CSF 5-HIAA than nondominant animals (Raleigh, Brammer, & McGuire, 1983), and dominant social status facilitated the behavioral effects of serotonergic agonists (Raleigh, Brammer, McGuire, & Yutwiler, 1985). Rhesus monkeys have been shown to have stable individual differences in CSF 5-HIAA correlated with adaptive social behavior (Higley et al., 1996). A rearing study of rhesus monkeys used structural equation modeling and found genetic influences accounting for CSF 5-HIAA concentrations (Higley et al., 1993) and interacting with environmental influences on CSF 5-HIAA (Higley & Linnoila, 1997). Path analysis in a study of adult human twins, siblings, and unrelated individuals suggested CSF 5-HIAA to have greater cultural than genetic heritability (Oxenstierna et al., 1986). Significant positive correlations between social competence and CSF 5-HIAA concentrations were seen in children and adolescents (Kruesi, Rapoport, et al., 1990).

Season

Seasonal impact on the serotonergic system has been less studied in children than in adults. In adults, seasonal variations have been repeatedly demonstrated in platelet 5-HT levels (Arendt, Wirz-Justice, & Bradtke, 1977; Wirz-Justice et al., 1977; Mann, McBride, Anderson, & Mieczkowski, 1992), in platelet 5-HT uptake (Swade & Coppen, 1980; Arora, Kregel, & Meltzer, 1984; Egrise, Rubinstein, Schoutens, Cantraine, & Mendelewicz, 1986), and in the major 5-HT metabolite in CSF, 5-HIAA (Brewerton, Berrettini, Nurnberger, & Linnoila, 1988; Czernansky, Faull, & Pfefferbaum, 1988). One study also demonstrated a seasonal variation in whole-blood 5-HT, with levels being highest in the winter and lowest in the summer (Mann et al., 1992).

Exceptions to seasonal variation have been reported. No significant variation in CSF 5-HIAA was seen in a study of 135 adult alcoholics (Roy, Adinott, DeJong, & Linnoila, 1991). In children, two studies examined the seasonal variation of the serotonergic measures. One study did not find the seasonal variation seen in most adult studies of CSF levels of 5-HT metabolites in the CSF of children and adolescents (Swedo et al., 1989). Platelet 5-HT did show seasonal variation in a pediatric sample (Brewerton, Flament, Rapoport, & Murphy, 1993). Neither study followed a within-subjects design; thus the apparent seasonal variation, or lack thereof, might instead have been due to differences between the individuals tested during the different seasons. Interestingly, a study of whole-blood 5-HT showed an interaction of season and 5-HT transporter promoter genotype, but this preliminary finding should be pursued in a study using a within-subjects design (Hanna et al., 1998).

Blood Contamination

During the course of a lumbar puncture, microscopic contamination of the CSF sample with blood is possible and not likely to be detected by visual inspection. Microscopic contamination does not significantly alter CSF amino acid concentrations in pediatric specimens (McFarlin, Kruesi, & Nadi, 1990); however, gross blood contamination will.

Assay Methodology

Older studies of CSF monoamine metabolites used fluorometric assays, which produced results that are less specific and do not correspond to those obtained with more recent methods that include gas chromatography–mass spectroscopy, high-pressure liquid chromatography (HPLC) with electrochemical detection (Jimerson, Gordon, Post, & Goodwin, 1978; Sjoquist & Johansson, 1978; Muskiet et al., 1979; Mefford et al., 1981), and HPLC with fluorometric detection (Anderson, Teff, & Young, 1987).

Laboratory Techniques

Once samples have been collected, they must be assayed immediately, processed immediately and stored, or stored immediately without processing. The only assays which are commonly performed immediately are those involving tissue function. For example, assays of platelet functions such as aggregation and 5-HT uptake must be performed on fresh platelets, because function is not retained after freezing and thawing of platelets. Processing before freezing is the most common procedure for blood components, because centrifugation will separate red blood cells (RBCs), white blood cells

(WBCs), platelets, and/or plasma, depending on the assay. Since CSF is acellular, it is usually frozen without processing. In addition, whole-blood measures such as whole-blood 5-HT do not require processing before freezing. One must never forget to label the samples carefully with indelible ink written on the tube, separately on tape, and protected with clear tape or similar permanent marking. In addition, if blood is collected in glass tubes, it is important to transfer it to plastic tubes (which will not crack upon freezing and thawing).

There are several levels of refrigeration/freezing. Most samples are kept on ice immediately after collection until transfer to the laboratory. However, few neurochemicals are stable for more than 2 hours without being frozen. Although many published protocols refer to freezing at $-20°C$, frost-free freezers operate by cycling to warmer temperatures and are not adequate. Most neurochemical samples are stable for months to years at $-70°C$. For protection of samples, CO_2 backup systems and remote alarms are necessary precautions. For storage of cell lines, storage at lower temperatures using ultra-low-temperature freezers or liquid nitrogen is preferred to maintain viability over time.

Development of neurochemical assays is a tedious task with several essential steps. When one is designing an assay or selecting a published assay, accuracy and precision must be optimized. Accuracy is analogous to validity, and precision is analogous to reliability. Accuracy is sometimes as difficult to determine as validity in a diagnostic interview. Comparison to previous assays is the usual standard of validity. However, precision is much easier to determine and is expressed as intra-assay and interassay coefficients of variation. Both measures should be less than 15%, with values less than 5% considered optimal. When a method is being developed, reliability is increased by reducing the steps needed to process samples while not sacrificing separation of molecules. Automation of processing will often increase precision. When detecting neurochemicals, improvement of signal-to-noise ratios will increase precision. In fact, the accurate and precise measurement of plasma 5-HT was made possible by the use of a microbore HPLC column and a dual emission–excitation monochromator fluorescence detector (Anderson, Feibel, & Cohen, 1987).

Although many laboratories may perform the same assay with good precision, if assays are performed in two different laboratories, they must be standardized between the laboratories. Since most samples can be maintained frozen and shipped overnight, it is usually easier to analyze all samples in an experiment at the same laboratory. If a laboratory is sending samples overnight, it is important to pack them in dry ice and to consult the carrier for details in identifying the dry ice and biological samples as hazardous. If samples are to be transported by a third party, it is good insurance to split the samples and retain an adequate amount of each sample in the originating laboratory, in case samples are lost during transport.

TISSUE SAMPLES

The major limitation in moving from the elegance of molecular and cellular investigation in bacteria to the study of children and adolescents is the availability of the material of most importance—brain tissue. This is rarely possible, so more accessible tissues are also discussed, with an emphasis on the strengths and weaknesses of each tissue type in the study of child and adolescent psychopathology. A discussion of the important ethical issues raised by differing levels of invasive biological procedures in children and adolescents is beyond the scope of this chapter; these issues have been reviewed elsewhere (Arnold et al., 1995).

Brain

Biopsy

Brain biopsy is the only way to obtain tissue from the CNS of living humans. Some pediatric patients undergo brain biopsy for assessment of possible *Herpes simplex* encephalitis or for surgical treatment of intractable epilepsy or tumors. However, this tissue is usually grossly pathological and not very helpful for studying neurochemical perturbation in the absence of gross neuropathology. Although "normal" tissue surrounding pathological tissue is usually taken out, this tissue is affected by having its usual afferent (input) and efferent (output) connections altered. One potential use of nonmalignant tissue from biopsy is the use of mRNA obtained from biopsy to screen for mutations in candidate proteins expressed in brain through reverse transcription of the mRNA to cDNA, as well to screen for mutations by single-stranded conformational polymorphism (SSCP) analysis (Orita, Iwahana, Kanazawa, Hayashi, & Sekiya, 1989). This is particularly helpful for neurochemical genes for which the genomic structure is not available. However, if the biopsy is obtained because of tumor, the mutation may have occurred during cell replication and be related to the tumor and unrelated to psychopathology. There is no advantage to obtaining DNA directly from brain tissue, except perhaps to study tissue-specific modification such as methylation.

Postmortem Tissue

Since brain tissue is rarely available from living patients, the only source of brain tissue from children and adolescents with psychopathology is from patients who have died. There are three major limitations to this tissue. The first is availability, because most child and adolescent psychopathologies do not decrease life span, and their onset is early in life by definition. However, for many psychopathological conditions such as depression, death by suicide or accident is increased. The best solution to the "problem" of few children and adolescents dying from their disorders shortly after onset of symptoms is to identify older patients with persistent disorders, such as Tourette's disorder, autistic disorder, ADHD, mood disorders, or obsessive–compulsive disorder. A more feasible strategy is the collection of all samples in a "brain bank." Several investigators are involved in collecting brains from patients with child and adolescent psychopathology. It will be important to collaborate in the referrals to such banks, so that such tissue may be most efficiently studied.

A second problem with postmortem studies is that patients who die have rarely been diagnosed by trained raters using reliable diagnostic instruments. In addition, medication use before death is often difficult to ascertain with certainty. This is related to the third problem—namely, that the circumstances of the death may alter neurochemistry, and certainly changes in neurochemicals occur rapidly after death. The best way of preventing postmortem neurochemical changes is immersion in liquid nitrogen, but this is rarely practical within seconds of death in humans.

In addition to studying levels of neurochemicals or enzymes by grinding up regions of the brain, autoradiographic analyses allow quantitation of levels of neurochemicals and receptors with histological resolution. This allows quantitation within regions of the brain, such as layers of the temporal and frontal cortex (Arango et al., 1990; Arango, Underwood, & Mann, 1992). Quantitation should be performed with stereological techniques.

In spite of these problems, several researchers have studied neurochemistry and/or neuropathology associated with child and adolescent psychopathology. Tryptophan, 5-HT, and 5-HIAA were decreased in most areas examined and glutamate was decreased in the three major projection areas of the subthalamus, in patients with Tourette's disorder (Anderson et al., 1992). In patients with autistic disorder, Purkinje cell counts have been shown to be reduced in the cerebellum (Ritvo et al., 1986; Kemper & Bauman, 1993; Bailey et al., 1998). In addition, increased cell-packing density has been found on postmortem examination of the hippocampal formation, amygdala, entorhinal cortex, mammillary body, and septum in autistic disorder in one study (Kemper & Bauman, 1993), but not another (Bailey et al., 1998). A postmortem study of suicide victims has revealed increased [^{125}I]-lysergic acid diethylamide (LSD)-labeled 5-HT$_2$ receptor binding sites in the frontal cortex and increased [^{125}I]-pindolol-labeled β-adrenergic receptor binding sites in the temporal and frontal cortices of victims compared to controls (Arango et al., 1990, 1992). In addition, a postmortem study of patients with schizophrenia, using postmortem neurochemical markers for cell type, suggests that developmental neuropathology in schizophrenia occurs during neuronal migration and/or programmed cell death during gestation and/or infancy (Akbarian et al., 1993).

When mRNA is obtained from postmortem studies, it may be used to study mutations as described above. Although quantitation of mRNA expression in tissues of interest would be helpful, this is often limited by rapid degradation of mRNA by endogenous RNAase.

Neuroimaging

Positron emission tomography studies offer the opportunity to use radioligands or pharmacological challenges to study neurochemical receptors and function. The risk of ionizing radiation is a limiting factor for some, but not all, studies of children and adolescents (Arnold et al., 1995).

Fetal Tissue

Fetal brain tissue may provide information about normal human neurochemical development, such as identification of the normal development of dopamine receptors in humans *in utero* (Kumar & Sastry, 1992; Unis, 1994). In addition, in disorders such as fragile X syndrome, identification of the disease genotype of the fetal tissue may be feasible. This may permit detailed neurochemical study during essential periods of neural development. However, use of fetal tissue raises ethical concerns (Kearney, Vawter, & Gervais, 1991; Kallenberg, Forslin, & Westerborn, 1993). There must be no connection between investigators using fetal tissue and the process of collection of tissue, to avoid possible interference with very sensitive issues regarding preservation of human life. If an investigator is a clinician, that clinician should not be permitted to work with any tissue or collaborate with other investigators on tissue obtained through any parents that the clinician has worked with, because of potential conflicts between counseling regarding termination of pregnancy and research interests.

Cerebrospinal Fluid

CSF has been relatively infrequently used as a window to the brain in child psychiatric studies. An earlier review questioned whether the risk–benefit ratio of CSF investigations in children and adolescents warranted the lumbar punctures needed to accomplish such studies (Ferguson & Bawden, 1988). One reason for this was the supposition that studies involving lumbar punctures were in some fashion far worse for children than procedures such as venipuncture, and thus posed ethical problems. Systematic studies of research lumbar punctures have found and replicated the finding that from a child's perspective, lumbar puncture does not differ significantly in noxiousness from venipuncture or electroencephalography (Kruesi, Swedo, Coffey, et al., 1988; Castellanos et al., 1994).

The merits and limitations of CSF monoamine metabolite studies have been reviewed (Potter & Manji, 1993). Historically, the hope was that changes in CSF metabolites would occur in patients and mirror the hypothesized specific pathophysiological changes associated with psychiatric disorders. However, several problems have diminished these expectations. The exact meaning and source of CSF concentrations of neurotransmitters and their metabolites remain to be clarified. Although significant correlations exist between CSF and brain 5-HIAA concentrations at autopsy (Stanley, Traskman-Bendz, & Dorovini-Zis, 1985), the correlation between the two compartments is lost with drug treatment (Anderson, Teff, & Young, 1987).

Given the uncertainty about exactly what CSF tells us, does the risk–benefit ratio warrant continued CSF studies? Yes. Evidence suggests that there is useful information to be gained from CSF—information that may further inform us and influence treatment. Independent studies have found that the balance of CSF HVA and 5-HIAA has clinical relevance in schizophrenia. Neuroleptic treatment in one study raised HVA and 5-HIAA levels, and the increase significantly correlated with reduction in schizophrenia symptoms (Kahn et al., 1993). Correlations between the metabolites were normalized in schizophrenics with neuroleptic treatment in another study (Hsiao et al., 1993). Schizophrenics with relatively low CSF HVA and 5-HIAA show better response to clozapine than to more classical neuroleptics (Pickar et al., 1992; Risch & Lewine, 1993). Low concentration of CSF 5-HIAA is a biological marker associated with violent suicide and impulsive aggression (Asberg et al., 1987; Coccaro et al., 1989; Brown & Linnoila, 1990; Kruesi et al., 1992). CSF HVA concentration was a significant predictor of stimulant drug response in 45 hyperactive boys (Castellanos et al., 1996). CSF samples from a variety of neurological and psychiatric illnesses helped explain the role of quinolinic acid and kynurenine pathway metabolism in inflammatory and noninflammatory neurological disease (Heyes et al., 1992). CSF concentrations of quinolinic acid, an endogenous N-methyl-D-aspartate receptor agonist, were found to be elevated in inflammatory brain diseases and are now hypothesized to be mediators of neuronal dysfunction. Therefore, strategies to attenuate the neurological effects of kynurenine pathway metabolites offer new approaches to therapy. Whether these CSF markers will play a significant role in processes that ameliorate the behavioral disturbances is yet to be determined. However, markers are valuable clues, and as such deserve continued extension and investigation. PKU was once such a marker. CSF 5-HIAA may have other prognostic importance: it predicts depression risk in patients with Parkinson's disease (Cummings, 1992).

Neurochemical Depletion

Still another approach to the study of neurochemistry is to alter CNS neurochemicals and study the effect on mood or cognition. For example, plasma tryptophan depletion can be precipitated by administration of a low-tryptophan diet for a day, followed by a tryptophan-free amino acid drink. Subsequent tryptophan transport across the blood–brain barrier is decreased, with a concomitant decrease in neuronal 5-HT synthesis. This challenge test led to a recurrence in depressive symptoms in patients with major depression who had had a remission in symptoms after pharmacological treatment (Delgado et al., 1990). Repetitive behaviors also worsened in adult subjects with autistic disorder after tryptophan depletion (McDougle et al., 1996).

Peripheral Neurochemical Measures

Many readers may feel that peripheral neurochemical measures do not warrant coverage in the study of neurochemistry in the last year of the 20th century. The chief advantage of peripheral measures is availability of many samples from well-characterized subjects. As we have noted above, lack of availability is the chief disadvantage of direct study of the brain. However, the chief disadvantage of peripheral tissues is obviously that they are not taken from the organ of interest. Therefore, peripheral neurochemical findings always require consideration of what mechanism of brain function is being modeled. For some measures the model is straightforward, such as the identification of mutations in DNA obtained from blood or saliva that would alter the function of proteins in the brain, or the finding of association and linkage of dopamine gene markers with ADHD (Cook et al., 1995; Cook, Stein, & Leventhal, 1997; Gill, Daly, Heron, Haw, & Fitzgerald, 1997; Smalley et al., 1998; Swanson et al., 1998; Waldman et al., 1998). For other measures, such as plasma NE, the analogy is direct. Plasma NE is highly correlated with CSF NE because the peripheral sympathetic nervous system is under CNS noradrenergic control. In contrast, a measure such as platelet 5-HT may have a direct analogy, but not the first one that comes to mind. For example, it may be more closely analogous to presynaptic 5-HT levels than to synaptic 5-HT levels. The most important aspect in the use of peripheral measures is that a model of the relationship to the brain must be considered hypothetical until data are obtained to confirm (or disconfirm) the model. Potential neural processes that may be modeled by use of peripheral tissues are neurochemical uptake, synthesis, steady-state levels, synaptic levels, presynaptic concentration, and/or signal transduction (Cook & Leventhal, 1996).

Not all peripheral measures are equally noninvasive. For example, although venipuncture to obtain blood is a routine practice in pediatric offices, inclusion of blood sampling in large-scale epidemiological studies of child and adolescent psychopathology is often not feasible because of cost, logistics, or the psychopathology investigators' valid concern that some subjects may drop out because of blood sampling. Saliva and urine sampling may have advantages in such studies.

Blood

The discussion of peripheral measures begins with blood, because it is the tissue that has been most often studied in neurochemical studies of psychopathology and because it provides multiple measures for study. However, several disadvantages must be highlighted. In addition to blood not being the brain, blood sampling requires venipuncture, which is uncomfortable. Moreover, although there are no definite federal guidelines, the amount of blood that can be drawn practically is limited to 10% of blood volume over an 8-week period. Blood volume may be estimated for children who are more than 1 month old by the following equation: Blood volume = 75 ml/kg body weight. Within these guidelines, the greatest practical risk to a subject is bruising at the site of venipuncture. However, researchers must be aware that once venipuncture has taken place, the needle and blood samples are biohazards. Although laboratory personnel handling blood products should be immunized against hepatitis B infection, each sample must still be handled carefully because of infection risk. The best safety precaution is to consider each sample to be potentially infected (with human immunodeficiency virus, other viruses such as hepatitis B or C, etc.).

Blood is a complex tissue, including cellular components (RBCs, or erythrocytes, WBCs, or leukocytes); cellular fragments (platelets); proteins, many of which bind neurochemicals; and free neurochemicals and hormones outside of cells and unbound to proteins. "Whole blood" refers to blood in which all of these components are present. "Plasma" refers to samples in which RBCs have been removed via exploitation of their greater density by centrifugation. There are several varieties of plasma, each of which is obtained by first collecting whole-blood samples in tubes containing anticoagulant. The first is platelet-rich plasma (PRP), which is obtained by simply removing RBCs and WBCs (lower two layers of three). If PRP is spun further, platelets may be removed, with the remaining top layer of straw-colored plasma being platelet-poor plasma (PPP). PPP also contains proteins, which may be removed by ultrafiltration through membranes that do not allow proteins to pass through; this results in ultrafiltrate PPP, which then contains only free neurochemicals and hormones. Serum is a commonly reported measure, which is obtained by collecting blood in tubes without anticoagulant and allowing the samples to clot. After centrifugation, the top straw-colored layer consists of the rough equivalent of PRP, with an important difference: Coagulation involves aggregation of platelets and release of the contents of platelets, including 5-HT, among other neurochemicals. Therefore, most of the platelets will not be intact, and neurochemicals from platelets will be contained in the serum. Each of the components of whole blood is discussed in more detail below.

Cellular Components of Blood (RBCs and WBCs).   RBCs are not commonly studied in child and adolescent psychopathology. Available measures include ouabain binding to study the density of Na^+-K^+ adensosine triphosphatase (ATPase). Reduction in the activity of this enzyme in Down's syndrome has been shown to be associated with reduced platelet 5-HT uptake, which is dependent on normal sodium transport by Na^+-K^+ ATPase. In addition, RBC proton T_1 relaxation time, a measure that may reflect tissue water content, has been studied in adults with episodic aggression (Kent et al., 1988).

WBCs may be subdivided into lymphocytes (which may be further subdivided by cell surface antigens into several subtypes), granulocytes, and monocytes. Lymphocytes are the most commonly used cells in child and adolescent psychopathology studies, primarily because of their functional response to stimulation in the study of immune function. Studies of lymphocyte response and subpopulations have been most commonly studied as evidence of autoimmunity in the pathophysiology of autistic disorder (Warren et al., 1990) and subgroups of obsessive–compulsive disorder or tic disorders (Murphy et al., 1997; Swedo et al., 1997). However, lymphocyte response to antigens and mitogens occurs through neurochemical processes using the same anterograde and retrograde signaling mechanisms as those used by neural cells to communicate. Therefore, all immune findings in child and adolescent psychopathology may occur because the same protein may be used by lymphocytes and neural cells for communication. For example, mitogen activation of lymphocytes leads to an increase in 5-HT$_{1A}$ receptor mRNA, stimulation of lymphocyte 5-HT$_{1A}$ receptors, and increased proliferation of T lymphocytes by inhibition of adenylyl cyclase (Aune, McGrath, Sarr, Bombara, & Kelley, 1993). Another example is that both lymphocytes and neural cells use *src*-related protein tyrosine kinases for signaling. Knockout of one of these proteins, *fyn*, has been shown to lead to altered T-cell receptor response (Stein, Lee, Rich, & Soriano, 1992), loss of hippocampal LTP, increased granule cell development in the dentate gyrus and pyramidal cells of the CA3 field of the hippocampus, and impaired spatial learning in mice (Grant et al., 1992).

Lymphocytes may also be transformed with Epstein–Barr virus in the laboratory to form a less differentiated lymphoblastoid cell that may be grown indefinitely and used as a source of DNA or in the study of signaling processes (Shearer et al., 1988). Caveats include the possibility that the process of dedifferentiation may result in the loss of mature cellular functions of interest. DNA may commonly be extracted from lymphocytes in whole blood for molecular genetic studies.

Cellular Fragments (Platelets). Platelets are fragments of megakaryocytes, which are large, multinucleated cells localized to the bone marrow. They retain a plasma membrane, mitochondria, cytoplasm, dense granules (which contain 5-HT and ATP and are analogous to 5-HT-containing synaptic vesicles), and concomitant cytoplasmic, plasma membrane, and vesicular proteins (including transporters, receptors, and tyrosine kinases). They do not have a nucleus and therefore do not contain DNA, but they do contain mRNA. They have been extensively studied in neurochemical studies of psychopathology because they use 5-HT in signaling processes. In the platelet, the function of 5-HT is to provide amplification of aggregation signals. For example, 5-HT increases release of 5-HT to create a positive feedback loop leading to platelet aggregation, which contributes to clot formation and contributes to vasoconstriction at the site of blood vessel injury. Although platelet 5-HT mechanisms may be implicated in cardiovascular disease, the study of platelet 5-HT mechanisms is an indirect model in the study of child and adolescent psychopathology. This is based on the homology of various platelet processes, such as 5-HT transport, with their neural counterparts. (See Figure 13.3 for an illustration of this model.) Many tissues in the body use signaling systems present in other tissue types. For example, 5-HT plasma membrane transport occurs in enterochromaffin cells of the gut (where peripheral 5-HT is synthesized), in megakaryocytes, in platelets, and in raphe neurons. The presence of similar processes between brain and peripheral tissues should not lead one to assume that identical proteins are involved, because peripheral mRNAs are often spliced differently than their brain counterparts derived from the same gene. However, in the case of the 5-HT transporter, the amino acid sequence (primary structure) of the 5-HT transporter protein is identical to that of the raphe neurons (Lesch, Wolozin, Murphy, & Riederer, 1993). Although this does not mean that the protein has the same secondary structure (shape) or is associated with the same lipids and proteins that regulate its function, changes in the primary structure (amino acid sequence) of the platelet 5-HT transporter would imply changes in the primary structure of the neural 5-HT transporter.

Study of the 5-HT plasma membrane transporter in child and adolescent psychopathology has been limited to study of platelet 5-HT uptake and radiolabeled ligand binding ([^{3}H]-imipramine and [^{3}H]-paroxetine) to the platelet 5-HT transporter. The presence of 5-HT transporter mRNA allows screening for mutations through screening of mRNA from patients with child and adolescent psychopathology. One way of doing this is through reverse transcription of the mRNA to cDNA and amplification of the cDNA by polymerase chain reaction, and then through screening of 300 base pair fragments of the cDNA by gel electrophoresis, which is sensitive to point mutations in the cDNA (Orita et al., 1989) or by sequencing. In addition, uptake kinetics and binding to the dense-granule 5-HT transporter may be studied (Chatterjee & Anderson, 1993).

One of the most frequently studied neurochemical measures in child and adolescent psychopathology has been the platelet concentration of 5-HT. Measurement of the amount of 5-HT in whole blood that has not been separated into a platelet fraction is the best estimate of platelet 5-HT content

Platelet Model

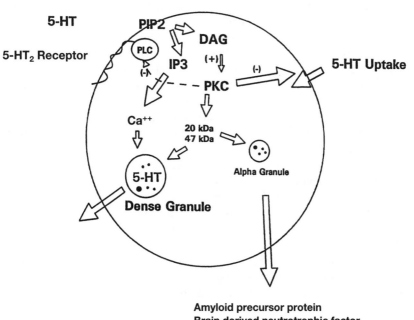

Amyloid precursor protein
Brain derived neutrotrophic factor
Epidermal growth factor
Transforming growth factor-beta 1
Beta-thromboglobulin, platelet factor 4

FIGURE 13.3. Platelet model of 5-HT receptor stimulation leading to an increase in the activity of phospholipase C (PLC), which cleaves phosphatidylinositiol bisphospate (PIP2) into two second messengers: inositol trisphosphate (IP3), which increases the activity of the third messenger Ca⁺⁺; and diacylglycerol (DAG), which increases the activity of the third messenger protein kinase C (PKC). PKC and increased Ca⁺⁺ lead to increased release of 5-HT. Platelets also contain alpha granules, which contain several proteins that have a role in CNS development.

in a given volume of blood, because of the high concentration of 5-HT in platelets. The amount of 5-HT in plasma outside of platelets makes a negligible contribution. For example, the mean whole-blood 5-HT level in parents of children with autistic disorder was 181 ng/ml, while the PPP free 5-HT level from the same subjects was 0.86 ng/ml (Cook, Leventhal, & Freedman, 1988a). Although this is the only study reporting a direct comparison of subjects with both measures, it is consistent with a greater than 100-fold difference between 5-HT concentration in whole blood (containing platelets) and in PPP collected in a manner to minimize platelet 5-HT release during processing and to maximize removal of platelets (Anderson, Feibel, & Cohen, 1987). The disadvantage of direct measurement of 5-HT in platelets is that it adds several steps that introduce laboratory error—some random due to pipetting errors, and some systematic due to differential yield of platelets from subjects with differences in platelet age and/or size. Although one may avoid systematic errors in collection of platelet membranes for radioligand binding studies by using the Corash method, in which several centrifugation steps are used to make sure that the yield of platelets is greater than 95% (Corash, 1980), this procedure may lead to platelet 5-HT release into the discarded fractions. After assay of 5-HT in whole blood, there are two options in reporting the data: reporting the amount of 5-HT in an amount of blood (usually in nanograms per milliliter), or obtaining a platelet count from the same blood and dividing the whole-blood 5-HT level present in a given volume of blood by the number of platelets in another sample of the same blood. This should be represented as a whole-blood 5-HT level per 10^8 platelets, and should not be confused with direct measurement of platelet 5-HT content. Again, representation without correction for platelet count has the advantage of not adding the error of platelet measurement. The platelet count of the patient group should be studied to document that it is not significantly different from that of the control group (Geller, Yuwiler, Freeman, & Ritvo, 1988).

The mechanism of normal regulation of whole-blood 5-HT levels has not been established in normal human subjects, although the rate of platelet 5-HT uptake has been shown to be positively correlated with whole-blood 5-HT levels in vervet monkeys (Brammer, McGuire, & Raleigh, 1987) and in parents of autistic children (Cook et al., 1993). In addition, whole-blood 5-HT levels were negatively correlated with the number of platelet [³H]-LSD-labeled 5-HT$_2$ receptor binding sites (Cook et al., 1993). Platelet [¹²⁵I]-LSD-labeled 5-HT$_2$ receptor binding sites have been shown to be increased by treatment with the 5-HT$_2$ antagonist mianserin (Whiteford, Jarvis, Stedman, Pond, & Csernansky, 1993). Although the findings were not significant because of small sample size, platelet 5-HT levels decreased after mianserin treatment, consistent with an expected inverse relationship between platelet 5-HT$_2$ receptor binding sites and levels of platelet 5-HT. Although increased 5-HT uptake would be expected to lead to increased platelet 5-HT content, the relationship between 5-HT$_2$ receptor binding site number and whole-blood 5-HT levels is not obvious, because there was no relationship between the binding site number and thrombin-stimulated 5-HT release. In addition, there was not a significant correlation between whole-blood 5-HT levels and [¹²⁵I]-spiroperidol-labeled 5-HT$_2$ receptor binding sites (Perry, Cook, Leventhal, Wainwright, & Freedman, 1991), suggesting that the relationship between platelet [³H]-LSD-labeled 5-HT$_2$ receptor binding sites and whole-blood 5-HT levels may be due to polymorphisms of the receptor or a different coupling state of the receptor to its associated G proteins (Cook et al.,

1993). Both alternatives are consistent with the finding of decreased augmentation by 5-HT of adenosine diphosphate (ADP)-induced platelet aggregation in autistic men compared to normal controls (McBride et al., 1989).

The relationship between the platelet and brain 5-HT_2 receptors is raised by the work described above and by the finding that the primary structure (amino acid composition) of the platelet and frontal cortical 5-HT_{2A} receptors are identical (Cook et al., 1994). Platelet and frontal cortical [^{125}I]-LSD-labeled 5-HT_2 receptor binding K_i were positively correlated ($r = .96$) in a study of adult neurosurgical patients (Elliott & Kent, 1989). In addition, platelet [^{125}I]-LSD-labeled 5-HT_2 receptor binding sites and 5-HT augmentation of ADP-induced platelet aggregation were both positively correlated with prolactin release after fenfluramine challenge (McBride et al., 1989). Another measure of 5-HT_2 receptor function in platelets is 5-HT-stimulated shape change of platelets, which involves changes in the platelet cytoskeleton that may be analogous to shape change in the neuronal growth cone (Brazell, McClue, & Stahl, 1988; McClue, Brazell, & Stahl, 1989).

Development has been shown to have a significant impact on normal levels of whole-blood 5-HT, with adolescent levels lower than preadolescent levels (Ritvo et al., 1971; Anderson, Freedman, et al., 1987; McBride et al., 1998). Determination of the factors leading to developmental regulation of platelet 5-HT levels may identify factors involved in differentiation of the CNS. Several of the cytokines involved in platelet development also have a role in development of the CNS. Gender differences have been found both for whole-blood 5-HT levels in normal controls (Cook, Leventhal, & Freedman, 1988b) and for PPP free 5-HT levels in autistic children, their parents, and their siblings (Cook et al., 1988a). Although African American children with autistic disorder had whole-blood 5-HT levels greater than those of European American children, healthy control African American children have also been found to have higher whole-blood 5-HT than European American healthy controls (McBride et al., 1998; Pfeffer et al., 1998). Diet does not appear to have an effect on whole-blood 5-HT levels (Anderson, Teff, & Young, 1984). In fact, administration of up to 100 mg/kg of the 5-HT precursor, L-tryptophan, had no effect on whole-blood 5-HT levels (Cook et al., 1992). In other studies, whole-blood 5-HT levels expressed per platelet (Brewerton et al., 1993) and per milliliter of blood (Mann et al., 1992) were both found to have seasonal variation. However, the whole blood was collected at different times of the year from different subjects, rather than from the same subjects at different times of the year. Diurnal effects have been reported for platelet 5-HT (milligrams of 5-HT per milligram of platelet protein; Wirz-Justice et al., 1977) and for whole-blood 5-HT (Pietraszek et al., 1992) in control adults, but have not been studied in children and adolescents.

Although platelet neurochemicals have emphasized 5-HT, platelet levels of NE, epinephrine, and dopamine have also been reported (Launay et al., 1987). In one study, platelet NE, epinephrine, and dopamine were decreased in children with autism, while NE and epinephrine were increased in plasma. Using whole blood or platelet-rich plasma would not be an appropriate way of estimating platelet NE, because approximately 30% of the whole-blood NE content would be contributed by the extraplatelet plasma NE compartment (Popp-Snijders, Geenen, & Heijden, 1989).

Several platelet functions may be studied as a model of cellular processes that are not directly related to monoamines. For example, the basal and stimulated production of second messengers (cAMP and inositol phosphates) may be studied (Cook et al., 1993). More recently, thrombin has been shown to lead to tyrosine phosphorylation and association of developmental regulatory proteins such as phosphatidylinositol-3-kinase, *src*-related proteins such as *fyn*, and ras-guanosine triphosphatase activating protein (Guinebault et al., 1993).

Platelets contain mitochondria, which contain MAO-B, which metabolizes dopamine and phenylethylamine (Youdim & Riederer, 1993). Although MAO-A is found in the brain but not in platelets, the amino acid sequence of MAO-B is identical in platelets and the brain (Chen, Wu, & Shih, 1993). Therefore, platelets may provide a measure of the adequacy of MAO-B inhibition by MAO-B inhibitors or nonspecific MAO inhibitors, but may not be an adequate indicator of the adequacy of MAO-A inhibition by specific MAO-A inhibitors such as clorgyline.

Cell-Free Plasma (PRP, PPP, Ultrafiltrate PPP, Serum).

Since contamination of plasma with WBCs, RBCs, or platelets may confound estimation of the circulating levels of neurochemicals, the ideal plasma sample is free of these components and free of components that may be released from cells or platelets during processing. The other main consideration in processing plasma is to decide whether to measure total plasma neurochemicals, or free plasma neurochemicals which are unbound to plasma proteins. This may be accomplished by ultrafiltration through filters that trap proteins because of their high molecular weight. The free plasma neurochemical fraction is the fraction that is biologically active at blood vessel or blood cell or platelet receptors (Anderson, Feibel, & Cohen, 1987).

Neurochemicals in plasma may be studied both in a resting state and in a stimulated state. The most studied plasma neurochemical is NE. However, plasma NE is state rather than a trait measure. In contrast to no or minimal changes in the trait measure (platelet 5-HT content) in relationship to season, time of day, activity, stress, or diet, plasma NE may double after a person changes from a lying to a standing position, or undergoes mental stress such as being asked to perform challenging arithmetic (Mefford et al., 1981). Therefore, in a study of resting plasma NE levels, subjects must lie supine for at least 20 minutes after the insertion of an intravenous catheter so that they may recover from the stress of needle insertion. For many studies of child and adolescent psychopathology, this is not possible. Stimulated NE values are obtained from subjects who are sitting or standing and may be subjected to mental stress such as challenging arithmetic problems. Ideally, stimulated measures are performed with subjects who have had stable baseline measures collected. The ideal measures of peripheral NE are the kinetics of distribution and metabolism of NE, determined by using compartmental analysis (Linares et al., 1987). This procedure requires administration of radioactively tagged NE and insertion of two intravenous catheters, which limits the feasibility of such a method for most studies of child and adolescent psychopathology.

Plasma MHPG probably represents a more stable measure than plasma NE, because it is a more abundant pool formed by metabolism of NE. Plasma dopamine is a very low and often undetectable measure. The dopamine metabolite, HVA, is more commonly studied as an estimate of dopamine function. Administration of debrisoquine has been attempted to increase the amount of plasma HVA that is represented by the CNS rather than the periphery (Riddle, Leckman, et al., 1986; Riddle et al., 1989). More recently, administration of 2-deoxyglucose has been employed as a metabolic stressor to stimulate plasma HVA production in the study of adult subjects with schizophrenia, but this method has not been employed in children and adolescents (Breier, Davis, Buchanan, Moricle, & Munson, 1993).

Epithelial Cells (Saliva, Skin, and Hair)

Epithelial cells are the most accessible of tissues. Saliva is the most accessible, because the cells that are constantly being shed from the buccal mucosa in a relatively intact state. In contrast, the outer layer of skin and outer portion of hair are hardened and lose much of their cell contents before becoming accessible, unless vigorous methods such as pulling hairs out by their roots are used. Cortisol has been studied in saliva to avoid blood sampling for psychoendocrine testing (see Dahl, Dorn, & Ryan, Chapter 12, this volume). It is also a source of DNA for study of microsatellite markers or for mutational screening. In fact, it is the preferred method for obtaining epidemiological data on genotypes (e.g., the number of males in the population with the fragile X mutation, or the prevalence of individuals in a population with amplification of the myotonic dystrophy gene). Such epidemiological data will be important to define the ranges of the phenotypes associated with these genotypes. For example, ascertainment of fragile X subjects only from residential placements with mentally retarded boys will obviously skew ascertainment toward a severe phenotype and will miss fragile X subjects with a milder phenotype in the community. Saliva may be collected directly into a cup; it may also be obtained by swabbing the inside of the mouth with cotton, or by rinsing the mouth with ½ ounce of normal saline solution (Lench, Stanier, & Williamson, 1988) or more palatable sugar solutions.

Hair may also be collected to acquire DNA. However, as noted above, this requires pulling one or more hair shafts out of the scalp from the roots (which will lead to more discomfort than saliva sampling, although it will usually be less uncomfortable than blood sampling). The disadvantage of relatively low yields of DNA from hair and saliva has been minimized by the development of polymerase chain reaction methods for amplification of DNA, which have been demonstrated to provide microsatellite genotyping information from small quantities of DNA (Higuchi, von Beroldingen, Sensabaugh, & Erlich, 1988).

Skin, although accessible, is of little value without biopsy, which is probably somewhere between a blood draw and a spinal tap in level of discomfort. Fibroblasts from such biopsies can be cultured, and cellular functions can be studied (Page, Yu, Fontanesi, & Nyhan, 1997).

Urine

Urine is also a relatively noninvasive means of sampling neurochemical metabolites, such as 5-HIAA, MHPG, and HVA. However, some children and adolescents may not cooperate fully with this procedure. A "spot" urine sample, or collection of a single void, rarely provides useful information unless one is screening for severe amino acidurias. Samples collected over a 24-hour period provide a more meaningful estimate of excretion rates of neurochemical metabolites, but collection of all urine over 24 hours is often challenging, particularly in outpatient studies. Most excretion rates are divided by excretion of creatinine. However, for at least excretion of HVA, HVA clearance was been found to be determined by urinary clearance rather than production of HVA (Potter, Hsiao, & Goldman, 1989).

CLOSING NOTE

There are several points to highlight in the use of neurochemical measures in child and adolescent psychopathology. The selection of a neurochemical measure for study in child and adolescent psychopathology usually requires a creative approach to studying the brain. However, if the brain is not directly studied, several important considerations must be considered in collection, analysis, and interpretation of findings. More importantly, the relevant neurochemistry to study in child and adolescent psychopathology is *developmental* neurochemistry.

REFERENCES

Adham, N., Gerald, C., Vaysse, P. J.-J., Weinshank, R., & Branchek, T. (1994). Pharmacological characterization of two splice variants of the cloned rat 5-HT$_4$ receptor coupled to stimulation of adenylate cyclase. *Society for Neuroscience Abstracts, 20,* 1266.

Akbarian, S., Bunney, W., Jr., Potkin, S., Wigal, S., Hagman, J., Sandman, C., & Jones, E. (1993). Altered distribution of nicotinamide–adenine dinucleotide phosphate–diaphorase cells in frontal lobe of schizophrenics implies disturbances of cortical development. *Archives of General Psychiatry, 50,* 169–177.

Anderson, G. M., Feibel, F. C., & Cohen, D. J. (1987). Determination of serotonin in whole blood, platelet-rich plasma, platelet-poor plasma and plasma ultrafiltrate. *Life Sciences, 40,* 1063–1070.

Anderson, G. M., Freedman, D. X., Cohen, D. J., Volkmar, F. R., Hoder, E. L., McPhedran, P., Minderaa, R. B., Hansen, C. R., & Young, J. G. (1987). Whole blood serotonin in autistic and normal subjects. *Journal of Child Psychology and Psychiatry, 28,* 885–900.

Anderson, G. M., Pollak, E. S., Chatterjee, D., Leckman, J. F., Riddle, M. A., & Cohen, D. J. (1992). Postmortem analysis of subcortical monoamines and amino acids in Tourette syndrome. *Advances in Neurology, 58,* 123–133.

Anderson, G. M., Teff, K. L., & Young, S. N. (1984). Effect of a meal on human whole blood serotonin. *Gastroenterology, 88,* 86–89.

Anderson, G. M., Teff, K. L., & Young, S. N. (1987). Serotonin in cisternal cerebrospinal fluid of the rat: Measurement and use as an index of functionally active serotonin. *Life Sciences, 40,* 2253–2260.

Arango, V., Ernsberger, P., Marzuk, P. M., Chen, J. S., Tierney, H., Stanley, M., Reis, D. J., & Mann, J. J. (1990). Autoradiographic demonstration of increased serotonin 5-HT2 and beta-adrenergic receptor binding sites in the brain of suicide victims. *Archives of General Psychiatry, 47,* 1038–1047.

Arango, V., Underwood, M. D., & Mann, J. J. (1992). Alterations in monoamine receptors in the brain of suicide victims. *Journal of Clinical Psychopharmacology, 12,* 8S–12S.

Arendt, J., Wirz-Justice, A., & Bradtke, J. (1977). Annual rhythm of serum melatonin in man. *Neuroscience Letters, 7,* 327–330.

Armstrong, R., & Montminy, M. (1993). Transynaptic control of gene expression. *Annual Review of Neuroscience, 16,* 17–29.

Arnold, L. E., Stoff, D. M., Cook, E., Jr., Cohen, D. J., Kruesi, M., Wright, C., Hattab, J., Graham, P., Zametkin, A., Castellanos, F. X., & Graham, P. (1995). Ethical issues in biological psychiatric research with children and adolescents. *Journal of the American Academy of Child and Adolescent Psychiatry, 34,* 929–939.

Arora, R. C., Kregel, L., & Meltzer, H. (1984). Seasonal variation in serotonin uptake in normal controls and depressed patients. *Biological Psychiatry, 19,* 795–804.

Asberg, M., Schalling, D., Traskman-Bendz, L., & Wagner, A. (1987). Psychobiology of suicide, impulsivity, and related phenomena. In H. Y. Meltzer (Ed.), *Psychopharmacology: The third generation of progress.* New York: Raven Press.

Aune, T., McGrath, K., Sarr, T., Bombara, M., & Kelley, K. (1993). Expression of 5HT1a receptors on activated human T cells: Regulation of cyclic AMP levels and T cell proliferation by 5-hydroxytryptamine. *Journal of Immunology, 151,* 1175–1183.

Azmitia, E. C., Griffin, W. S., Marshak, D. R., Van Eldik, L. J., & Whitaker-Azmitia, P. M. (1992). S100 beta and serotonin: A possible astrocytic-neuronal link to neuropathology of Alzheimer's disease. *Progress in Brain Research, 94,* 459–473.

Bailey, A., Luthert, P., Dean, A., Harding, B., Janota, I., Montgomery, M., Rutter, M., & Lantos, P. (1998). A clinicopathological study of autism. *Brain, 121,* 889–905.

Bard, J., Zgombick, J., Adham, N., Vaysse, P., Branchek, T., & Weinshank, R. (1993). Cloning of a novel human serotonin receptor (5-HT$_7$) positively coupled to adenylate cyclase. *Journal of Biological Chemistry, 268,* 23422–23426.

Berrettini, W. H., Nurnberger, J. I., Scheinin, M., Seppala, T., Linnoila, M., Narrow, W., Simmons-Alling, S., & Gershon, E. S. (1985). Cerebrospinal fluid and plasma monoamines and their metabolites in euthymic bipolar patients. *Biological Psychiatry, 20*, 257–269.

Bertilsson, L., & Asberg, M. (1984). Amime metabolites in the cerebrospinal fluid as measure of central neurotransmitter function: Methodological aspects. In E. Usdin, M. Asberg, L. Bertilsson, & F. Sjoqvist (Eds.), *Frontiers in biochemical and pharmocological research in depression.* New York: Raven Press.

Bowers, M. B., Heninger, G. R., & Gerbode, F. A. (1969). CSF 5-HIAA and HVA in psychiatric patients. *International Journal of Neuropharmacology, 8*, 255–262.

Brammer, G. L., McGuire, M. T., & Raleigh, M. J. (1987). Vervet monkey (*Cercopithecus aethiops sabaeus*) whole blood serotonin level is determined by platelet uptake sites. *Life Sciences, 41*, 1539–1546.

Brazell, C., McClue, S. J., Preston, G. C., King, B., & Stahl, S. M. (1988). 5-Hydroxytryptamine (5-HT)-induced shape change in human platelets determined by computerized data acquisition then correlation of [125I]-LSD binding at 5-HT$_2$ receptors. *Blood Coagul Fibinolysis, 2*, 17–24.

Breier, A., Davis, O., Buchanan, R., Moricle, L., & Munson, R. (1993). Effects of metabolic perturbation on plasma homovanillic acid in schizophrenia: Relationship to prefrontal cortex volume. *Archives of General Psychiatry, 50*, 541–550.

Brewerton, T., Flament, M., Rapoport, J., & Murphy, D. (1993). Seasonal effects on platelet 5-HT content in patients with OCD and controls. *Archives of General Psychiatry, 50*, 409.

Brewerton, T. D., Berrettini, W. H., Nurnberger, J. I., & Linnoila, M. (1988). Analysis of seasonal fluctuations of CSF monoamine metabolites and neuropeptides in normal controls: Findings with 5HIAA and HVA. *Psychiatry Research, 23*, 257–265.

Brown, G. L., & Linnoila, M. I. (1990). CSF serotonin metabolite (5-HIAA) studies in depression, impulsivity, and violence. *Journal of Clinical Psychiatry, 51*, 31–41.

Bunzow, J., Van Tol, H., Grandy, D., Albert, P., Salon, J., Christie, M., Machida, C., Neve, K., & Civelli, O. (1988). Cloning and expression of a rat D$_2$ dopamine receptor cDNA. *Nature, 336*, 783–787.

Butler, I. J., Koslow, S. H., Seifert, W. E., Jr., Caprioli, R. M., & Singer, H. S. (1979). Biogenic amine metabolism turnover in Tourette's syndrome. *Annals of Neurology, 6*, 37–39.

Castellanos, F., Elia, J., Kruesi, M., Gulotta, C., Mefford, I., Potter, W., Ritchie, G., & Rapoport, J. (1994). Cerebrospinal fluid monoamine metabolites in boys with attention-deficit hyperactivity disorder. *Psychiatry Research, 52*, 305–316.

Castellanos, F., Elia, J., Kruesi, M., Marsh, W. L., Gulotta, C., Potter, W., Ritchie, G., Hamburger, S., & Rapoport, J. (1996). Cerebrospinal fluid homovanillic acid predicts behavioral response to stimulants in 45 boys with attention deficit hyperactivity disorder. *Neuropsychopharmacology, 14*, 125–137.

Chatterjee, D., & Anderson, G. M. (1993). The human platelet dense granule: Serotonin uptake, tetrabenazine binding, phospholipid and ganglioside profiles. *Archives of Biochemistry Biophysics, 302*, 439–446.

Chen, K., Wu, H. F., & Shih, J. C. (1993). The deduced amino acid sequences of human platelet and frontal cortex monoamine oxidase B are identical. *Journal of Neurochemistry, 61*, 187–190.

Chen, K., Yang, W., Grimsby, J., & Shih, J. C. (1992). The human 5-HT2 receptor is encoded by a multiple intron–exon gene. *Brain Research Molecular Brain Research, 14,* 20–26.

Coccaro, E. F., Siever, L. J., Klar, H. M., Maurer, G., Cochrane, K., Cooper, T. B., Mohs, R. C., & Davis, K. L. (1989). Serotonergic studies in patients with affective and personality disorders: Correlates with suicidal and impulsive aggressive behavior. *Archives of General Psychiatry, 46,* 587–599.

Cohen, D. J., Caparulo, B. K., Shaywitz, B. A., & Bowers, M. B. J. (1977). Dopamine and serotonin metabolism in neuropsychiatrically disturbed children: CSF homovanillic acid and 5-hydroxyindoleacetic acid. *Archives of General Psychiatry, 34,* 545–550.

Cohen, D. J., Shaywitz, B. A., Caparulo, B., Young, J. G., & Bowers, M. B. J. (1978). Chronic, multiple tics of Gilles de la Tourette's disease: CSF acid monoamine metabolites after probenecid administration. *Archives of General Psychiatry, 35,* 245–250.

Cook, E. H., Anderson, G., Heninger, G., Fletcher, K. E., Freedman, D. X., & Leventhal, B. L. (1992). Tryptophan loading in hyperserotonemic and normoserotonemic adults. *Biological Psychiatry, 31,* 525–528.

Cook, E. H., Arora, R., Anderson, G., Berry-Kravis, E., Yan, S.-Y., Yeoh, H., Sklena, P., Charak, D., & Leventhal, B. (1993). Platelet serotonin studies in hyperserotonemic relatives of children with autistic disorder. *Life Sciences, 52,* 2005–2015.

Cook, E. H., Fletcher, K. E., Wainwright, M., Marks, N., Yan, S.-Y., & Leventhal, B. L. (1994). Primary structure of the human platelet serotonin 5-HT$_{2A}$ receptor: Identity with frontal cortex serotonin 5-HT$_{2A}$ receptor. *Journal of Neurochemistry, 63,* 465–469.

Cook, E. H., & Leventhal, B. L. (1992). Neuropsychiatric disorders of childhood and adolescence. In S. C. Yudofsky & R. E. Hales (Eds.), *Textbook of neuropsychiatry.* Washington, DC: American Psychiatric Press.

Cook, E. H., & Leventhal, B. (1996). The serotonin system in autism. *Current Opinions in Pediatrics, 8,* 348–354.

Cook, E. H., Leventhal, B. L., & Freedman, D. X. (1988a). Free serotonin in plasma: Autistic children and their first-degree relatives. *Biological Psychiatry, 24,* 488–491.

Cook, E. H., Leventhal, B. L., & Freedman, D. X. (1988b). Serotonin and measured intelligence. *Journal of Autism and Developmental Disorders, 18,* 553–559.

Cook, E., Stein, M., Krasowski, M., Cox, N., Olkon, D., Kieffer, J., & Leventhal, B. (1995). Association of attention deficit disorder and the dopamine transporter gene. *American Journal of Human Genetics, 56,* 993–998.

Cook, E. H., Stein, M. A., & Leventhal, B. L. (1997). Family-based association of the dopamine transporter gene in attention deficit disorder. In K. Blum & E. P. Noble (Eds.), *Handbook of psychiatric genetics.* New York: CRC Press.

Corash, L. (1980). Platelet heterogeneity. *Psychopharmacology Bulletin, 16,* 65–67.

Cotecchia, S., Schwinn, D., Randall, R., Lefkowitz, R., Caron, M., & Kobilka, B. (1988). Molecular cloning and expression of the cDNA for the hamster α_1-adrenergic receptor. *Proceedings of the National Academy of Sciences USA, 85,* 7159–7163.

Cowdry, R. W., Ebert, M. H., van Kammen, D. P., Post, R. M., & Goodwin, F. K. (1983). Cerebrospinal fluid probenecid studies: A reinterpretation. *Biological Psychiatry, 18,* 1287–1299.

Cox, N., Baker, L., & Spielman, R. (1988). Insulin gene sharing in sib pairs with insulin-dependent diabetes mellitus: No evidence for linkage. *American Journal of Human Genetics, 42,* 167–172.

Crews, C., & Erikson, R. (1993). Extracellular signals and reversible protein phosphorylation: What to Mek of it all. *Cell, 74,* 215–217.

Cummings, J. L. (1992). Depression and Parkinson's disease: A review. *American Journal of Psychiatry, 149,* 443–454.

Czernansky, J. G., Faull, K. F., & Pfefferbaum, A. (1988). Seasonal changes in CSF monoamine metabolites in psychiatric patients: What is the source? *Psychiatry Research, 25,* 361–363.

Dearry, A., Gingrich, J., Falardeau, P., Fremeau, R., Jr., Bates, M., & Caron, M. (1990). Molecular cloning and expression of the gene for a human D_1 dopamine receptor. *Nature, 347,* 72–76.

Delgado, P., Charney, D., Price, L., Aghajanian, G., Landis, H., & Heninger, G. (1990). Serotonin function and the mechanism of antidepressant action: Reversal of antidepressant-induced remission by rapid depletion of plasma tryptophan. *Archives of General Psychiatry, 47,* 411–418.

Dickson, B., Sprenger, F., Morrison, D., & Hafen, E. (1992). Raf functions downstream of Ras1 in the sevenless signal transduction pathway. *Nature, 360,* 600–603.

Dixon, R. A., Kobilka, B. K., Benovic, J. L., Dohlman, H. G., Frielle, T., Bolanowski, M. A., Bennett, C. D., Rands, E., Diehl, R. E., Mumford, R. A., Slater, E. E., Sigal, I. S., Caron, M. G., Lefkowitz, R. J., & Strader, C. D. (1986). Cloning of the gene and cDNA for mammalian β-adrenergic receptor and homology with rhodopsin. *Nature, 321,* 75–79.

Egan, S. E., Giddings, B. W., Brooks, M. W., Buday, L., Sizeland, A. M., & Weinberg, R. A. (1993). Association of Sos Ras exchange protein with Grb2 is implicated in tyrosine kinase signal transduction and transformation. *Nature, 363,* 45–51.

Egrise, D., Rubinstein, M., Schoutens, A., Cantraine, F., & Mendelewicz, J. (1986). Seasonal variation of platelet serotonin uptake and ^3H-imipramine binding in normal and depressed subjects. *Biological Psychiatry, 21,* 283–293.

Elliott, J. M., & Kent, A. (1989). Comparison of [125I]iodolysergic acid diethylamide binding in human frontal cortex and platelet tissue. *Journal of Neurochemistry, 53,* 191–196.

Emorine, L., Marullo, S., Briend-Sutren, M.-M., Patey, G., Tate, K., Delavier-Klutchko, C., & Strosberg, A. (1989). Molecular characterization of the human β3-adrenergic receptor. *Science, 245,* 1128–1131.

Erdmann, J., Shimron-Abarbanell, D., Cichon, S., Albus, M., Maier, W., Lichtermann, D., Minges, J., Reuner, U., Franzek, E., Ertl, M. A., et al. (1995). Systematic screening for mutations in the promoter and the coding region of the 5-HT1A gene. *American Journal of Medical Genetics (Neuropsychiatric Genetics), 60,* 393–399.

Erdmann, J., Shimron-Abarbanell, D., Rietschel, M., Albus, M., Maier, W., Koerner, J., Bondy, B., Chen, K., Shih, J. C., Knapp, M., Propping, P., & Nothen, M. M. (1996). Systematic screening for mutations in the human serotonin–2A (5-HT2A) receptor gene: Identification of two naturally occurring receptor variants and association analysis in schizophrenia. *Human Genetics, 97,* 614–619.

Erlander, M. G., Lovenberg, T. W., Baron, B. M., de Lecea, L., Danielson, P. E., Racke, M., Slone, A. L., Siegel, B. W., Foye, P. E., Cannon, K., Burns, D. E., & Sutcliffe, G. J. (1993). Two members of a distinct subfamily of 5-hydroxytryptamine receptors differentially expressed in rat brain. *Proceedings of the National Academy of Sciences USA, 90,* 3452–3456.

Escover, H., Malitz, S., & Wilkins, B. (1961). Clinical profiles of paid normal subjects volunteering for hallucinogen studies. *American Journal of Psychiatry, 117,* 910–915.

Eysenck, S. B. G., Easting, G., & Pearson, P. R. (1984). Age norms for impulsiveness, venturesomeness and empathy in children. *Personality and Individual Differences, 5,* 315–321.

Fargin, A., Raymond, J., Lohse, M., Kobilka, B., Caron, M., & Lefkowitz, R. (1988). The genomic clone G–21 which resembles the β-adrenergic receptor sequence encodes the 5-HT$_{1A}$ receptor. *Nature, 335,* 358–360.

Faustman, W., Elliott, P., Ringo, D., & Faull, K. (1993). CSF 5-HIAA and atmospheric pressure: Failure to replicate. *Biological Psychiatry, 33,* 61–63.

Ferguson, H. B., & Bawden, H. N. (1988). Psychobiological measures. In M. Rutter, A. H. Tuma & I. S. Lann (Eds.), *Assessment and diagnosis in child psychopathology.* New York: Guilford Press.

Foguet, M., Hoyer, D., Pardo, L., Parekh, A., Kluxen, F., Kalkman, H., Stühme, W., & Lübbert, H. (1992). Cloning and functional characterization of the rat stomach fundus serotonin receptor. *EMBO Journal, 11,* 3481–3487.

Frielle, T., Collins, S., Daniel, K., Caron, M., Lefkowitz, R., & Kobilka, B. (1987). Cloning of the cDNA for the β$_1$-adrenergic receptor. *Proceedings of the National Academy of Sciences USA, 85,* 9494–9498.

Garelis, E., Young, S. N., Lal, S., & Sourkes, T. L. (1974). Monoamine metabolites in lumbar CSF: The question of their origin in relation to clinical studies. *Brain Research, 79,* 1–8.

Gelernter, J., & Freimer, M. (1994). PstI RFLP at the SERT locus. *Human Molecular Genetics, 3,* 383.

Gelernter, J., Rao, P., Pauls, D., Hamblin, M., Sibley, D., & Kidd, K. (1995). Assignment of the 5HT7 receptor gene (HTR7) to chromosome 10q and exclusion of linkage with Tourette syndrome. *Genomics, 26,* 207–209.

Geller, E., Yuwiler, A., Freeman, B. J., & Ritvo, E. (1988). Platelet size, number, and serotonin content in blood of autistic, childhood schizophrenic, and normal children. *Journal of Autism and Developmental Disorders, 18,* 119–126.

Gerald, C., Adham, N., Kao, H. T., Olsen, M. A., Laz, T. M., Schechter, L. E., Bard, J. A., Vaysse, P. J. J., Hartig, P. R., Branchek, T. A., & Weinshank, R. L. (1995). The 5-HT4 receptor: Molecular cloning and pharmacological characterization of two splice variants. *EMBO Journal, 14,* 2806–2815.

Gibbons, R. D., Davis, J. M., & Hedeker, D. R. (1990). A comment on the selection of "healthy controls" for psychiatric experiments. *Archives of General Psychiatry, 47,* 785–786.

Giese, K. P., Fedorov, N. B., Filipkowski, R. K., & Silva, A. J. (1998). Autophosphorylation at Thr286 of the alpha calcium-calmodulin kinase II in LTP and learning. *Science, 279,* 870–873.

Gill, M., Daly, G., Heron, S., Haw, Z., & Fitzgerald, M. (1997). Confirmation of association between attention deficit hyperactivity disorder and a dopamine transporter polymorphism. *Molecular Psychiatry, 2,* 311–313.

Giros, B., Martres, M., Sokoloff, P., & Schwartz, J. (1990). Gene cloning of the human dopaminergic D$_3$ receptor and chromosome identification. *Comptes Rendus de l'Academie des Sciences, 311,* 501–508.

Giroud, M., Dumas, R., Dauvergne, M., D'Athis, P., Rochette, L., Beley, A., & Bralet, J. (1990). 5-Hydroxyindoleacetic acid and homovanillic acid in cerebrospinal fluid of children with febrile convulsions. *Epilepsia, 31,* 178–181.

Goldman, D., Lappalainen, J., Ozaki, N., Nakhai, B., Pesonen, U., Koulu, M., Giblin, B.,

Nielsen, D., Linnoila, M., & Dean, M. (1994). Polymorphism and genetic mapping of six human serotonin receptor genes. *Society for Neuroscience Abstracts, 20,* 1266.

Goldman, D., Nielsen, D., Okada, M., Adamson, M., Lappalainen, J., Nalhotra, N., Pesonen, U., Koulu, M., Eggert, M., Virkkunen, M., et al. (1996). Molecular genetics of impaired impulse control and early onset alchoholism. *Biological Psychiatry, 39,* A212.

Grailhe, R., Amlaiky, N., Ghavami, A., Ramboz, S., Yocca, F., Mahle, C., Margouris, C., Perrot, F., & Hen, R. (1994). Human and mouse 5-HT_{5A} and 5-HT_{5B} receptors: Cloning and functional expression. *Society for Neuroscience Abstracts, 20,* 1160.

Grandy, D., Marchionni, M., Makam, H., Stofko, R., Alfano, M., Frothingham, L., Fischer, J., Burke-Howie, K., Bunzow, J., Server, A., & Civelli, O. (1989). Cloning of the cDNA and a gene for a human D_2 dopamine receptor. *Proceedings of the National Academy of Sciences USA, 86,* 9762–9766.

Grandy, D., Zhang, Y., Bouvier, C., Zhou, Q.-Y., Johnson, R., Allen, L., Buck, K., Bunzow, J., Salon, J., & Civelli, O. (1991). Multiple D_5 dopamine receptor genes: A functional receptor and two pseudogenes. *Proceedings of the National Academy of Sciences USA, 88,* 9175–9179.

Grant, S. G., O'Dell, T. J., Karl, K. A., Stein, P. L., Soriano, P., & Kandel, E. R. (1992). Impaired long-term potentiation, spatial learning, and hippocampal development in fyn mutant mice. *Science, 258,* 1903–1910.

Grasbeck, R. (1981). Health as seen from the laboratory. In R. Grasbeck & T. Alstrom (Eds.), *Reference values in laboratory medicine: The current state of the art.* New York: Wiley.

Guinebault, C., Payrastre, B., Sultan, C., Mauco, G., Breton, M., Levy-Toledano, S., Plantavid, M., & Chap, H. (1993). Tyrosine kinases and phosphoinositide metabolism in thrombin-stimulated human platelets. *Biochemical Journal, 292,* 851–856.

Guthrie, S. K., Berrettini, W., Rubinow, D. R., Nurnberger, J. I., Bartko, J. J., & Linnoila, M. (1986). Different neurotransmitter metabolite concentrations in CSF samples from inpatient and outpatient normal volunteers. *Acta Psychiatrica Scandinavica, 73,* 315–321.

Habel, A., Yates, C. M., McQueen, J. K., Blackwood, D., & Elton, R. A. (1981). Homovanillic acid and 5-hydroxyindoleacetic acid in lumbar cerebrospinal fluid in children with afebrile and febrile convulsions. *Neurology, 31,* 488–491.

Hanna, G. L., Himle, J. A., Curtis, G. C., Koram, D. Q., Weele, J. V. V., Leventhal, B. L., & Cook, E. H., Jr. (1998). Serotonin transporter and seasonal variation in blood serotonin in families with obsessive–compulsive disorder. *Neuropsychopharmacology, 18,* 102–111.

Hartig, P. R., Branchek, T. A., & Weinshank, R. L. (1992). A subfamily of 5-HT_{1D} receptor genes. *TiPS, 13,* 152–159.

Heyes, M. P., Saito, K., Crowley, J., Davis, L. E., Demitrack, M. A., Der, M., Dilling, L. A., Elia, J. E., Kruesi, M. J. P., Lackner, A., et al. (1992). Quinolinic acid and kynurenine pathway metabolism in inflammatory and non-inflammatory neurologic disease. *Brain, 115,* 1249–1273.

Higley, J. D., King, S. T., Hasert, M. F., Champoux, M., Suomi, S. J., & Linnoila, M. (1996). Stability of interindividual differences in serotonin function and its relationship to severe aggression and competent social behavior in rhesus macaque females. *Neuropsychopharmacology, 14,* 67–76.

Higley, J. D., & Linnoila, M. (1997). Low central nervous system serotonergic activity is traitlike and correlates with impulsive behavior: A nonhuman primate model investigating genetic and environmental influences on neurotransmission. *Annals of the New York Academy of Sciences, 836,* 39–56.

Higley, J. D., Thompson, W. W., Champoux, M., Goldman, D., Hasert, M. F., Kraemer, G. W., Scanlan, J. M., Suomi, S. J., & Linnoila, M. (1993). Paternal and maternal genetic and environmental contributions to cerebrospinal fluid monoamine metabolites in rhesus monkeys (*Macaca mulatta*). *Archives of General Psychiatry, 50,* 615–623.

Higuchi, R., von Beroldingen, C., Sensabaugh, G., & Erlich, H. (1988). DNA typing from single hairs. *Nature, 332,* 543–546.

Hsiao, J. K., Colison, J., Bartko, J. J., Doran, A. R., Konicki, P. E., Potter, W. Z., & Pickar, D. (1993). Monoamine neurotransmitter interactions in drug-free and neuroleptic-treated schizophrenics. *Archives of General Psychiatry, 50,* 606–614.

Jessell, T., & Kandel, E. (1993). Synaptic transmission: A bidirectional and self-modifiable form of cell–cell communication. *Cell/Neuron, 72*(Suppl. 10), S1–S30.

Jessell, T., Kandel, E., Lewin, B., & Reid, L. (Eds.). (1993). Signaling at the synapse. *Cell/Neuron, 72*(Suppl. 10), S1–S149.

Jimerson, D. C., & Berrettini, W. (1985). *Cerebrospinal fluid amine metabolite studies in depression: Research update.* Berlin: Springer-Verlag.

Jimerson, D. C., Gordon, E. K., Post, R. M., & Goodwin, F. K. (1978). Homovanillic acid in human CSF: Comparison of fluorimetry and gas chromatography–mass spectrometry. *Communications in Psychopharmacology, 2,* 343–349.

Julius, D., Huang, K. N., Livelli, T. J., Axel, R., & Jessell, T. M. (1990). The 5HT2 receptor defines a family of structurally distinct but functionally conserved serotonin receptors. *Proceedings of the National Academy of Sciences USA, 87,* 928–932.

Julius, D., MacDermott, A., Axel, R., & Jessel, T. (1988). Molecular characterization of a functional cDNA encoding the serotonin 1C receptor. *Science, 241,* 558–564.

Kahn, R. S., Davidson, M., Knott, P., Stern, R. G., Apter, S., & Davis, K. (1993). Effects of neuroleptic medication on cerebrospinal fluid monoamine metabolite concentrations in schizophrenia: Serotonin–dopamine interactions as a target for treatment. *Archives of General Psychiatry, 50,* 599–605.

Kallenberg, K., Forslin, L., & Westerborn, O. (1993). The disposal of the aborted fetus—new guidelines: Ethical considerations in the debate in Sweden. *Journal of Medical Ethics, 19,* 32–36.

Kaufman, M., Hartig, P., & Hoffman, B. (1995). Serotonin 5-HT$_{2C}$ receptor stimulates cyclic GMP formation in choroid plexus. *Journal of Neurochemistry, 64,* 199–205.

Kearney, W., Vawter, D. E., & Gervais, K. G. (1991). Fetal tissue research and the misread compromise. *Hastings Center Report, 21,* 7–12.

Kemper, T. L., & Bauman, M. L. (1993). The contribution of neuropathologic studies to the understanding of autism. *Neurologic Clinics, 11,* 175–187.

Kent, T., Brown, C., Bryant, S., Barratt, E., Felthous, A., & Rose, R. (1988). Blood uptake of serotonin in episodic aggression: Correlation with red blood cell proton T_1 and impulsivity. *Psychopharmacology Bulletin, 24,* 454–457.

Kimelberg, H., & Katz, D. (1985). High-affinity uptake of serotonin into immunocytochemically identified astrocytes. *Science, 228,* 889–891.

Kirwin, P. D., Anderson, G. M., Chappell, P. B., Saberski, L., Leckman, J. F., Geracioti, T. D., Heninger, G. R., Price, L. H., & McDougle, C. J. (1997). Assessment of diurnal variation of cerebrospinal fluid tryptophan and 5-hydroxyindoleacetic acid in healthy human females. *Life Sciences, 60,* 899–907.

Kling, M. A., DeBellis, M. D., O'Rourke, D. K., Listwak, S. J., Geracioti, T. D., McCutcheon, I. E., Kalogeras, K. T., Oldfield, E. N., & Gold, P. W. (1994). Diurnal variation of cerebrospinal releasing hormome in healthy volunteers. *Journal of Clinical Endocrinology and Metabolism, 79,* 233–239.

Kobilka, B., Matsui, H., Kobilka, T., Yang-Feng, T., Franke, U., Caron, M., Lefkowitz, R., & Regan, J. (1987). Cloning, sequencing, and expression of the gene coding for the human platelet α₂-adrenergic receptor. *Science, 238,* 650–656.

Kohen, R., Metcalf, M. A., Khan, N., Druck, T., Huebner, K., Lachowicz, J. E., Meltzer, H. Y., Sibley, D. R., Roth, B. L., & Hamblin, M. W. (1996). Cloning, characterization, and chromosomal localization of a human 5-HT6 serotonin receptor. *Journal of Neurochemistry, 66,* 47–56.

Kruesi, M. J. P., Hibbs, E. D., Zahn, T. P., Keysor, C. S., Hamburger, S. D., Bartko, J. J., & Rapoport, J. L. (1992). A 2-year prospective follow-up study of children and adolescents with disruptive behavior disorders: Prediction by cerebrospinal fluid 5-hydroxyindoleacetic acid, homovanillic acid, and autonomic measures? *Archives of General Psychiatry, 49,* 429–435.

Kruesi, M. J. P., & Jacobsen, T. (1998). Serotonin and human violence: Do environmental mediators exist? In A. Raine, D. Farrington, P. Brennan, & S. Mednick (Eds.), *Biosocial bases of violence.* New York: Plenum Press.

Kruesi, M. J. P., Lenane, M. C., Hibbs, E. D., & Major, J. (1990). Normal controls and biological reference values in child psychiatry: Defining normal. *Journal of the American Academy of Child and Adolescent Psychiatry, 29,* 449–452.

Kruesi, M. J. P., & Rapoport, J. L. (1992). Psychoactive agents. In S. Yaffee & J. Aranda (Eds.), *Pediatric pharmacology.* Philadelphia: W.B. Saunders.

Kruesi, M. J. P., Rapoport, J. L., Hamburger, S., Hibbs, E., Potter, W. Z., Lenane, M., & Brown, G. L. (1990). Cerebrospinal fluid monoamine metabolites, aggression, and impulsivity in disruptive behavior disorders of children and adolescents. *Archives of General Psychiatry, 47,* 419–426.

Kruesi, M. J. P., Swedo, S. E., Coffey, M. L., Hamburger, S. D., Leonard, H., & Rapoport, J. L. (1988). Objective and subjective side effects of research lumbar punctures in children and adolesecents. *Psychiatry Research, 25,* 59–63.

Kruesi, M. J. P., Swedo, S. E., Hamburger, S. D., Potter, W. Z., & Rapoport, J. L. (1988). Concentration gradient of CSF monoamine metabolites in children and adolescents. *Biological Psychiatry, 24,* 507–514.

Kruesi, M. J. P., Swedo, S. E., Leonard, H. L., Rubinow, D. R., & Rapoport, J. L. (1990). CSF somatostatin in childhood psychiatric disorders: A preliminary investigation. *Psychiatry Research, 33,* 277–284.

Kumar, B. V., & Sastry, P. S. (1992). Dopamine receptors in human foetal brains: Characterization, regulation and ontogeny of [3H]spiperone binding sites in striatum. *Neurochemistry International, 20,* 559–566.

Kursar, J., Nelson, D., Wainscott, D., Cohen, M., & Baez, M. (1992). Molecular cloning, functional expression, and pharmacological characterization of a novel serotonin receptor (5-hydroxytryptamine₂F) from rat stomach receptor. *Molecular Pharmacology, 42,* 549–557.

Lake, C. R., Wood, J. H., Ziegler, M. G., Ebert, M. H., & Kopin, I. J. (1978). Probenecid induced norepinephrine elevations in plasma and CSF. *Archives of General Psychiatry, 35,* 237–240.

Lam, S., Shen, Y., Nguyen, T., Messier, T. L., Brann, M., Comings, D., George, S. R., & BF, O. D. (1996). A serotonin receptor gene (5HT1A) variant found in a Tourette's syndrome patient. *Biochemical and Biophysical Research Communications, 219,* 853–858.

Lappalainen, J., Zhang, L., Dean, M., Oz, M., Ozaki, N., Yu, D. H., Virkkunen, M., Weight, F., Linnoila, M., & Goldman, D. (1995). Identification, expression, and pharmacology of a Cys_{23}-Ser_{23} substitution in the human 5-HT_{2C} receptor gene (HTR2C). *Genomics, 27,* 274–279.

Lasagna, L., & von Felsinger, J. M. (1954). The volunteer subject in research. *Science, 120,* 186–190.

Launay, J., Bursztejn, C., Ferrari, P., Dreux, C., Braconnier, A., Zarifian, E., Lancrenon, S., & Fermanian, J. (1987). Catecholamine metabolism in infantile autism: A controlled study of 22 autistic children. *Journal of Autism and Developmental Disorders, 17,* 333–347.

Le Coniat, M., Choi, D. S., Maroteaux, L., Launay, J. M., & Berger, R. (1996). The 5-HT2B receptor gene maps to 2q36.3–2q37.1. *Genomics, 32,* 172–173.

Lench, N., Stanier, P., & Williamson, R. (1988). Simple non-invasive method to obtain DNA for gene analysis. *Lancet, i,* 1356–1358.

Lesch, K.-P., Bengel, D., Heils, A., Sabol, S. Z., Greenberg, B. D., Petri, S., Benjamin, J., Müller, C. R., Hamer, D. H., & Murphy, D. L. (1996). Association of anxiety-related traits with a polymorphism in the serotonin transporter gene regulatory region. *Science, 274,* 1527–1531.

Lesch, K.-P., Wolozin, B. L., Murphy, D. L., & Riederer, P. (1993). Primary structure of the human platelet serotonin uptake site: Identity with the brain serotonin transporter. *Journal of Neurochemistry, 60,* 2319–2322.

Levy, F., Gudermann, T., Birnbaumer, M., Kaumann, A., & Birnbaumer, L. (1994). Assignment of the gene encoding the 5-HT1E serotonin receptor (S31)(locus HTR1E) to human chromosome 6q14–q15. *Genomics, 22,* 637–640.

Linares, O. A., Jacquez, J. A., Zech, L. A., Smith, M. J., Sanfield, J. A., Morrow, L. A., Rosen, S. G., & Halter, J. B. (1987). Norepinephrine metabolism in humans: Kinetic analysis and model. *Journal of Clinical Investigation, 80,* 1332–1341.

Lomasney, J., Cotecchia, S., Lorenz, W., Leung, W.-Y., Schwinn, D., Yang-Feng, T., Brownstein, M., Lefkowitz, R., & Caron, M. (1991). Molecular cloning and expression of the cDNA for the α_{1A}-adrenergic receptor. *Journal of Biological Chemistry, 266,* 6365–6369.

Lovenberg, T., Erlander, M., Baron, B., Racke, M., Slone, A., Siegel, B., Craft, C., Burns, J., Danielson, P., & Sutcliffe, J. (1993). Molecular cloning and functional expression of rat and human 5-HT_{1E}-like 5-hydroxytryptamine receptor genes. *Proceedings of the National Academy of Sciences USA, 90,* 2184–2188.

Mann, J., McBride, P., Anderson, G., & Mieczkowski, T. (1992). Platelet and whole blood serotonin content in depressed inpatients: Correlations with acute and life-time psychopathology. *Biological Psychiatry, 32,* 243–257.

Maricq, A. V., Peterson, A. S., Brake, A. J., Myers, R. M., & Julius, D. (1991). Primary structure and functional expression of the 5HT-3 receptor, a serotonin-gated ion channel. *Science, 254,* 432–437.

Matthes, H., Boschert, U., Amlaiky, N., Grailhe, R., Plassat, J., Muscatelli, F., Mattei, M., & Hen, R. (1993). Mouse 5-hydroxytryptamine$_{5A}$ and 5-hydroxytryptamine$_{5B}$ receptors define a new family of serotonin receptors: Cloning, functional expression, and chromosomal localization. *Molecular Pharmacology, 43,* 313–319.

Mazer, C., Muneyyirci, J., Taheny, K., Raio, N., Borella, A., & Whitaker-Azmitia, P.

(1997). Serotonin depletion during synaptogenesis leads to decreased synaptic density and learning deficits in the adult rat: A possible model of neurodevelopmental disorders with cognitive deficits. *Brain Research, 760,* 68–73.

McAllister, G., Charlesworth, A., Snodin, C., Beer, M., Noble, A., Middlemiss, D., Iversen, L., & Whiting, P. (1992). Molecular cloning of a serotonin receptor from human brain (5-HT$_{1E}$): A fifth 5-HT$_1$-like subtype. *Proceedings of the National Academy of Sciences USA, 89,* 5517–5521.

McBride, P. A., Anderson, G. M., Hertzig, M. E., Snow, M. E., Thompson, S. M., Khait, V. D., Shapiro, T., & Cohen, D. J. (1998). Effects of diagnosis, race, and puberty on platelet serotonin levels in autism and mental retardation. *Journal of the American Academy of Child and Adolescent Psychiatry, 37,* 767–776.

McBride, P. A., Anderson, G. M., Hertzig, M. E., Sweeney, J. A., Kream, J., Cohen, D. J., & Mann, J. J. (1989). Serotonergic responsivity in male young adults with autistic disorder. *Archives of General Psychiatry, 46,* 205–212.

McClue, S. J., Brazell, C., & Stahl, S. M. (1989). Hallucinogenic drugs are partial agonists of the human platelet shape change response: A physiological model of the 5-HT2 receptor. *Biological Psychiatry, 26,* 297–302.

McDougle, C., Naylor, S., Cohen, D., Aghajanian, G., Heninger, G., & Price, L. (1996). Effects of tryptophan depletion in drug-free adults with autistic disorder. *Archives of General Psychiatry, 53,* 993–1000.

McFarlin, K. E., Kruesi, M. J. P., & Nadi, N. S. (1990). Red blood cell contamination and amino acid concentration in the cerebrospinal fluid of children. *Psychiatry Research, 33,* 99–101.

Mefford, I. N., Ward, M. M., Miles, L., Taylor, B., Chesney, M. A., Keegan, D. L., & Barchas, J. D. (1981). Determination of plasma catecholamines and free 3,4-dihydroxyphenolacetic acid in continuously collected human plasma by high performance liquid chromatography with electrochemical detection. *Life Sciences, 28,* 477–483.

Meyerhof, W., Obermüller, F., Fehr, S., & Richter, D. (1993). A novel rat serotonin receptor: Primary structure, pharmacology, and expression pattern in distinct brain regions. *DNA and Cell Biology, 12,* 401–409.

Miyake, A., Mochizuki, S., Takemoto, Y., & Akuzawa, S. (1995). Molecular cloning of human 5-hydroxytryptamine3 receptor: Heterogeneity in distribution and function among species. *Molecular Pharmacology, 48,* 407–416.

Moir, A. T. B., Ashcroft, G. W., Crawford, T. B. B., Eccleston, D., & Guldberg, H. C. (1970). Cerebral metabolites in cerebrospinal fluid as a biochemical approach to the brain. *Brain, 93,* 357–368.

Monsma, F., Jr., Mahan, L., McVittie, L., Gerfen, C., & Sibley, D. (1990). Molecular cloning and expression of a D$_1$ dopamine receptor linked to adenylyl cyclase activation. *Proceedings of the National Academy of Sciences USA, 87,* 6723–6727.

Monsma, F., Jr., Shen, Y., Ward, R., Hamblin, M., & Sibley, D. (1993). Cloning and expression of a novel serotonin receptor with high affinity for tricyclic psychotropic drugs. *Molecular Pharmacology, 43,* 320–327.

Murphy, T. K., Goodman, W. K., Fudge, M. W., Williams, R. C., Jr., Ayoub, E. M., Dalal, M., Lewis, M. H., & Zabriskie, J. B. (1997). B lymphocyte antigen D8/17: A peripheral marker for childhood-onset obsessive–compulsive disorder and Tourette's syndrome? *American Journal of Psychiatry, 154,* 402–407.

Muscettola, G., Wehr, T., & Goodwin, F. K. (1977). Effect of diet on urinary MHPG excretion in depressed patients and normal control subjects. *American Journal of Psychiatry, 134,* 914–916.

Muskiet, F. A., Jeuring, H. J., Korf, J., Sedvall, G., Westerink, B. H., Teelken, A. W., & Wolthers, B. G. (1979). Correlations between a fluorimetric and mass fragmentographic method for the determination of 3-methoxy–4-hydroxyphenylacetic acid and two mass fragmentographic methods for the determination of 3-methoxy–4-hydroxyphenylethylene glycol in cerebrospinal fluid. *Journal of Neurochemistry, 32,* 191–194.

Nakhai, B., Nielsen, D., Linnoila, M., & Goldman, D. (1995). Two naturally occurring amino acid substitutions in the human 5HT1A receptor: 5HT1A–22 Gly-Ser and 5HT1A–28 Ile-Val. *Biochemical and Biophysical Research Communications, 210,* 530–536.

Needlman, R., Zuckerman, B., Anderson, G., Mirochnick, M., & Cohen, D. (1993). Cerebrospinal fluid monoamine precursors and metabolites in human neonates following in utero cocaine exposure: A preliminary study. *Pediatrics, 92,* 55–60.

Nicoletti, F., Raffaele, R., Falsaperla, A., & Paci, R. (1981). Circadian variation in 5-hydroxyindoleacetic acid levels in human cerebrospinal fluid. *European Neurology, 20,* 9–12.

Nordin, C. (1989). Gradients of monoamine metabolites in relation to position of the lumbar puncture needle. *Biological Psychiatry, 25,* 513–516.

Nordin, C. (1991). CSF spinal gradients of 5-HIAA [Letter]. *Biological Psychiatry, 29,* 302–303.

Nordin, C., Swedin, A., & Zachau, A. (1992). CSF 5-HIAA and atmospheric pressure [Letter]. *Biological Psychiatry, 31,* 644–645.

Nöthen, M., Erdmann, J., Shimron-Abarbanell, D., & Propping, P. (1994). Identification of genetic variation in the human serotonin 1Dβ receptor gene. *Biochemical and Biophysical Research Communications, 205,* 1194–1200.

Orita, M., Iwahana, H., Kanazawa, H., Hayashi, K., & Sekiya, T. (1989). Detection of polymorphisms of human DNA by gel electrophoresis as single-stranded conformation polymorphisms. *Proceedings of the National Academy of Sciences USA, 86,* 2766–2770.

Oxenstierna, G., Edman, G., Iselius, L., Oreland, L., Ross, S. B., & Sedvall, G. (1986). Concentrations of monoamine metabolites in the cerebrospinal fluid of twins and unrelated individuals: A genetic study. *Journal of Psychiatric Research, 20,* 19–29.

Ozaki, N., Rosenthal, N., Pesonen, U., Lappalainen, J., Felman-Naim, S., Schwartz, P., Turner, E., & Goldman, D. (1996). Two naturally occurring amino acid substitutions of the 5-HT$_{2A}$ receptor: Similar prevalence in patients with seasonal affective disorder and controls. *Biological Psychiatry, 40,* 1267–1272.

Pacholczyk, T., Blakely, R. D., & Amara, S. G. (1991). Expression cloning of a cocaine- and antidepressant-sensitive human noradrenaline transporter. *Nature, 350,* 350–354.

Page, T., Yu, A., Fontanesi, J., & Nyhan, W. L. (1997). Developmental disorder associated with increased cellular nucleotidase activity. *Proceedings of the National Academy of Sciences USA, 94,* 11601–11606.

Perry, B. D., Cook, E. H., Leventhal, B. L., Wainwright, M. S., & Freedman, D. X. (1991). Platelet 5-HT$_2$-serotonin receptor binding sites in autistic children and their first-degree relatives. *Biological Psychiatry, 30,* 1–10.

Pfeffer, C. R., McBride, P. A., Anderson, G. M., Kakuma, T., Fensterheim, L., & Khait, V. (1998). Peripheral serotonin measures in prepubertal psychiatric inpatients and normal children: Associations with suicidal behavior and its risk factors. *Biological Psychiatry, 44,* 568–577.

Pickar, D., Owen, R. R., Litman, R. E., Konicki, P. E., Gutierrez, R., & Rapaport, M. H. (1992). Clinical and biologic response to clozapine in patients with schizophrenia. *Archives of General Psychiatry, 49,* 345–353.

Pietraszek, M., Urano, T., Sumiyoshi, K., Takada, Y., Takada, A., Ohara, K., Kondo, N., & Ohara, K. (1992). Diurnal variations of whole blood serotonin content in patients with depression and neurosis. *Journal of Neurology, Neurosurgery and Psychiatry, 55,* 336.

Plassat, J.-L., Amlaiky, N., & Hen, R. (1993). Molecular cloning of a mammalian serotonin receptor that activates adenylate cyclase. *Molecular Pharmacology, 44,* 229–236.

Pliszka, S., Rogeness, G., Renner, P., Sherman, J., & Broussard, T. (1988). Plasma neurochemistry in juvenile offenders. *Journal of the American Academy of Child and Adolescent Psychiatry, 27,* 588–594.

Pollin, W., & Perlin, S. (1958). Psychiatric evaluation of "normal control" volunteers. *American Journal of Psychiatry, 115,* 129–133.

Popp-Snijders, C. P., Geenen, B., & Heijden, V. D. (1989). Serum noradrenaline is composed of plasma and platelet noradrenaline. *Annals of Clinical Biochemistry, 26,* 191–192.

Post, R. M., Kotin, J., Goodwin, F. K., & Gordon, E. K. (1973). Psychomotor activity and cerebrospinal fluid amine metabolites in affective illness. *American Journal of Psychiatry, 130,* 67–72.

Potter, W., Hsiao, J., & Goldman, S. (1989). Effects of renal clearance on plasma concentrations of homovanillic acid. *Archives of General Psychiatry, 46,* 558–562.

Potter, W., & Manji, H. (1993). Are monoamine metabolites in cerebrospinal fluid worth measuring? *Archives of General Psychiatry, 50,* 653–656.

Pulver, A. E., Bartko, J. J., & McGrath, J. A. (1988). The power of analysis: Statistical perspectives. Part 1. *Psychiatry Research, 23,* 295–299.

Purves, D., & Lichtman, J. W. (1985). *Principles of neural development.* Sunderland, MA: Sinauer Associates.

Raleigh, M. J., Brammer, G. L., & McGuire, M. T. (1983). Male dominance, serotonergic systems, and the behavioral and physiological effects of drugs in vervet monkeys (*Cercopithecus aethiops sabaeus*). In K. Miczek (Ed.), *Ethnopharmacology: Primate models of neuropsychiatric disorders.* New York: Alan R. Liss.

Raleigh, M. J., Brammer, G. L., McGuire, M. T., & Yuwiler, A. (1985). Dominant social status facilitates the behavioral effects of serotonergic agonists. *Brain Research, 348,* 274–282.

Regan, J., Kobilka, T., Yang-Feng, T., Caron, M., & Lefkowitz, R. (1988). Cloning and expression of a human kidney cDNA for a novel α_2-adrenergic receptor. *Proceedings of the National Academy of Sciences USA, 85,* 6301–6305.

Reiss, A. L., Freund, L. S., Baumgardner, T. L., Abrams, M. T., & Denckla, M. B. (1995). Contribution of the FMR1 gene mutation to human intellectual dysfunction. *Nature Genetics, 11,* 331–334.

Riddle, M. A., Anderson, G. M., McIntosh, S., Harcherik, D. F., Shaywitz, B. A., & Cohen, D. J. (1986). Cerebrospinal fluid monoamine precursor and metabolite levels in children treated for leukemia: Age and sex effects and individual variability. *Biological Psychiatry, 21,* 69–83.

Riddle, M. A., Jatlow, P. I., Anderson, G. M., Cho, S. C., Hardin, M. T., Cohen, D. J., & Leckman, J. F. (1989). Plasma debrisoquin levels in the assessment of reduction of plasma homovanillic acid: The debrisoquin method. *Neuropsychopharmacology, 2,* 123–129.

Riddle, M. A., Leckman, J. F., Cohen, D. J., Anderson, M., Ort, S. I., Caruso, K. A., & Shaywitz, B. A. (1986). Assessment of central dopaminergic function using plasma-free homovanillic acid after debrisoquin administration. *Journal of Neural Transmission, 67,* 31–43.

Risch, S. C., & Lewine, R. R. (1993). Low cerebrospinal fluid homovanillic acid–5-hydroxyindoleacetic acid ratio predicts clozapine efficacy: A replication. *Archives of General Psychiatry, 50,* 670.

Ritvo, E. R., Freeman, B. J., Scheibel, A. B., Duong, T., Robinson, H., Guthrie, D., & Ritvo, A. (1986). Lower Purkinje cell counts in the cerebella of four autistic subjects: Initial findings of the UCLA–NSAC autopsy research report. *American Journal of Psychiatry, 143,* 862–866.

Ritvo, E., Yuwiler, A., Geller, E., Plotkin, S., Mason, A., & Saeger, K. (1971). Maturational changes in blood serotonin levels and platelet counts. *Biochemical Medicine, 5,* 90–96.

Rosengren, L. E., Ahlsen, G., Belfrage, M., Gillberg, C., Haglid, K. G., & Hamberger, A. (1992). A sensitive ELISA for glial fibrillary acidic protein: Application in CSF of children. *Journal of Neuroscience Methods, 44,* 113–119.

Rothpearl, A. B., Mohs, R. C., & Davis, K. L. (1981). Statistical power in biological psychiatry. *Psychiatry Research, 5,* 257–266.

Roy, A., Adinoff, B., DeJong, J., & Linnoila, M. (1991). Cerebrospinal fluid variables among alcoholics lack seasonal variation. *Acta Psychiatrica Scandinavica, 84,* 579–582.

Rozakis-Adcock, M., Fernley, R., Wade, J., Pawson, T., & Bowtell, D. (1993). The SH2 and SH3 domains of mammalian Grb2 couple the EGF receptor to the Ras activator mSos1. *Nature, 363,* 83–85.

Ruat, M., Traiffort, E., Arrang, J. M., Tardivel-Lacombe, J., Diaz, J., Leurs, R., & Schwartz, J. C. (1993). A novel rat serotonin (5-HT6) receptor: Molecular cloning, localization and stimulation of cAMP accumulation. *Biochemical and Biophysical Research Communications, 193,* 268–276.

Rubinow, D. R. (1986). Cerebrospinal fluid somatostatin and psychiatric illness. *Biological Psychiatry, 21,* 341–365.

Saudou, F., Amara, D., Dierich, A., LeMeur, M., Ramboz, S., Segu, L., Buhot, M.-C., & Hen, R. (1994). Enhanced aggressive behavior in mice lacking 5-HT$_{1B}$ receptor. *Science, 265,* 1875–1878.

Schanen, N. C., Scherer, S. W., Tsui, L. C., & Francke, U. (1996). Assignment of the 5-hydroxytryptamine (serotonin) receptor 5A gene (HTR5A) to human chromosome band 7q36.1. *Cytogenetics and Cell Genetics, 72,* 187–188.

Schmidt, M. E., Kruesi, M. J. P., Elia, J., Borcherding, B., Elin, R., Hoseini, J., McFarlin, K. E., & Hamburger, S. D. (1994). The effect of dextroamphetamine and methylphenidate on calcium and magnesium in hyperactive boys. *Psychiatry Research, 54,* 199–210.

Schmuck, K., Ullmer, C., Engels, P., & Lübbert, H. (1994). Cloning and functional characterization of the human 5-HT$_{2B}$ serotonin receptor. *FEBS Letters, 342,* 85–90.

Schwinn, D. A., Lomasney, J. W., Lorenz, W., Szklut, P. V., Fremeau, R. T., Yang-Feng, T. L., Caron, M. G., Lefkowitz, R. J., & Cotecchia, S. (1990). Molecular cloning and expression of the cDNA for a novel alpha 1-adrenergic receptor subtype. *Journal of Biological Chemistry, 265,* 8183–8189.

Seifert, W. E., Foxx, J. F., & Butler, I. J. (1980). Age effect on dopamine and serotonin metabolite levels in cerebrospinal fluid. *Annals of Neurology, 8,* 38–42.

Shaywitz, B. A., Cohen, D. J., & Bowers, M. B. J. (1977). CSF monoamine metabolites in children with minimal brain dysfunction: Evidence for alteration of brain dopamine. A preliminary report. *Journal of Pediatrics, 90,* 67–71.

Shearer, W. T., Patke, C. L., Gilliam, E. B., Rosenblatt, H. M., Barron, K. S., & Orson, F. M. (1988). Modulation of a human lymphoblastoid B cell line by cyclic AMP: Ig secretion and phosphatidylcholine metabolism. *Journal of Immunology, 141,* 1678–1686.

Sheng, M., Thompson, M. A., & Greenberg, M. E. (1991). CREB: A Ca(2+)-regulated transcription factor phosphorylated by calmodulin-dependent kinases. *Science, 252,* 1427–1430.

Shetty, T., & Chase, T. N. (1976). Central monoamines and hyperkinesis of childhood. *Neurology, 26,* 1000–1002.

Shimada, S., Kitayama, S., Lin, C., Patel, A., Nanthakumar, E., Gregor, P., Kuhar, M., & Uhl, G. (1991). Cloning and expression of a cocaine-sensitive dopamine transporter complementary DNA. *Science, 254,* 576–578.

Siegel, G., Agranoff, B., & Albers, R. (1998). *Basic neurochemistry: Molecular, cellular, and medical aspects* (6th ed.). Baltimore: Williams & Wilkins.

Siever, L., Kraemer, H., Sack, R., Angwin, P., Berger, P., Zarcone, V., Barchas, J., & Brodie, K. H. (1975). Gradients of biogenic amine metabolites in cerebrospinal fluid. *Diseases of the Nervous System, 36,* 13–16.

Silva, A. J., Paylor, R., Wehner, J. M., & Tonegawa, S. (1992). Impaired spatial learning in α-calcium-calmodulin kinase II mutant mice. *Science, 257,* 206–211.

Silva, A. J., Stevens, C. F., Tonegawa, S., & Wang, Y. (1992). Deficient hippocampal long-term potentiation in α-calcium-calmodulin kinase II mutant mice. *Science, 257,* 201–206.

Singer, H. S., Butler, I. J., Tune, L. E., Seifert, W. E., Jr., & Coyle, J. T. (1982). Dopaminergic dysfunction in Tourette syndrome. *Annals of Neurology, 12,* 361–366.

Sjoquist, B., & Johansson, B. (1978). A comparison between fluorometric and mass fragmentographic determinations of homovanillic acid and 5-hydroxyindoleacetic acid in human cerebrospinal fluid. *Journal of Neurochemistry, 31,* 621–625.

Sjostrom, R. (1972). Steady state levels of probenecid and their relation to acid monoamine metabolites in human cerebrospinal fluid. *Psychopharmacologia, 25,* 96–100.

Smalley, S., Bailey, J., Palmer, C., Cantwell, D., McGough, J., Del'Homme, M., Asarnow, J., Woodward, J., Ramsey, C., & Nelson, S. (1998). Evidence that the dopamine D4 receptor is a susceptibility gene in attention deficit hyperactivity disorder. *Molecular Psychiatry, 3,* 427–430.

Snyder, S. H. (1992). Nitric oxide: First in a new class of neurotransmitters. *Science, 257,* 494–496.

Sokoloff, P., Giros, B., Martres, M., Bouthenet, M., & Schwartz, J. (1990). Molecular cloning and characterization of a novel dopamine receptor (D_3) as target for neuroleptics. *Nature, 347,* 146–151.

Stanley, M., Traskman-Bendz, L., & Dorovini-Zis, K. (1985). Correlations between aminergic metabolites simultaneously obtained from human CSF and brain. *Life Sciences, 37,* 1279–1286.

Stein, P. L., Lee, H. M., Rich, S., & Soriano, P. (1992). p59fyn mutant mice display differential signaling in thymocytes and peripheral T cells. *Cell, 70,* 741–750.

Sunahara, R., Guan, H., O'Dowd, B., Seeman, P., Laurier, L., Ng, G., George, S., Torchia, J., Van Tol, H., & Niznik, H. (1991). Cloning of the gene for a human dopamine D_5 receptor with higher affinity for dopamine than D_1. Nature, 350, 614–619.

Sunahara, R. K., Niznik, H. B., Weiner, D. M., Storman, T. M., Brann, M. R., Kennedy, J. L., Gelertner, J. E., Rozmahel, R., Yang, Y., Israel, Y., Seeman, P., & O'Dowd, B. F. (1990). Human dopamine D_1 receptor encoded by an intronless gene on chromosome 5. Nature, 347, 80–83.

Swade, C., & Coppen, A. (1980). Seasonal variations in biochemical factors related to depressive illness. Journal of Affective Disorders, 2, 249–255.

Swanson, J. M., Sunohara, G. A., Kennedy, J. L., Regino, R., Fineberg, E., Wigal, T., Lerner, M., Williams, L., LaHoste, G. J., & Wigal, S. (1998). Association of the dopamine receptor D4 (DRD4) gene with a refined phenotype of attention deficit hyperactivity disorder (ADHD): A family-based approach. Molecular Psychiatry, 3, 38–41.

Swedo, S. E., Kruesi, M. J. P., Leonard, H. L., Hamburger, S. D., Cheslow, D. L., Stipetic, M., & Potter, W. Z. (1989). Lack of seasonal variation in pediatric lumbar cerebrospinal fluid neurotransmitter metabolite concentrations. Acta Psychiatrica Scandinavica, 80, 644–649.

Swedo, S. E., Leonard, H. L., Kruesi, M. J., Rettew, D. C., Listwak, S. J., Berrettini, W., Stipetic, M., Hamburger, S., Gold, P. W., Potter, W. Z., et al. (1992). Cerebrospinal fluid neurochemistry in children and adolescents with obsessive–compulsive disorder. Archives of General Psychiatry, 49, 29–36.

Swedo, S. E., Leonard, H. L., Mittleman, B. B., Allen, A. J., Rapoport, J. L., Dow, S. P., Kanter, M. E., Chapman, F., & Zabriskie, J. (1997). Identification of children with pediatric autoimmune neuropsychiatric disorders associated with streptococcal infections by a marker associated with rheumatic fever. American Journal of Psychiatry, 154, 110–112.

Tecott, L., Sun, L., Akana, S., Strack, A., Lowenstein, D., Dallman, M., & Julius, D. (1995). Eating disorder and epilepsy in mice lacking 5-HT_{2C} serotonin receptors. Nature, 374, 542–546.

Tiberi, M., Jarvie, K., Silvia, C., Falardeau, P., Gingrich, J., Godinot, N., Bertrand, L., Yang-Feng, T., Fremeau, R., Jr., & Caron, M. (1991). Cloning, molecular characterization and chromosomal assignment of a gene encoding a second D_1 dopamine receptor subtype: Differential expression pattern in rat brain compared to the D_{1A} receptor. Proceedings of the National Academy of Sciences USA, 88, 7491–7495.

Uetz, P., Adelatty, F., Villaroel, A., Rappold, G., Weiss, B., & Koenen, M. (1994). Organisation of the murine 5-HT3 receptor gene and assignment to human chromosome 11. FEBS Letters, 339, 302–306.

Unis, A. (1994). Ontogeny of [^{3}H]-SCH 23390 and [^{3}H]-YM 09151-2 binding sites in human fetal forebrain. Biological Psychiatry, 35, 562–569.

Vacha, J. (1978). Biology and the problem of normality. Scientia, 113, 823–846.

Van Tol, H., Bunzow, J., Guan, H., Sunahara, R., Seeman, P., Niznik, H., & Civelli, O. (1991). Cloning of the gene for a human dopamine D_4 receptor with high affinity for the antipsychotic clozapine. Nature, 350, 610–614.

Vandenbergh, D. J., Persico, A. M., Hawkins, A. L., Griffin, C. A., Li, X., Jabs, E. W., & Uhl, G. R. (1992). Human dopamine transporter gene (DAT1) maps to chromosome 5p15.3 and displays a VNTR. Genomics, 14, 1104–1106.

Wagner, J. J., Terman, G. W., & Chavkin, C. (1993). Endogenous dynorphins inhibit excitatory neurotransmission and block LTP induction in the hippocampus. *Nature, 363,* 451–454.

Waldman, I., Rowe, D., Abramowitz, A., Kozel, S., Mohr, J., Sherman, S., Cleveland, H., Sanders, M., Gard, J., & Stever, C. (1998). Association and linkage of the dopamine transporter gene and attention-deficit hyperactivity disorder in children: Heterogeneity owing to diagnostic subtype and severity. *American Journal of Human Genetics, 63,* 1767–1776.

Warren, R. P., Yonk, L. J., Burger, R. A., Cole, P., Odell, J. D., Warren, W. L., White, E., & Singh, V. K. (1990). Deficiency of suppressor–inducer (CD4+CD45RA+) T cells in autism. *Immunological Investigations, 19,* 245–251.

Weinshank, R., Adham, N., Macchi, M., Olsen, M., Branchek, T., & Hartig, P. (1991). Molecular cloning and characterization of high affinity dopamine receptor ($D_{1\beta}$) and its pseudogene. *Journal of Biological Chemistry, 266,* 22427–22435.

Weinshank, R., Zgombick, J., Macchi, M., Adham, N., Lichtblau, H., Branchek, T., & Hartig, P. (1990). Cloning, expression and pharmacological characterization of a human α_{2B}-adrenergic receptor. *Molecular Pharmacology, 38,* 681–688.

Weiss, B., Mertz, A., Schroeck, E., Koenen, M., & Rappold, G. (1995). Assignment of a human homolog of the mouse Htr3 receptor gene to chromosome 11q23.1–q23.2. *Genomics, 29,* 304–305.

Weisz, J. R., Weiss, B., & Donenberg, G. R. (1992). The lab versus the clinic. Effects of child and adolescent psychotherapy. *American Psychologist, 47,* 1578–1585.

Whitaker-Azmitia, P. M., Murphy, R., & Azmitia, E. C. (1990). Stimulation of astroglial 5-HT1A receptors releases the serotonergic growth factor, protein S–100, and alters astroglial morphology. *Brain Research, 528,* 155–158.

Whiteford, H., Jarvis, M., Stedman, T., Pond, S., & Csernansky, J. (1993). Mianserin-induced up-regulation of serotonin receptors on normal human platelets *in vivo. Life Sciences, 53,* 371–376.

Winkel, P., & Statland, B. E. (1984). The theory of reference values. In J. B. Henry (Ed.), *Clinical diagnosis and management by laboratory methods.* Philadelphia: W.B. Saunders.

Wirz-Justice, A., Lichtsteiner, M., & Feer, H. (1977). Diurnal and seasonal variations in human platelet serotonin in man. *Journal of Neural Transmission, 41,* 7–15.

Youdim, M., & Riederer, P. (1993). Dopamine metabolism and neurotransmission in primate brain in relationship to monoamine oxidase A and B inhibition. *Journal of Neural Transmission (Basic Neurosciences and Genetics), 91,* 181–195.

Yuwiler, A., Ritvo, E. R., Bald, D., Kipper, D., & Koper, A. (1971). Examination of circadian rhythmicity of blood serotonin and platelets in autistic and non-autistic children. *Journal of Autism and Childhood Schizophrenia, 1,* 421–435.

Zhou, Q.-Y., Grandy, D., Thambi, L., Kushner, J., Van Tol, H., Cone, R., Pribnow, D., Salon, J., Bunzow, J., & Civelli, O. (1990). Cloning and expression of human and rat D_1 dopamine receptors. *Nature, 347,* 76–80.

Index

385